The Basics of Cancer Immunotherapy

Haidong Dong • Svetomir N. Markovic
Editors

The Basics of Cancer Immunotherapy

Second Edition

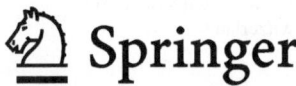 Springer

Editors
Haidong Dong
Department of Urology and Immunology
Mayo Clinic College of Medicine
Rochester, MN, USA

Svetomir N. Markovic
Division of Hematology/Oncology
Mayo Clinic
Rochester, MN, USA

ISBN 978-3-031-59474-8   ISBN 978-3-031-59475-5   (eBook)
https://doi.org/10.1007/978-3-031-59475-5

Cover image: The image shows a region of interest (ROI) of a primary met (Lymph node metastasis) from a patient who relapsed with immunotherapy. The patient had no response to the immune checkpoint blocker. This is one facet of that tumor-immune interface. Credit: Markovic Lab, Mayo Clinic (https://dimi-lab.github.io/)

This Springer imprint is published by the registered company Springer Nature Switzerland AG
The registered company address is: Gewerbestrasse 11, 6330 Cham, Switzerland

If disposing of this product, please recycle the paper.

Acknowledgements

We are grateful to the pioneers, our mentors/mentees, and colleagues in the field of cancer immunology and immunotherapy. We dedicate our book to our patients and their families for fighting cancer with us. Our research has been supported by the National Institute of Health, the National Cancer Institute, and the Mayo Foundation. We appreciate Sarah Lawler for the administration support and Crystal Lin for graphing figures of some chapters. We apologize for not being able to cite all the excellent studies and clinical trials in this field due to space limitations.

Contents

About the Editors

Haidong Dong is a tumor immunologist who co-discovered B7-H1 (PD-L1) in 1998 at Mayo Clinic, USA. His research is on mechanisms of cancer immunity and developments of cancer immunotherapy.

Svetomir N. Markovic is a medical oncologist and physician scientist at Mayo Clinic who specializes in the care of patients with metastatic melanoma. His research is focused on melanoma immune biology and immunotherapy.

Chapter 1
Basic Concepts in Cancer Immunology and Immunotherapy

Laura M. Rogers and Haidong Dong

Abstract Our immune system works in our bodies to prevent cancer cells from developing into full-blown disease, and yet cancer cells can evolve and escape our immune system. Cancer immunotherapy can help our immune system regain its ability to find and destroy cancer cells. In this chapter, we introduce and explain some basic concepts and processes of how our immune system controls cancer cells and how cancer cells escape immune control. Research on the interactions between immune cells and cancer cells has helped us identify therapeutic targets and develop new immunotherapies. We discuss the success of existing therapies and highlight current challenges and opportunities for future improvement.

Keywords Cancer · Adaptive immunity · Innate immunity · Immune checkpoints · Immunotherapy

Introduction

Cancer immunotherapy has revolutionized the field of oncology, offering new hope for patients by harnessing the power of the immune system to combat cancer. Unlike traditional cancer treatments like chemotherapy and radiation that directly target cancer cells, immunotherapies enhance the body's natural defense mechanisms (immune system) to recognize and destroy cancer cells. Understanding basic concepts of cancer immunology is vital in developing effective immunotherapies. This

L. M. Rogers
Department of Immuniology, Mayo Clinic, Rochester, MN, USA

H. Dong (✉)
Department of Urology and Immunology, Mayo Clinic College of Medicine, Rochester, MN, USA
e-mail: Dong.haidong@mayo.edu

© The Author(s), under exclusive license to Springer Nature Switzerland AG 2024
H. Dong, S. N. Markovic (eds.), *The Basics of Cancer Immunotherapy*,
https://doi.org/10.1007/978-3-031-59475-5_1

chapter explains how the immune system recognizes cancer cells and how cancer cells evade the immune system and discusses the current and future of cancer immunotherapy.

Why Do We Have Cancer?

Cancer is a cellular disease resulting from the uncontrolled growth of proliferative cells. A massive amount of cancer cells can accumulate in one part of the body or spread throughout the body by a process called metastasis. Contrary to normal cells, cancer cells have lost control of their proliferation; nothing can stop them until they take over the whole body. Normal cells are programmed to follow a precise and tightly controlled process of growth, division, and death. This regulation ensures that new cells are produced when needed and that damaged or old cells are eliminated. When mutations occur in specific genes, they can lead to uncontrolled cell growth, resulting in the formation of cancers. These mutations can arise due to various factors, such as exposure to carcinogens, lifestyle choices, and inherited genetic predispositions, which collectively increase the risk of developing cancer. Cancer is the result of a multistep process that involves the accumulation of multiple genetic mutations over time. However, not all mutations or errors in our cells will lead to cancer. We have both internal and external checking systems to monitor what happens to the cells in our bodies. If all these checking systems fail, cancer cells will proliferate and take control. The disease spreads throughout the body, eventually resulting in death if not treated.

Cancer-causing mutations are classified as oncogenes. Oncogenes are a group of genes that, when mutated or overexpressed, can promote the development of cancer via uncontrolled cell proliferation. Examples of oncogenes include mutated HER2, EGFR, and KRAS. On the other hand, tumor suppressor genes are a class of genes that play a critical role in preventing the development of cancer. Unlike oncogenes, which promote cell growth and division, tumor suppressor genes act as "brakes" in the cell cycle, regulating cell proliferation and preventing the formation of cancers. When functioning correctly, tumor suppressor genes help maintain genomic stability, repair damaged DNA, and promote cell death when necessary. Mutations or inactivation of these genes can lead to uncontrolled cell growth and an increased risk of cancer development. Examples of tumor suppressors include BRCA1 and BRCA2, PTEN, and TP53. Loss of tumor suppressor gene function is a critical step in the progression of many cancers. Basically, normal cells are programmed to die if they detect any mutations within their genes that they cannot correct. If cancer cells escape this internal check, they will face an external check that is mediated by the immune system (Fig. 1.1a).

The external checking system—our immune system—has developed the ability to check for tiny changes in our cells. A robust and efficient immune system can recognize and eliminate abnormal or cancerous cells before they grow into cancers. Because cancer cells arise due to genetic mutations, they display abnormal proteins

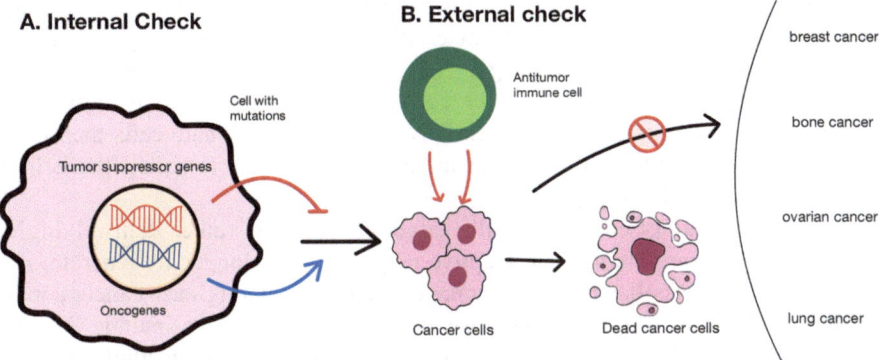

Fig. 1.1 The internal and external check systems that prevent the development of cancer as a disease. (**a**) Oncogenes in mutant cells would promote a conversion of normal cell to become cancer cells, but tumor suppressor genes inhibit this process. (**b**) Immune cells with antitumor activity identify and destroy mutant cancer cells to prevent them to form cancer disease in multiple organs.

on their surface or produce unique molecules that are not present in normal cells. These alterations make cancer cells different from healthy cells, and immune cells have specific "eyes" to identify these changes in cancer cells. The "eyes" of immune cells are receptors that function to detect specific changes in cancer cells. Once our immune cells detect these altered proteins on the surfaces of the cancer cells, they will recognize them, become activated, and eventually destroy the cancer cells. If our immune system can recognize these changes inside any cancer cells, the cancer cells cannot accumulate and develop into a disease. Therefore, cancer is ultimately a disease caused by unlimited growth of cancer cells that escaped the attack of immune system (Fig. 1.1b).

How Does the Immune System Protect Us from Cancer?

Many of us may have cancerous cells in our bodies, but most of us do not develop cancer as a disease. Our immune system prevents spontaneously generated cancer cells from developing into cancers. This phenomenon has been reproduced in animal models and prompted the theory of "immune surveillance," that is, an intact and functional immune system is required to detect and destroy cancer cells before they become cancer as a disease. To that end, our current immunotherapy has been developed to boost the immune system to find and destroy cancer cells. The success of this therapy provides direct evidence that we have pre-existing immune responses to cancer in our body, but at times, they do not function as well as they should. However, once we give them a booster, they will do a great job in attacking cancer.

There are two main components of the immune system involved in recognizing cancer called innate and adaptive immunities. Innate immunity serves as the first response against mutated cells and helps damaged tissue repair itself. Innate cells, such as natural killer (NK) cells and macrophages, detect "danger signals" associated with cellular stress and damage. These signals are called danger-associated molecular patterns (DAMPs). Cancer cells release DAMPs, which alert innate immune cells to the presence of potentially harmful cells. Innate cells then begin clearing damaged cells while sending inflammatory signals to solicit the help of adaptive immune cells (Fig. 1.2).

Adaptive immunity can specifically target cancer cells rather than relying on generalized patterns. Though an adaptive response takes longer to generate, it is associated with less collateral tissue damage and improved long-term cancer control through generation of immune memory. Adaptive immune cells include B and T cells, both of which have antigen receptors that confer target specificity through antigen recognition. Antigens are small protein fragments from cancer cells that are presented on the cell surface in complex with major histocompatibility complex

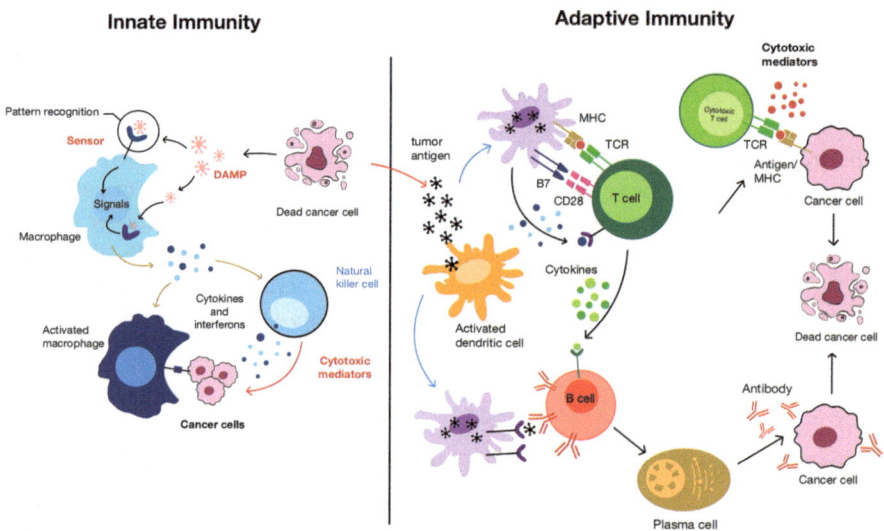

Fig. 1.2 Innate and adaptive immune system in control of cancer. Although cancer cells can grow without limitation, some of them will die due to insufficient nutrients during their rapid growth. Once they die, they release danger-associated molecule patterns (DAMP) that can be sensed by pattern recognition receptor (sensor) in innate immune cells (macrophages) and activate macrophages. Activated macrophages release cytokines or interferons to activate other macrophages to "eat" cancer cells or activate natural killer (NK) cells to kill cancer cells via cytotoxic mediators. Adaptive immune cells (B cells or T cells) are activated by dendritic cells (antigen-presenting cells) that take up tumor antigens from dead cancer cells. Activated dendritic cells present tumor antigen in MHC complex to prime T cells through T cell receptor (TCR). Primed T cells are activated via co-stimulation signals of B7/CD28 and cytokines that promote T cell growth. Dendritic cells also present antigen to B cells that will also be activated by cytokines released from activated T helper cells. Some of the activated T cells become cytotoxic T cells that can specifically kill cancer cells with the same antigen that primed them. Activated B cells become plasma cells that produce antigen-specific antibody that can bind to tumor cells to direct cancer destruction

(MHC) molecules (human MHC is also called HLA, human leukocyte antigen), and the antigen receptors on B and T cells can recognize when these are abnormal. If activated by an abnormal cancer antigen, B cells produce antibodies that can bind to cancer cells and mark them for destruction by other components of the immune system. Similarly, T cells can scan the surface of cells and can recognize cancer-specific antigens as "foreign" or abnormal, triggering a cytotoxicity (cell killing) process against the cancer cell (Fig. 1.2).

Since an immune (T or B) cell only can recognize a tiny part of an antigen and only a few cells have this specificity, the efficiency of the immune system in responses to any altered proteins or pathogens could be very low. To increase efficiency but not compromise specificity, diversity is granted to the immune system. This diversity is achieved at the genetic level to produce a battery of different kinds of receptors or antibodies for recognizing different antigens and a panel of different HLA for presenting different antigens.

Why Does the Immune System Fail to Control Cancer Cells?

Despite the immune system's surveillance, cancer cells can develop strategies to evade detection and destruction, allowing them to continue growing and spreading. This enigma of co-existing progressive cancers and antitumor immune cells in patients with advanced cancer was first described as the Hellström paradox. Since then, multiple evasion mechanisms have been speculated in an immunosuppressive microenvironment that allows cancer cells to thrive and evade immune detection. Overcoming these evasion strategies is a key focus in cancer immunotherapy research. Some common ways by which cancer cells evade the immune system and the therapeutic strategies scientists have invented to overcome these are discussed in the following paragraphs.

Cancer cells do their best to hide from the detection of immune system. In some cases, immune cells are not properly alerted to the presence of cancer cells. This may occur when cancer cells disrupt antigen presentation, preventing immune cells from recognizing them as threats (Fig. 1.3). Further, individual cancer cells display different antigens, that is, antigen heterogeneity, making it more challenging for the immune system to kill all the cells at one time point. Thus, antigen heterogeneity (variants in their expression) and antigen downregulation (decreased expression) allow some cancer cells to escape immune attack. Additionally, cancer cells can hide from an immune attack via immune exclusion. Immune exclusion is a buildup of physical barriers to exclude the infiltration of immune cells in the tumor micro-environment. Thus, even if immune cells are alerted to the presence of cancer cells, they may not be able to penetrate into the tumor tissues.

Cancer cells also take the advantage of the brakes in the immune system. Immune checkpoints are regulatory mechanisms in the immune system that help maintain a balance between the activation and suppression of immune responses. They prevent the immune system from becoming excessively active, which could lead to

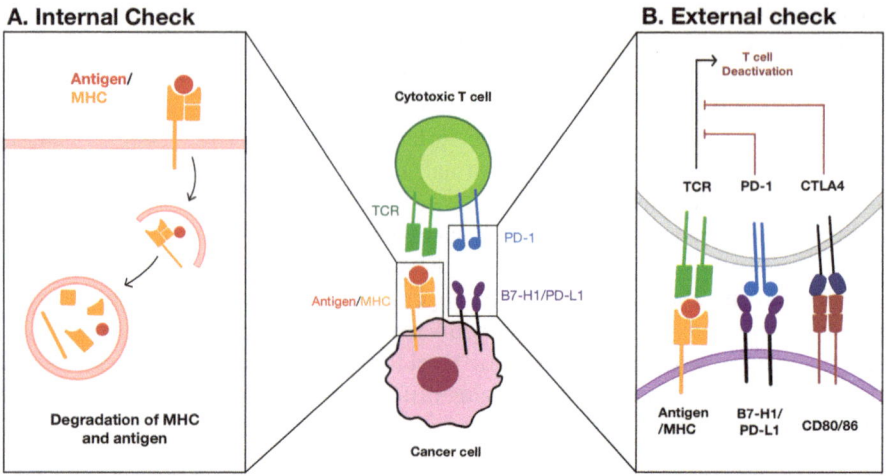

Fig. 1.3 Mechanisms of cancer immune evasion. (**a**) Cancer cells can hide themselves from downregulation of their tumor antigen expression. This can be done via degradation of antigen/MHC (major histocompatibility complex that can present antigen) within cancer cells. (**b**) Cancer cells increase their expression of B7-H1 (PD-L1) that binds to PD-1 expressed by activated T cells. Like CTLA-4, another immune checkpoint molecule, PD-1, impairs the antitumor activity of activated T cells

autoimmune reactions but that hinder their antitumor functions. Cancer cells express immune checkpoint molecules to actively turn down the immune responses against them. One important molecule expressed by cancer cells is called B7-H1 (also named PD-L1) which was discovered at the Mayo Clinic in 1998. PD-L1 binds to PD-1, one of the immune checkpoint molecules like CTLA-4, which restrains the immune responses to cancer cells (Fig. 1.3). Therefore, it is no surprise that high expression of PD-L1 predicts poor survivorship of patients with renal cell carcinoma, lung cancer, ovarian cancer, and some other cancers. The discovery of B7-H1 expressed by human cancer cells not only explains a reason underlying the Hellström paradox but also opens a door for us to develop new therapeutics in cancer therapy.

Strategies to Harness the Immune System to Fight Cancer Cells

Cancer immunotherapy works through the immune system to control cancer; therefore, its direct target is the immune cells rather than the cancer cells. Cancer immunotherapy is aimed at restoring or enhancing the capability of immune cells to recognize and destroy cancer cells, and the therapeutic effects will be determined by the extent to which the immune cells eliminate cancer cells. One of the ideal scenarios is that enough tumor-reactive immune cells are generated and able to move

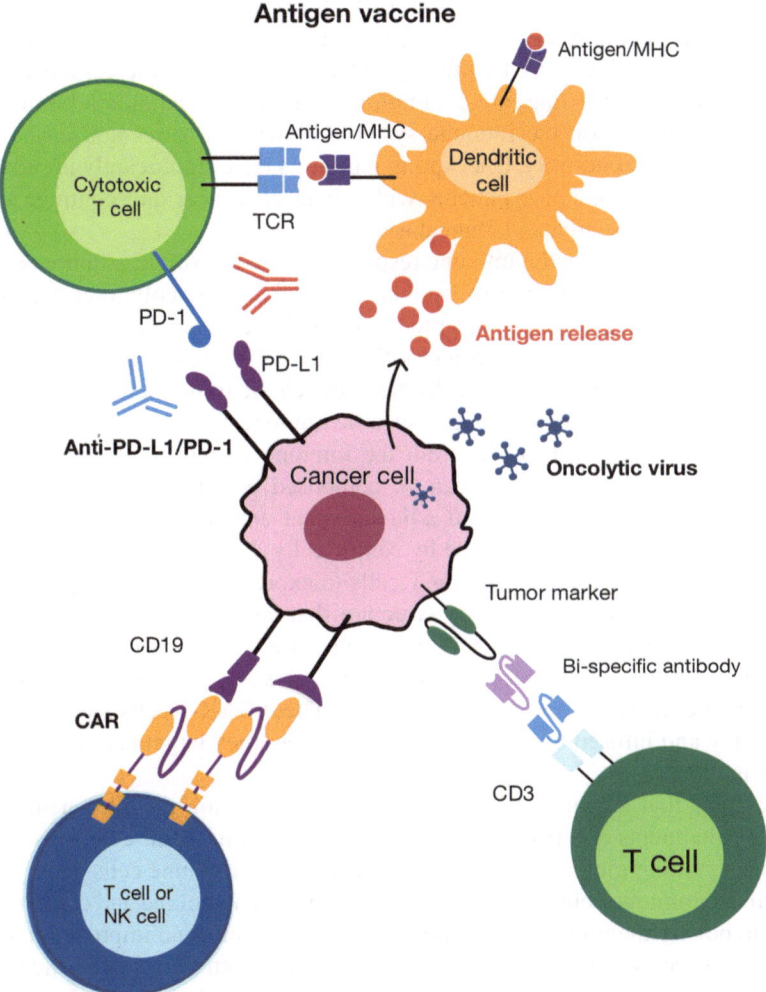

Fig. 1.4 Cancer immunotherapy aimed to improve the immune cells to fight cancer. The immune suppressive signals of PD-1 can be blocked by anti-PD-1 or anti-PD-L1 antibodies (immune checkpoint inhibitors) to remove the "brakes" on antitumor activity of cytotoxic T cells. Tumor vaccines provide new antigens (neoantigens) to dendritic cells for them to prime more effective T cells. Oncolytic viruses specifically infect and destroy cancer cells to release tumor antigen that can further be used by dendritic cells to activate T cells or B cells. CAR-T cells use surface "antibody" to recognize tumor antigens (like CD19) and are activated via CAR signals that direct them to kill cancer cells. Bispecific antibodies can bind tumor marker and CD3 (T cell marker) at the same time and then link cancer cells and T cells together and activate T cells to kill cancer cells

to cancer sites where they can destroy cancer cells. Since PD-L1 (B7-H1) expressed by cancer cells suppresses this process, therapeutically targeting the interaction of PD-1 and PD-L1 using antibodies that block this contact will be able to restore the antitumor function of immune cells (Fig. 1.4). Immune checkpoint inhibitors are drugs designed to block the interaction between checkpoint receptors (like PD-1) and their ligands (like PD-L1), thereby unleashing the immune response against cancer cells. By inhibiting these inhibitory signals, checkpoint inhibitors help "release the brakes" on the immune system, allowing it to recognize and attack cancer cells more effectively. Checkpoint inhibitors have significantly improved the outcomes and prognosis for patients with advanced cancer and continue to be a focus of ongoing research and clinical trials.

To boost a tumor-specific immune response that will result in a tumor rejection, scientists have engineered innovative therapies including oncolytic viruses, cancer vaccines, and chimeric antigen receptor T (CAR-T) cell therapy. Oncolytic viruses are designed to selectively infect and kill cancer cells while leaving healthy cells unharmed. As the infected cancer cells die, they release tumor-specific antigens that will further stimulate a tumor antigen-specific immune response against the cancer. Cancer vaccines are designed to train the immune system to recognize specific tumor antigens. These vaccines can be composed of tumor-specific antigens or immune-stimulating agents (called adjuvant) that enhance the immune response against a specific antigen expressed by cancer cells (Fig. 1.4). CAR-T cell therapy involves engineering a patient's own T cells to express chimeric antigen receptors (CARs) that comprise an antibody structure that can recognize a specific tumor antigen and a signaling constructure that can activate T cells. Once the CARs bind to a tumor antigen expressed by cancer cells, the CAR-T cells are activated and release cytotoxic mediators to kill cancer cells. These CAR-T cells are produced out of the body and infused back into the patient, where they target and destroy cancer cells (Fig. 1.4).

Therapies that aim to enhance immune cell infiltration include chemokine or cytokine treatments and bispecific antibodies. Chemokines and cytokines are both immune signaling molecules. Chemokines can recruit immune cells and cytokines can activate immune cells. Researchers are exploring chemokine and cytokine treatments to bolster the immune response against cancer cells and improve tumor penetration. Bispecific antibodies are designed to bind to both cancer cells and immune cells, bringing them into proximity to enhance immune cell-mediated destruction of cancer cells (Fig. 1.4).

Advantages and Side Effects of Cancer Immunotherapy

Immunotherapy offers several advantages over treatments designed to target a specific genetic mutation in cancers. Immunotherapy can be effective against a wide range of cancer types because it targets the immune system, which has the potential to recognize and attack multiple antigens present on cancer cells, providing a more comprehensive approach to tackling cancer heterogeneity (genetic variants). Immunotherapy has shown the potential for long-lasting responses, with some patients experiencing durable remissions even after completing the treatment. This is because immunotherapy can generate a pool of immune cells that can "remember" tumor antigens and respond quickly once cancer cells come back (recurrence).

However, like all cancer treatments, immunotherapy can be associated with certain side effects. Immunotherapy works by enhancing the immune system's activity, which can lead to immune-related adverse events. These side effects occur when the immune system attacks healthy tissues and organs in addition to cancer cells. Skin rash is one of the most common side effects of immunotherapy. It can range from mild to severe and may present as redness, itching, or blistering. Other side effects include neurological and cardiological toxicities, gastrointestinal upset, fatigue, and flu-like symptoms. It is important to note that while some of these side effects can be serious, most are manageable and resolved with appropriate management and treatment. Physicians closely monitor patients undergoing immunotherapy to detect any side effects early and provide prompt intervention. Research is ongoing to better understand and minimize these side effects while maximizing therapeutic benefits.

Future of Cancer Immunotherapy

The landscape of cancer immunotherapy is continually evolving, and breakthroughs have led to the approval of multiple immunotherapies for cancer treatment worldwide. These drugs have revolutionized the treatment of cancer and have significantly improved outcomes for many patients. Despite the significant successes and promise of cancer immunotherapy, there are several limitations and challenges. Addressing these limitations requires continued research and innovation in cancer immunotherapy. Active areas of research include the following:

1. Response rate variability: The response to immunotherapy can vary significantly among different patients and cancer types. While some patients experience remarkable and durable responses, others may show little to no benefit from immunotherapy.
2. Combination therapy complexity: Identifying the most effective combinations of immunotherapies with other treatments, such as chemotherapy, radiation therapy, or targeted therapies, requires extensive research. The optimal sequencing and timing of these treatments are still being explored.
3. Toxicities and immune-related adverse events: Immunotherapy can lead to immune-related adverse events (IRAEs), as the immune system may attack healthy tissues and organs, causing autoimmune-like side effects. While most IRAEs are manageable, they can be severe and even life-threatening in some cases.
4. Biomarker identification: Predicting which patients will respond to immunotherapy remains a challenge. Biomarkers will help inform healthcare providers making treatment decisions and reduce the financial burden associated with ineffective treatments.

Conclusion

Cancer immunotherapy has reshaped the landscape of cancer treatment, offering new possibilities for patients worldwide. A deeper understanding of cancer immunology (the interaction between immune cells and cancer cells at molecular levels), achieved with scientific research, will continue to advance this promising field by discovery of new therapeutic targets. The collaboration between researchers, healthcare providers, and patients will pave the way for innovative and personalized approaches that promise to transform cancer into a manageable, and maybe even curable, disease.

Chapter 2
Immune Checkpoint Inhibitors in Oncology

Katherine Smith and Svetomir N. Markovic

Abstract In this chapter, we explore the evolution and current state of immune checkpoint inhibitors (ICIs) in cancer treatment, focusing on their mechanism of action, FDA-approved agents, and novel immune checkpoints. Understanding ICIs is critical since ICIs have revolutionized the treatment for many solid tumors and some hematological malignancies after the first approvals in the early 2010s. First, we review concepts to help gain an understanding of immunotherapy in general, such as monoclonal antibodies and immune checkpoints. We then focus on the current ICI treatment landscape, including the use of ipilimumab, nivolumab, pembrolizumab, and relatlimab in the metastatic, adjuvant, and neoadjuvant settings. Additionally, we discuss new upcoming treatment targets. Finally, we review the side effects of ICI treatments, also known as immune-related adverse events (irAEs), and special circumstances where ICIs should be used with caution. At the end of the chapter, the reader will gain insight on general concepts in immunotherapy and obtain an understanding on the current standard of care regimens using ICIs.

Keywords Immune checkpoint inhibitors · Immunotherapy · PD-1 · PD-L1 · LAG-3 · Novel immune checkpoints · Immune-related adverse events

Introduction

Unlike traditional chemotherapy, which affects the replication of both cancer and healthy cells, immunotherapy empowers the immune system to eliminate cancer with more precision. The immune system is typically thought of in the acute illness setting—protecting us from bacteria and viruses. However, the immune system

K. Smith (✉)
Division of Medical Oncology, Mayo Clinic, Rochester, MN, USA
e-mail: smith.katherine3@mayo.edu

S. N. Markovic
Division of Hematology/Oncology, Mayo Clinic, Rochester, MN, USA

keeps us safe from any invaders, including cancer. The problem is that cancer cells can develop ways to evade the immune system and avoid detection. Immunotherapy, and more specifically immune checkpoint inhibitors (ICIs), helps patients' immune systems better recognize and destroy cancer cells (Robert, 2020).

Targeted immunotherapy began in the 1990s with the development of mono-clonal antibodies (mAb). Before this, immunotherapies broadly activated the immune system with bacterial toxins or cytokines (Carlson et al., 2020; Pettenati & Ingersoll, 2018; Raeber et al., 2023). mAbs target a specific receptor expressed on a cell surface. After the antibody binds to the receptor, the immune system kills the cell through antibody-dependent cell-mediated cytotoxicity (ADCC), complement-mediated cytotoxicity (CDC), and antibody-dependent phagocyto-sis (ADP); however, there is also likely an element of direct cell killing from the drug itself (Pierpoint et al., 2018). The first approved mAb was rituximab, an anti-CD-20 antibody, meaning the antibody binds to CD-20, a receptor found on B lymphocyte cells and some hematologic malignancies (Fig. 2.1). After

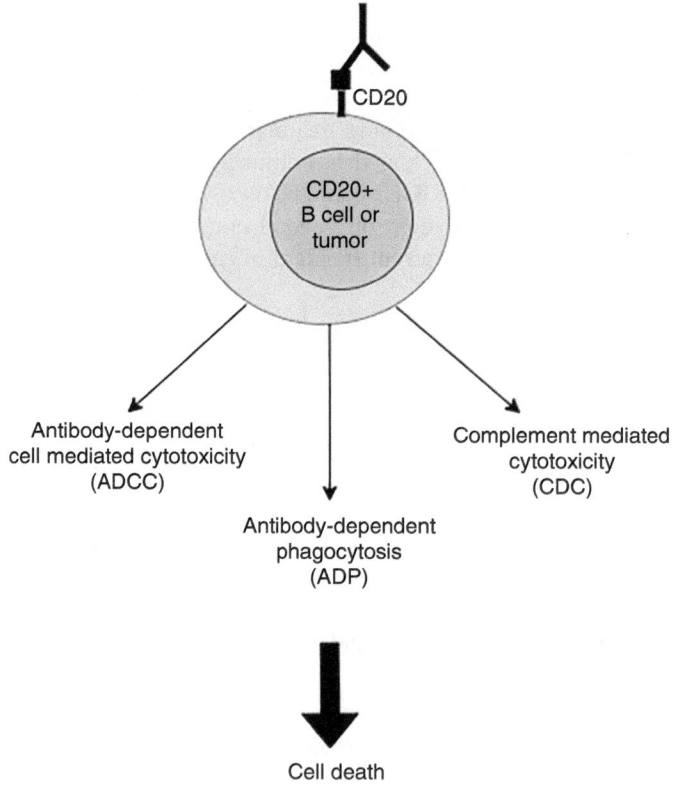

Fig. 2.1 Illustration of a monoclonal antibody (mAb). Rituximab is a mAb targeted to CD-20. After binding, cell death results from antibody-dependent cell-mediated cytotoxicity (ADCC), antibody-dependent phagocytosis (ADP), and complement-medicated cytotoxicity (CDC). Direct cell lysis from the drug may play a role in cell death as well

approval in 1997, rituximab became known as the first targeted cancer immuno-therapy and is now used widely in oncology, hematology, and rheumatology. Other mAbs that followed rituximab and are used in cancer care today include, but are not limited to, bevacizumab (anti-VEGF-A, vascular endothelial growth factor), ramucirumab (anti-VEGFR-2), trastuzumab (anti-HER2, human epidermal growth factor receptor family), pertuzumab (anti-HER2), and obinutuzumab (anti-CD-20). More recently, mAbs have been modified to (1) carry a chemotherapy payload to create targeted antibody-drug conjugates (ADCs) that directly brings chemotherapy to the targeted cell and (2) carry a second mAB that directs T cells to the tumor, also known as bispecific T cell engagers (BiTEs) (Khongorzul et al., 2020; Shanshal et al., 2023).

Shortly after the incorporation of targeted mAbs, immune checkpoint inhibitors (ICIs) came to the immunotherapy scene in the 2010s (Robert, 2020). To understand ICIs, we must first grasp the concept of immune checkpoints, which are proteins expressed on the surface of normal cells. When immune cells bind to immune checkpoints, the immune cells receive feedback that this cell is normal (Bagchi et al., 2021; Vaddepally et al., 2020). Immune checkpoints serve as the "brakes" of our immune system and prevents destruction of healthy tissue. When this process goes awry, patients develop autoimmune diseases (i.e., rheumatoid arthritis, lupus, psoriasis, ulcerative colitis, etc.) due to immune cells destroying tissues usually seen as "self."

Cancer cells express immune checkpoints on their surface to evade detection by the immune system. Immune checkpoint *inhibitors* are antibodies (mAbs) that work by binding to the immune checkpoints thus allowing immune cells to then "see" the cancer. The immune system can then develop tumor-specific T cells that can recognize and destroy tumor cells (Wei et al., 2018). In other words, ICIs "release the brakes" of the immune system (Fig. 2.2).

The ICI era began with ipilimumab, which was approved for melanoma in 2011 (Robert, 2020). Now, there are many ICI drug approvals as single agents (monotherapy) or in combinations with other ICIs, chemotherapy, or tyrosine kinase inhibitors (TKIs). With FDA approvals spanning various solid tumors and some hematological malignancies, over 40% of cancer patients are eligible for ICI treatment. As research progresses, the FDA continues to greenlight new ICI indications, expanding their use to different diseases and in earlier stages of treatment (Haslam et al., 2020). Understanding the rapidly evolving landscape of immuno-oncology (IO), particularly with the integration of ICIs, is critical for both patients and clinicians since these medications are now commonly used in oncology. Our review will focus on (1) ICIs that are FDA approved for use in standard of care treatment and (2) ICI side effects. We will briefly discuss novel upcoming therapies.

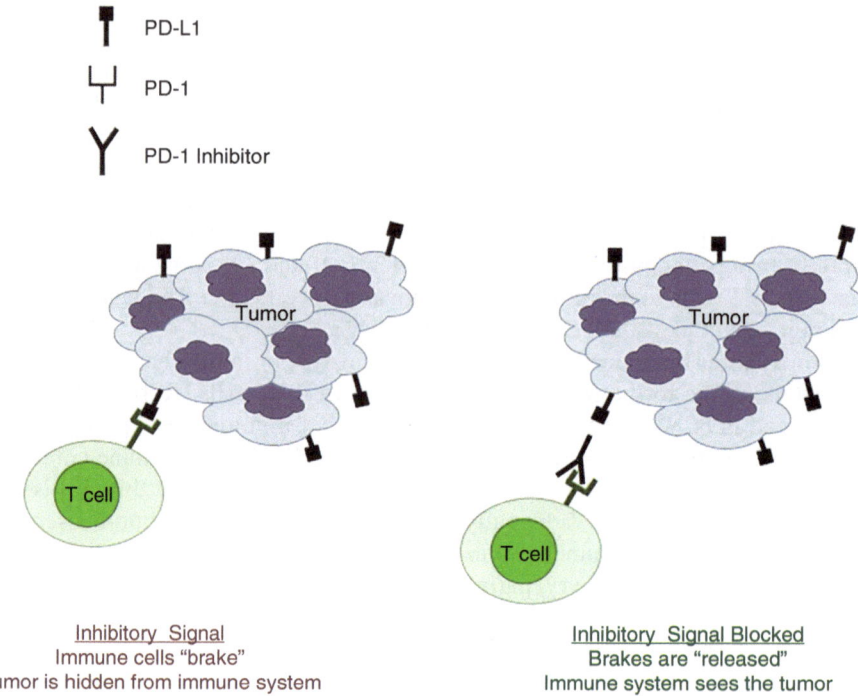

Fig. 2.2 Illustration of immune checkpoints and immune checkpoint inhibitors (ICIs). In this example, PD-L1 is expressed on tumor cells and PD-1 is expressed on a T cell. (**a**) When PD-1 bind to PD-L1, the T cell receives an inhibitory signal that downregulates the T cell. The tumor remains hidden from the T cell. (**b**) ICIs are antibodies that block the interaction between PD-1 and PD-L1; thus there are no inhibitory signals, and the T cell can then recognize the tumor cells. The T cell can become activated, replicate, and eventually eliminate the tumor cells

Currently Approved Immune Checkpoint Inhibitors

CTLA-4 (Cytotoxic T-Lymphocyte-Associated Protein 4) Inhibitors

CTLA-4 is an immunoglobulin receptor normally expressed on effector and regulatory T cells. When CTLA-4 binds to its counterpart, B7 (located on lymphocytes, dendritic cells, and monocytes), then T cell activation is downregulated (Chambers et al., 2001; Collins et al., 2005). Ipilimumab is an anti-CTLA-4 antibody that blocks this interaction, thus allowing for T cell activation. While ipilimumab has some activity against cancer on its own, this medication is most effective when used in combination with another ICI called nivolumab, which targets PD-1 (discussed further below) (Larkin et al., 2015). Ipilimumab plus nivolumab (also known as ipi/nivo) is now used in many different metastatic solid tumors, including melanoma, non-small-cell lung cancer (NSCLC), kidney cancer (RCC or renal cell cancer), mesothelioma, liver cancer, esophageal squamous cell cancer, and colorectal cancer with specific markers (MSI-H, microsatellite instability high, or dMMR, mismatch repair deficient) ("interactive dosing guide") (Table 2.1).

Table 2.1 Current FDA-approved immune checkpoint inhibitors (ICIs)

Immune checkpoint	Drug	Indication		
		Advanced disease	Adjuvant	Neoadjuvant
CTLA-4	Ipilimumab[a]	Melanoma NSCLC Mesothelioma HCC RCC ESCC CRC (MSI-H or dMMR)	—	—
PD-1	Nivolumab	Melanoma NSCLC Head/neck cancer, SCC RCC Urothelial ESCC CRC (MSI-H or dMMR) Hodgkin's lymphoma	Melanoma Urothelial Esophageal and GEJ junction	NSCLC[b]
	Pembrolizumab	Melanoma NSCLC Head/neck SCC RCC Urothelial Gastric or GEJ CRC (MSI-H or dMMR) Cervical Endometrial (MSI-H or dMMR) Merkel cell Skin cancer, SCC Hodgkin's lymphoma Primary mediastinal lymphoma Any tumor with TMB-H, MSI-H, dMMR	Melanoma, stage 2b-3 NSCLC, stage 1B-3A Breast cancer, triple negative, stage 2–3 RCC	Breast cancer, triple negative, stages 2–3[b]
	Cemiplimab	Skin cancer, SCC Skin cancer, basal cell NSCLC	—	—
	Dostarlimab	dMMR solid tumors Endometrial cancer[b]		

(continued)

Table 2.1 (continued)

Immune checkpoint	Drug	Indication		
		Advanced disease	Adjuvant	Neoadjuvant
PD-L1	Atezolizumab	NSCLC SCLC Liver cancer Melanoma	NSCLC	—
	Durvalumab	NSCLC SCLC Cholangiocarcinoma Liver cancer	NSCLC	—
	Avelumab	Merkel cell Urothelial	—	—
LAG-3	Relatlimab	Melanoma[c]	—	—

NSCLC non-small-cell lung cancer, *SCLC* small-cell lung cancer, *SCC* squamous cell cancer, *HCC* hepatocellular cancer (liver cancer), *RCC* renal cell, arcinoma (kidney cancer), *ESCC* esophageal squamous cell cancer, *CRC* colorectal cancer, *GEJ* gastroesophageal junction, *MSI-H* microsatellite instability high, *dMMR* deficient mismatch repair, *TMB-H* tumor mutational burden high
[a]All ipilimumab regimens are in combination with the PD-1 inhibitor, nivolumab. The dosing and treatment schedules vary based on the disease.
[b]In combination with chemotherapy
[c]In combination with nivolumab

PD-1 (Programmed Death—1) Inhibitors

The next round of ICI approvals were for anti-PD-1 drugs with pembrolizumab making its debut in 2014 for metastatic melanoma, closely followed by nivolumab in 2015. PD-1, located on naïve and activated T cells, interacts with its counterparts PD-L1 and PD-L2 (programmed death ligand 1 or 2). PD-L1 and PD-L2 are expressed on macrophages, monocytes, and dendritic cells but also on tumor cells (Patsoukis et al., 2020). As with all immune checkpoints, the interaction between PD-1 and PD-L1 will downregulate the immune system, so PD-1 blockade allows for immune activation.

Both pembrolizumab and nivolumab have garnered approvals across nearly all solid tumors and some hematological malignancies (such as Hodgkin's lymphoma and primary mediastinal B cell lymphoma (Keytruda. Package Insert. 2024; Opdivo. Package Insert. 2024). These drugs are used in the first-line treatment setting and beyond, either as monotherapy or in combination with other modalities, like chemotherapy and oral tyrosine kinase inhibitors (TKIs). Pembrolizumab's approval extends beyond tumor type and now incorporates the biomarkers MSI-H, dMMR, and high tumor mutational burden (TMB-H) (Marabelle et al., 2020; Le et al., 2020; Geoerger et al., 2020). In addition to pembrolizumab and nivolumab, cemiplimab and dostarlimab are newer PD-1 inhibitors, approved in 2018 and 2021, respectively. Cemiplimab currently has applications in the treatment of metastatic NSCLC, metastatic cutaneous squamous cell carcinoma, and advanced basal cell carcinoma.

Dostarlimab is used in dMMR solid tumors and in combination with chemotherapy for advanced endometrial cancer (Oaknin et al., 2022; Mirza et al., 2023) (Table 2.1).

While most PD-1 inhibitor approvals are in the metastatic setting, recent years have witnessed approvals for earlier stages of disease. The first use of PD-1 inhibitors in early-stage cancers was in the adjuvant setting or the time after surgery. Currently, pembrolizumab can be used in high-risk stage 2 or 3 melanoma, non-small-cell lung cancer (NSCLC), and stage 2–3 triple-negative breast cancer to decrease the risk of recurrence (Lao et al., 2022; O'Brien et al., 2022; Schmid et al., 2020). Now PD-1 inhibitors are being moved even earlier in the treatment course to the neoadjuvant setting (i.e., before surgery). There are several promising studies showing that neoadjuvant PD-1 inhibitors can induce complete pathological responses within the tumor at the time of surgery, providing valuable insights into patients' response to future treatment and predicting long-term outcomes. As of 2023, neoadjuvant indications are in breast cancer and NSCLC only, but there are numerous studies in progress (Mittendorf et al., 2022).

PD-L1 (Programmed Death Ligand 1)

As discussed above, PD-L1 is found on tumor cells (in addition to macrophages, monocytes, and dendritic cells), and its counterpart is PD-1. There are three PD-L1 inhibitors used routinely: atezolizumab, durvalumab, and avelumab. Atezolizumab has indications in NSCLC, small-cell lung cancer (SCLC), liver cancer, and melanoma. Durvalumab is approved for use in NSCLC, SCLC, cholangiocarcinoma (gallbladder and bile duct cancer), and liver cancer. Additionally, durvalumab has made its way to the adjuvant setting for NSCLC as well. Avelumab is mostly used in Merkel cell carcinoma and urothelial cancer (Chang et al., 2021) (Table 2.1).

LAG-3 (Lymphocyte Activation Gene—3) Inhibitors

From 2011 to 2022, the only immune checkpoints successfully targeted with ICIs were CTLA-4, PD-1, and PD-L1. In 2022, LAG-3 became the newest immune checkpoint to have an FDA-approved drug. LAG-3 is found on immune cells, including activated CD4+ and CD8+ T lymphocytes, and natural kill (NK) cells and can be co-expressed with other immune checkpoints, including PD-L1. This immune checkpoint binds to its counterpart major histocompatibility complex 2 (MHCII) on antigen-presenting cells (APCs), leading to an inhibitory signal (Maruhashi et al., 2020). Relatlimab is a LAG-3 inhibitor used in combination with nivolumab, the PD-1 inhibitor, in metastatic melanoma patient (Tawbi et al., 2022) (Table 2.1). The novel combination has a lower toxicity profile compared to ipi/nivo, so it is often used in patients who may not be able to tolerate ipi/nivo. Time to progression improved in the initial study leading to FDA approval, but overall survival (OS, or how long patients live) has not been seen yet. There are numerous ongoing studies of relatlimab and nivolumab in many tumor types in metastatic, adjuvant, and neoadjuvant settings.

Overall, the currently approved ICIs target the immune checkpoints CTLA-4, PD-1, PD-L1, and LAG-3. Most approvals are in the advanced or metastatic setting, but now ICIs are being used in the earlier stages of disease to prevent recurrence and progression to metastatic disease. Use in the adjuvant setting occurs after surgical removal of the primary tumor. Use in the neoadjuvant setting, or before surgery, is a new concept starting to gain momentum. Note the ICIs listed in this table are often used in combination with other therapies, such as chemotherapy and tyrosine kinase inhibitors.

Novel Immune Checkpoint Inhibitors

In addition to the aforementioned immune checkpoints (CTLA-4, PD-1, PD-L1, LAG-3), there are several additional immune checkpoints still under study and do not have therapeutic inhibitors for use in the clinic yet (Marin-Acevedo et al., 2021). These checkpoints include the following:

- B7-H3/4
- BTLA (B and T lymphocyte attenuator)
- ICOS (inducible T cell costimulatory)
- NKG2A (NK group protein 2 A)
- PVRIG (poliovirus receptor-related immunoglobulin domain) or CD122R
- TIM-3 (T cell immunoglobulin-3)
- TIGIT (T cell immunoglobulin and ITM domain)
- VISTA (V-domain Ig suppressor of T cell activation)

Of these immune checkpoints, TIGIT is the only one with inhibitors that are far enough through regulatory processes to be studied in human trials. TIGIT is expressed on activated T cell (CD4+ and CD8+) and NK cells and binds to poliovirus receptor (PVR), also known as CD 155, an adhesion molecule on dendritic cells and macrophages. Other binding counterparts for TIGIT are poliovirus receptor-related 2 (PVRL2), also known as CD112 and CD226. TIGIT inhibitors with published results include vibostolimab, etigilimab, and tiragolumab; however, there are no FDA-approved TIGIT inhibitors. Tiragolumab initially seemed promising in early studies, but phase 3 data did not support clinical efficacy. There are several other TIGIT inhibitors under study, such as domvanalimab, etigilimab, ociperlimab, and others (Rosseau et al., 2023).

Immune-Related Adverse Events

While ICIs have revolutionized cancer care and help many patients, there are still side effects to consider. These side effects, also known as immune-related adverse events or irAEs, are due to immune system overactivation causing damage to normal tissue. irAEs are very different from the side effects seen with traditional chemotherapy. Chemotherapy side effects occur as a result of decreased normal cell replication due to a direct effect from the medication. irAEs happen because the immune system now recognizes normal tissues as foreign, thus leading to autoimmune symptoms from immune destruction of "self". Since immune cells can travel to any part of the body, irAEs can occur in any organ system (Table 2.2). Common occurrences include rash (dermatitis), thyroiditis, and hepatitis. Often irAEs are mild to moderate, but sometimes events can be severe even, especially when vital organs are involved, such as the lungs (pneumonitis) or heart (myocarditis) (Schneider et al., 2021).

ICI side effects are difficult to predict—they can manifest at any point during treatment and are not related to the dose of medication (Sullivan & Weber, 2022). IrAEs can occur after one cycle, multiple cycles, or never at all. In contrast, chemotherapy toxicity follows predictable patterns based on the drugs' metabolism and elimination from the body. Since ICIs activate immune cells, which have memory, the risk of irAEs does not go away when the drug is stopped (Ghisoni et al., 2021).

Table 2.2 Overview of immune-related adverse events (irAEs)

irAE	Signs/symptoms
Dermatitis	Rash and itching
Thyroiditis	Low or high thyroid hormone
Hepatitis	Elevated liver enzymes
Pneumonitis	Respiratory symptoms Changes on imaging
Colitis	Diarrhea
Inflammatory arthritis	Swollen joints
Adrenal insufficiency	Low blood pressure Low adrenal hormones
Hypophysitis	Low pituitary hormones
Pancreatitis	Diabetes, type 1
Nephritis	Kidney damage elevated creatinine
Myocarditis	Heart damage
Myositis	Sore muscles Elevated creatine kinase
Cytopenias	Low blood counts
Uveitis and scleritis	Inflammation in the eyes
Encephalitis Aseptic meningitis	Neurological changes

The incidence of irAEs varies widely with estimates of up to 40% for treatment with one ICI and >60% for regimens containing ipilimumab (Martins et al., 2019). Specific patterns and the timing of irAEs depend on the tumor type and the class of ICI (Khoja et al., 2017). Once an irAE is identified, treatment involves supportive care for very mild cases (grade 1) or steroids for moderate (grades 2–3) to severe (grade 4) cases. The goal of steroid therapy is to dampen the overactive immune response. In some instances, irAEs are steroid refractory, necessitating additional immunosuppressive medications (Schneider et al., 2021). Since irAEs are complex, with the potential to occur at any time and affect any organ, it is essential to promptly notify a clinician of any new side effects, since irAEs can be severe and require timely intervention.

Special Circumstances

While ICIs have changed the treatment landscape in many cancers, there are certain scenarios where ICIs may cause harm, including preexisting autoimmune diseases and patients with transplanted organs.

Patients with History of Autoimmune Disorders

A prior diagnosis of an autoimmune disease has historically excluded patients from clinical trials investigating ICIs since they are at risk for flare of their disease from the ICI treatment. These patients may be at higher risk of cancer due to chronic inflammation and need for immunosuppressive medications, but there is a lack of clinical trial data to know how to best utilize ICIs in this population. The risk of an autoimmune disease flare is up to 75% for diseases such as rheumatoid arthritis, psoriasis, and polymyalgia rheumatica (Tison et al., 2022). To some patients, this may be an acceptable risk, while others may have debilitating symptoms during a flare. Ultimately, the decision of whether or not to pursue ICI treatment is shared between patient and clinician. If ICIs are used in patients with autoimmune disease, toxicity is still managed with steroids.

Solid-Organ Transplant Recipients

Patients with prior organ transplantation require ongoing immunosuppression to avoid rejection of the donated organ. Since ICIs essentially increase the immune system, there is a very high chance of organ rejection. Approximately 40% of liver transplant patients and 20% of cardiac transplant patients treated with ICIs experience rejection. Given the extremely high mortality of rejecting a vital organ, ICIs are typically avoided in transplant patients. If a patient has a kidney transplant, then they could trial ICIs knowing the risk of rejection and lifelong dialysis is nearly 50% (Murakami et al., 2020; Kumar et al., 2020). These patients should closely follow with transplant nephrology for adjustment of immunosuppression.

Conclusion

ICIs represent a revolutionary shift in cancer treatment. By blocking the inhibitory signals that regulate and suppress immune cells, ICIs enable the immune system to recognize and destroy cancer cells more effectively. These medications are commonly used in advanced solid tumors and are now moving to the adjuvant and neo-adjuvant settings. Trials exploring combinations of ICIs with other treatments and novel immune checkpoints are paving the way for expanded therapeutic options.

Take-Home Messages for Patients

- ICIs have a well-established and crucial role in the treatment of numerous tumor types. Most indications are in advanced or metastatic disease, but use in localized cancer is increasing.
- Current FDA-approved ICIs target PD-1, PD-L1, CTLA-4, and LAG-3.
- Side effects from ICIs, known as irAEs, are autoimmune symptoms from over-activation of the immune system leading to damage of normal tissues. Compared to chemotherapy side effects, irAEs are difficult to predict. Treatment usually involves steroids.
- Numerous clinical trials are actively investigating combinations of ICIs with other treatments, novel ICIs, and moving ICIs to the adjuvant and neoadjuvant settings.

References

Bagchi, S., Yuan, R., & Engleman, E. G. (2021). Immune checkpoint inhibitors for the treatment of cancer: Clinical impact and mechanisms of response and resistance. *Annual Review of Pathology, 16*, 223–249. https://doi.org/10.1146/annurev-pathol-042020-042741

Carlson, R. D., Flickinger, J. C., Jr., & Snook, A. E. (2020). Talkin' toxins: From Coley's to modern cancer immunotherapy. *Toxins (Basel), 12*(4), 241. https://doi.org/10.3390/toxins12040241

Chambers, C. A., Kuhns, M. S., Egen, J. G., & Allison, J. P. (2001). CTLA-4-mediated inhibition in regulation of T cell responses: Mechanisms and manipulation in tumor immunotherapy. *Annual Review of Immunology, 19*, 565–594. https://doi.org/10.1146/annurev.immunol.19.1.565

Chang, E., Pelosof, L., Lemery, S., Gong, Y., Goldberg, K. B., Farrell, A. T., et al. (2021). Systematic review of PD-1/PD-L1 inhibitors in oncology: From personalized medicine to public health. *The Oncologist, 26*(10), e1786–e1799. https://doi.org/10.1002/onco.13887

Collins, M., Ling, V., & Carreno, B. M. (2005). The B7 family of immune-regulatory ligands. *Genome Biology, 6*(6), 223. https://doi.org/10.1186/gb-2005-6-6-223

Geoerger, B., Kang, H. J., Yalon-Oren, M., Marshall, L. V., Vezina, C., Pappo, A., et al. (2020). Pembrolizumab in paediatric patients with advanced melanoma or a PD-L1-positive, advanced, relapsed, or refractory solid tumour or lymphoma (KEYNOTE-051): Interim analysis of an open-label, single-arm, phase 1-2 trial. *The Lancet Oncology, 21*(1), 121–133. https://doi.org/10.1016/S1470-2045(19)30671-0

Ghisoni, E., Wicky, A., Bouchaab, H., et al. (2021). Late-onset and long-lasting immune-related adverse events from immune checkpoint-inhibitors: An overlooked aspect in immunotherapy. *European Journal of Cancer, 149*, 153–164. https://doi.org/10.1016/j.ejca.2021.03.010

Haslam, A., Gill, J., & Prasad, V. (2020). Estimation of the percentage of US patients with cancer who are eligible for immune checkpoint inhibitor drugs. *JAMA Network Open, 3*(3), e200423. https://doi.org/10.1001/jamanetworkopen.2020.0423

Keytruda. Package Insert. Merck. 2024. Available at: https://www.merck.com/product/usa/pi_circulars/k/keytruda/keytruda_pi.pdf

Khoja, L., Day, D., Wei-Wu Chen, T., et al. (2017). Tumour- and class-specific patterns of immune-related adverse events of immune checkpoint inhibitors: A systematic review. *Annals of Oncology, 28*(10), 2377–2385. https://doi.org/10.1093/annonc/mdx286

Khongorzul, P., Ling, C. J., Khan, F. U., Ihsan, A. U., & Zhang, J. (2020). Antibody-drug conjugates: A comprehensive review. *Molecular Cancer Research, 18*(1), 3–19. https://doi.org/10.1158/1541-7786.MCR-19-0582

Kumar, V., Shinagare, A. B., Rennke, H. G., Ghai, S., Lorch, J. H., Ott, P. A., & Rahma, O. E. (2020). The safety and efficacy of checkpoint inhibitors in transplant recipients: A case series and systematic review of literature. *The Oncologist, 25*(6), 505–514. https://doi.org/10.1634/theoncologist.2019-0659

Lao, C. D., Khushalani, N. I., Angeles, C., & Petrella, T. M. (2022). Current state of adjuvant therapy for melanoma: Less is more, or more is better? *American Society of Clinical Oncology Educational Book, 42*, 738–744.

Larkin, J., Chiarion-Sileni, V., Gonzalez, R., et al. (2015). Combined nivolumab and ipilimumab or monotherapy in untreated melanoma. *The New England Journal of Medicine, 373*(1), 23–34. https://doi.org/10.1056/NEJMoa1504030

Le, D. T., Kim, T. W., Van Cutsem, E., et al. (2020). Phase II open-label study of pembrolizumab in treatment-refractory, microsatellite instability-high/mismatch repair-deficient metastatic colorectal cancer: KEYNOTE-164. *Journal of Clinical Oncology, 38*(1), 11–19. https://doi.org/10.1200/JCO.19.02107

Marabelle, A., Le, D. T., Ascierto, P. A., et al. (2020). Efficacy of pembrolizumab in patients with noncolorectal high microsatellite instability/mismatch repair-deficient cancer: Results from the phase II KEYNOTE-158 study. *Journal of Clinical Oncology, 38*(1), 1–10. https://doi.org/10.1200/JCO.19.02105

Marin-Acevedo, J. A., Kimbrough, E. O., & Lou, Y. (2021). Next generation of immune checkpoint inhibitors and beyond. *Journal of Hematology & Oncology, 14*(1), 45. https://doi.org/10.1186/s13045-021-01056-8

Martins, F., Sofiya, L., Sykiotis, G. P., et al. (2019). Adverse effects of immune-checkpoint inhibitors: epidemiology management and surveillance. *Nature Reviews Clinical Oncology, 16*(9), 563–580. https://doi.org/10.1038/s41571-019-0218-0

Maruhashi, T., Sugiura, D., Okazaki, I. M., & Okazaki, T. (2020). LAG-3: From molecular functions to clinical applications. *Journal for Immunotherapy of Cancer, 8*(2), e001014. https://doi.org/10.1136/jitc-2020-001014

Mirza, M. R., Chase, D. M., Slomovitz, B. M., et al. (2023). Dostarlimab for primary advanced or recurrent endometrial cancer. *The New England Journal of Medicine, 388*(23), 2145–2158. https://doi.org/10.1056/NEJMoa2216334

Mittendorf, E. A., Burgers, F., Haanen, J., & Cascone, T. (2022). Neoadjuvant immunotherapy: Leveraging the immune system to treat early-stage disease. *American Society of Clinical Oncology Educational Book, 42*, 189–203.

Murakami, N., Mulvaney, P., Danesh, M., Abudayyeh, A., et al. (2020). Immune checkpoint inhibitors in solid organ transplant consortium. A multi-center study on safety and efficacy of immune checkpoint inhibitors in cancer patients with kidney transplant. *Kidney International, 100*(1), 196–205. https://doi.org/10.1016/j.kint.2020.12.015

O'Brien, M., Paz-Ares, L., Marreaud, S., et al. (2022). Pembrolizumab versus placebo as adjuvant therapy for completely resected stage IB-IIIA non-small-cell lung cancer (PEARLS/ KEYNOTE-091): An interim analysis of a randomised, triple-blind, phase 3 trial. *The Lancet Oncology, 23*(10), 1274–1286. https://doi.org/10.1016/S1470-2045(22)00518-6

Oaknin, A., Gilbert, L., Tinker, A. V., et al. (2022). Safety and antitumor activity of dostarlimab in patients with advanced or recurrent DNA mismatch repair deficient/microsatellite instability-high (dMMR/MSI-H) or proficient/stable (MMRp/MSS) endometrial cancer: Interim results from GARNET—a phase I, single-arm study. *Journal for Immunotherapy of Cancer, 10*, e003777. https://doi.org/10.1136/jitc-2021-003777

Opdivo. Package Insert. Bristol Myers Squibb. 2024. Available at https://packageinserts.bms.com/ pi/pi_opdivo.pdf

Patsoukis, N., Wang, Q., Strauss, L., & Boussiotis, V. A. (2020). Revisiting the PD-1 pathway. *Science Advances, 6*(38), eabd2712. https://doi.org/10.1126/sciadv.abd2712

Pettenati, C., & Ingersoll, M. A. (2018). Mechanisms of BCG immunotherapy and its outlook for bladder cancer. *Nature Reviews. Urology, 15*(10), 615–625. https://doi.org/10.1038/ s41585-018-0055-4

Pierpont, T. M., Limper, C. B., & Richards, K. L. (2018). Past, present, and future of Rituximab-the world's first oncology monoclonal antibody therapy. *Frontiers in Oncology, 8*, 163. https:// doi.org/10.3389/fonc.2018.00163

Raeber, M. E., Sahin, D., Karakus, U., & Boyman, O. (2023). A systematic review of interleukin-2-based immunotherapies in clinical trials for cancer and autoimmune diseases. *eBioMedicine, 90*(104539). https://doi.org/10.1016/j.ebiom.2023.104539

Robert, C. (2020). A decade of immune-checkpoint inhibitors in cancer therapy. *Nature Communications, 11*(1), 3801. https://doi.org/10.1038/s41467-020-17670-y

Rousseau, A., Parisi, C., & Barlesi, F. (2023). Anti-TIGIT therapies for solid tumors: A systematic review. *ESMO Open, 8*(2), 101184. https://doi.org/10.1016/j.esmoop.2023.101184

Schmid, P., Cortes, J., Pusztai, L., et al. (2020). Pembrolizumab for early triple-negative breast cancer. *The New England Journal of Medicine, 382*(9), 810–821. https://doi.org/10.1056/ NEJMoa1910549

Schneider, B. J., Naidoo, J., Santomasso, B. D., et al. (2021). Management of immune-related adverse events in patients treated with immune checkpoint inhibitor therapy: ASCO guideline update. *Journal of Clinical Oncology, 39*(36), 4073–4126. https://doi.org/10.1200/ JCO.21.01440

Shanshal, M., Caimi, P. F., Adjei, A. A., & Ma, W. W. (2023). T-Cell engagers in solid cancers-current landscape and future directions. *Cancers (Basel), 15*(10), 2824. https://doi.org/10.3390/ cancers15102824

Sullivan, R. J., & Weber, J. S. (2022). Immune-related toxicities of checkpoint inhibitors: Mechanisms and mitigation strategies. *Nature Reviews. Drug Discovery, 21*(7), 495–508. https://doi.org/10.1038/s41585-018-0055-4

Tawbi, H. A., Schadendorf, D., Lipson, E. J., et al. (2022). Relatlimab and nivolumab versus nivolumab in untreated advanced melanoma. *The New England Journal of Medicine, 386*(1), 24–34. https://doi.org/10.1056/NEJMoa2109970

Tison, A., Garaud, S., Chiche, L., Cornec, D., & Kostine, M. (2022). Immune-checkpoint inhibitor use in patients with cancer and pre-existing autoimmune diseases. *Nature Reviews Rheumatology, 8*(11), 641–656. https://doi.org/10.1038/s41584-022-00841-0

Vaddepally, R. K., Kharel, P., Pandey, R., et al. (2020). Review of indications of FDA-approved immune checkpoint inhibitors per NCCN guidelines with the level of evidence. *Cancers (Basel), 12*(3), 738. https://doi.org/10.3390/cancers12030738

Wei, S. C., Duffy, C. R., & Allison, J. P. (2018). Fundamental mechanisms of immune checkpoint blockade therapy. *Cancer Discovery, 8*(9), 1069–1086. https://doi.org/10.1158/2159-8290. CD-18-0367

Chapter 3
Immunotherapies for Cancer: Bi-specific T Cell Engagers (BiTEs)

Richard C. Godby, Alex Niu, and Jonas Paludo

Abstract Bi-specific T cell engagers (BiTEs) are immunologically active molecules with dual specificity, concurrently binding to a tumor-associated antigen and CD3 on T cells. This approach brings cytotoxic T cells and tumor cells into close proximity, thereby intensifying immunological responses against neoplastic cells. Originally employed in the context of minimal residual disease in B-cell precursor acute lymphoblastic leukemia, various novel BiTEs have been approved or are currently in development for the management of multiple hematologic and solid malignancies. BiTEs may also present logistical advantages over chimeric antigen receptor T cell (CAR-T) therapies, as they circumvent the intricate procedures associated with autologous T cell genetic engineering and eliminate the necessity for supplementary cytotoxic chemotherapy while harnessing endogenous immune potential. As evidenced by an expanding spectrum of indications and demonstrated efficacy, BiTEs emerge as a promising anticancer therapy, capitalizing on the intricacies of the immune system while evading the logistical challenges associated with CAR-T therapies.

Keywords Bi-specific T cell engagers · BiTEs · T cell signaling · Epcoritamab · Glofitamab · Mosunetuzumab · Teclistamab · Blinatumomab · Tebentafusp · Cytokine release syndrome (CRS) · Immune effector cell-associated neurotoxicity syndrome (ICANS)

R. C. Godby · A. Niu · J. Paludo (✉)
Division of Hematology, Mayo Clinic, Rochester, MN, USA
e-mail: paludo.jonas@mayo.edu

© The Author(s), under exclusive license to Springer Nature Switzerland AG 2024
H. Dong, S. N. Markovic (eds.), *The Basics of Cancer Immunotherapy*,
https://doi.org/10.1007/978-3-031-59475-5_3

Introduction

Bi-specific T cell engagers (BiTEs) are immunologically active molecules with dual specificity—binding both to a unique tumor-associated antigen and CD3, an essential component of the T cell receptor complex. This approach focuses on bringing the tumor cell into close proximity to cytotoxic T cells, thus increasing immunological activity against the tumor (Fig. 3.1). BiTEs were initially introduced with blinatumomab in the treatment of minimal residual disease (MRD)-positive B-cell precursor acute lymphoblastic leukemia after initial induction and consolidation (Topp et al., 2011). The positive results of this study in 2011 opened the door for further investigation, and since then, there have been many additional landmark studies evaluating the use of BiTEs with substantially more clinical trials. These "off-the-shelf" products have logistical advantages over chimeric antigen receptor T cell (CAR-T) therapies as they do not require the same collection and manufacturing hurdles in order to genetically engineer autologous T cells and also obviate the need for additional cytotoxic chemotherapy while harnessing the potential of the patient's own immune system.

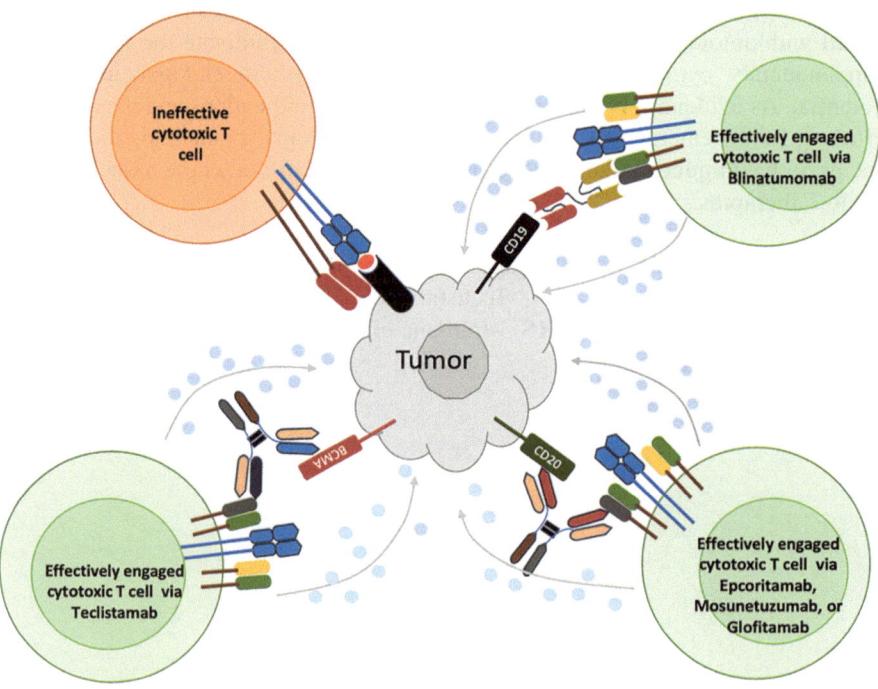

Fig. 3.1 Representation of currently FDA-approved BiTE technologies, which promote effective immune cytotoxicity by simultaneously engaging the CD3 portion of the T cell receptor complex and a surface tumor antigen of interest (e.g., CD19, CD20, BCMA)

T Cell Signaling and BiTEs

Typically, innate and adaptive arms of the immune system collaborate to achieve immunosurveillance and safeguard against harmful agents, including malignancies and microbes (Chaplin, 2010). The adaptive immune system consists of various cell types, among which T cells are particularly noteworthy as a vehicle for cancer therapeutics due to their crucial roles in both immune coordination and as IECs with inherently robust cytotoxic functionality. T cell effector functions rely on proper engagement of TCRs with antigen presentation via the major histocompatibility complex (MHC), such as that from the antigen-presenting cells (APC) or nucleated tumor cells (Fig. 3.1). TCR complexes are comprised of a diverse range of elements, encompassing both extracellular and intracellular components (Shah et al., 2021). Additional elements and further discussion of T cell immunology can be found in Chap. 1.

T cell dysfunction has the potential to manifest in various circumstances, such as anergy from suboptimal antigen stimulation, exhaustion caused by persistent over stimulation, and senescence from repeated stimulation (Xia et al., 2019). Malignant cells often employ various mechanisms to evade immune destruction and impair the proper functioning of T cells. These include upregulation of immunosuppressive ligands (e.g., PD-L1), loss of MHC expression, and changes in the tumor microenvironment (TME) that lead to immune suppression and exhaustion (Ansell, 2020). Some of these immune escape mechanisms have been targeted by many of the most impactful advances in hematology and oncology, such as immune checkpoint inhibitors to disinhibit T cell effector functions and reverse some dysfunctional states as well as CAR-T cell technologies to provide cytotoxic activity in a directed manner independent of MHC antigen presentation.

BiTEs are designed to augment T cell activities and facilitate interactions with cancer cells. This is achieved through engineering BiTEs to have multi-antigenic specificity, usually with a common T cell antigen (e.g., CD3) and an antigen commonly found on the tumor cell type (e.g., CD20). Once properly engaged with the tumor cell, the T cell becomes activated and initiates cytotoxic activity (Fig. 3.1).

Approved Products and Indications

Currently, there are several commercial BiTE products available for various malignancies (Table 3.1). Non-Hodgkin B-cell lymphomas utilize epcoritamab-bysp, glofitamab-gxbm, and mosunetuzumab-axgb. Multiple myeloma (MM), a plasma cell dyscrasia, utilizes teclistamab-cqyx. B-precursor acute lymphoblastic leukemia uses blinatumomab. Uveal melanoma uses tebentafusp-tebn. There are many several clinical trials underway expected to result in additional approvals.

Epcoritamab-bysp was initially evaluated in the EPCORE study. It is a BiTE targeted against CD20 and CD3 (Fig. 3.1). In this trial, adults with relapsed or

Table 3.1 Approved products and indications

	Epcoritamab-bysp	Glofitamab-gxbml	Mosunetuzumab-axgb	Blinatumomab	Teclistamab-cqyx	Tebentafusp
Relapsed/refractory follicular lymphoma ≥ 2 prior lines of therapy			x			
Relapsed/refractory large B-cell lymphoma: DLBCL (NOS) ≥ 2 prior lines of therapy	x	x				
Relapsed/refractory large B-cell lymphoma arising from indolent lymphoma ≥ 2 prior lines of therapy	x					
Relapsed/refractory large B-cell lymphoma arising from follicular lymphoma ≥ 2 prior lines of therapy	x	x				
Relapsed/refractory large B-cell lymphoma: high-grade ≥ 2 prior lines of therapy	x					
Relapsed/refractory B-cell ALL: Ph-negative adolescent and young adult or Ph-negative adult				x		
Relapsed/refractory B-cell ALL: Ph-positive adolescent and young adult or Ph-positive adult				x		
Relapsed/refractory multiple myeloma after ≥ four prior lines of therapy, including an immunomodulatory agent, a proteasome inhibitor, and an anti-CD38 monoclonal antibody					x	
Uveal melanoma, unresectable or metastatic, HLA-A*02:01 positive						x

refractory (R/R) CD20+ large B-cell lymphoma and at least two prior lines of therapy (including anti-CD20 therapies) were treated with epcoritamab. Specifically, this trial enrolled patients with diffuse large cell lymphoma (DLBCL) and other aggressive non-Hodgkin lymphomas, including primary mediastinal large B-cell lymphoma, high-grade B-cell lymphoma, and follicular lymphoma grade 3B. Interestingly, in the EPCORE study, 38.9% of patients had received prior CAR-T cell treatment. At a median follow-up of 10.7 months, the overall response (OR) rate was 63.1%, of which 38.9% had a complete response (CR). The median duration of response was 12.0 months (Thieblemont et al., 2023). Currently approved indications for epcoritamab are outlined in Table 3.1.

Glofitamab-gxbm was evaluated in patients with R/R DLBCL, who had received at least two previous lines of therapy. It is a BiTE targeted against CD20 and CD3 (Fig. 3.1). Similar to the EPCORE study, 33% of patients had previously received CAR-T treatment. Results showed that at a median follow-up of 12.6 months, 39% of the patients achieved a CR. In addition, results were consistent among the 33% of patients who had previously received CAR-T therapy (35% of whom had a CR). The median time to a CR was 42 days and 78% of patients who had achieved a CR maintained that response at 12 months of follow-up (Dickinson et al., 2022). Currently approved indications for glofitamab are outlined in Table 3.1.

Mosunetuzumab-axgb was evaluated in a single-arm phase 2 study, enrolling adult patients with R/R follicular lymphoma (grades 1–3A) who had received at least two prior lines of treatment, including an anti-CD20 therapy and an alkylating agent. It is a BiTE targeted against CD20 and CD3 (Fig. 3.1). The study demonstrated that at a median follow-up of 18.3 months, a CR was observed in 60% of patients. This CR rate was significantly higher than the historical control CR rate with copanlisib of 14% (which is currently approved for R/R follicular lymphoma in the third-line setting) (Budde et al., 2022). Currently approved indications for mosunetuzumab are outlined in Table 3.1.

Blinatumomab is perhaps the most well-known BiTE as it achieved the first FDA approval of a BiTE. It is a BiTE targeted against CD19 and CD3 (Fig. 3.1). In 2011, a phase II clinical study was conducted to determine the efficacy of blinatumomab in adults with MRD-positive B-lineage ALL after induction and consolidation chemotherapy. The study demonstrated that at a median observation time of 405 days, 78% of patients were in ongoing hematologic remission (Topp et al., 2011). This was further validated with the BLAST study, which enrolled a relatively higher number of patients. In this study, adults with B-cell precursor ALL in hematologic CR, but with positive MRD, received at least one cycle of blinatumomab. Of note, after the initial cycle of blinatumomab, patients could move onto allogeneic stem cell transplant if deemed appropriate. The study demonstrated that 78% of patients achieved MRD negativity after one cycle of blinatumomab. In a secondary endpoint analysis of 110 patients with Ph-negative ALL in hematologic remission, the relapse-free survival (RFS) at 18 months was 54% after all treatments (of which included at least one cycle of blinatumomab). Median OS in the study was found to be 36.5 months (Gökbuget et al., 2018). Since the BLAST study, there have been many more assessments of blinatumomab. One of the most pivotal studies was the

TOWER study published in 2017. In this multi-institutional phase 3 trial, patients over the age of 18, who were refractory to primary induction chemotherapy or to salvage chemotherapy, had a first relapse with the first remission lasting less than 12 months, a second or more relapse, or relapse at any time after allogeneic stem cell transplantation and were randomized to either blinatumomab or standard of care. The TOWER study demonstrated improved median OS with blinatumomab versus standard of care (7.7 vs. 4.0 months). Event-free survival was also higher with blinatumomab than standard of care (six-month estimates, 31% vs. 12%). And finally, remission rates within 12 weeks after treatment were significantly higher in the blinatumomab group than in the standard of care group. Currently approved indications for blinatumomab are outlined in Table 3.1.

Teclistamab-cqyx is the sole BiTE that is approved in the treatment of MM. It is a BiTE targeted against B-cell maturation antigen (BCMA) and CD3 (Fig. 3.1). Approval was achieved via the MajesTEC-1 trial in 2022. In this study, patients with R/R multiple myeloma after at least three systemic therapies, of which must have included triple-class exposure to an immunomodulatory drug, a proteasome inhibitor, and an anti-CD38 antibody, were treated with teclistamab. With a median follow-up of 14.1 months, the OR rate was 63.0%, with 39.4% having a CR. A total of 26.7% of patients were found to have MRD negativity. The median duration of response was 18.4 months with the median duration of progression-free survival of 11.3 months (Moreau et al., 2022). Currently approved indications for teclistamab are outlined in Table 3.1.

Tebentafusp-tebn is currently the only BiTE approved for treatment of a solid tumor, uveal melanoma. More specifically, it is used for unresectable or metastatic uveal melanoma. It uniquely binds to gp100 loaded into the HLA-A*02:01 molecule and brings it into proximity with CD3-expressing cells. It first gained approval in January 2022 based upon a phase 3 clinical trial demonstrating improved OS at 1 year (73% vs. 59% in control) (Nathan et al., 2021). Currently approved indications for tebentafusp-tebn are outlined in Table 3.1.

Adverse Events and Limitations

Cytokine Release Syndrome (CRS)

After administration of BiTE products, there is potential for rapid activation and cytotoxic activity resulting in large amounts of cytokine release (van de Donk & Zweegman, 2023). Clinically, this may manifest with fevers, hypotension, and hypoxia which are used to grade the CRS in a similar fashion to that of CAR-T and subsequently guide treatment (Lee et al., 2019; NCCN, 2023; van de Donk & Zweegman, 2023). This seems to be dependent on route of administration and pharmacokinetics of the product, with the highest rates occurring shortly after relatively larger intravenous dosing (van de Donk & Zweegman, 2023). Each therapy has product-specific recommendations for management of CRS, but in addition to supportive care, treatments if clinically warranted may include anti-IL6 therapy (e.g., tocilizumab) and dexamethasone (NCCN, 2023; van de Donk & Zweegman, 2023).

Immune Effector Cell-Associated Neurotoxicity Syndrome (ICANS)

After administration of BiTE products, there is potential for rapid activation and cytotoxic activity resulting in large amounts of cytokine release that may also disrupt the blood-brain barrier (van de Donk & Zweegman, 2023). Clinically, this may manifest with depressed consciousness, seizures, motor changes, and cerebral edema which are used to grade the ICANS in a similar fashion to that of CAR-T and subsequently guide treatment (Lee et al., 2019; Santomasso et al., 2021; NCCN, 2023). This occurs relatively infrequently for products not targeting CD19 (van de Donk & Zweegman, 2023). Each therapy has product-specific recommendations for management of ICANS, but in addition to supportive care, treatments if clinically warranted may include dexamethasone with the possible addition of antiepileptics; anti-IL6 therapy is usually added only for the simultaneous presence of CRS (NCCN, 2023; van de Donk & Zweegman, 2023).

Infections

Patients receiving BiTE therapies often experience infections that can arise from various etiologies. By the time patients are eligible for BiTEs, they have already been exposed to cytotoxic chemotherapy, and many BiTEs may lead to T cell exhaustion. Furthermore, another consequence of many approved BiTE products is hypogammaglobulinemia, predisposing to additional infectious complications (van de Donk & Zweegman, 2023).

Future Directions

Although BiTEs have been around for years, a rapidly growing list of indications with clear efficacy solidifies this technology as a cornerstone of hematology and oncology treatments in the future. There are several ongoing studies and ideas for technological advancements to further expand this armamentarium and enhance outcomes. For instance, from tri-specific engagers and sequencing of engagers to alternative and/or combinatorial targets of cell engagement in addition to T cells are interesting areas of research. Additionally, given that these "off-the-shelf" products have logistical advantages over CAR-T therapies and obviate the need for additional cytotoxic chemotherapy, they will continue to further the fields of both hematology and oncology by harnessing the potential of the immune system.

References

Ansell, S. M. (2020). Fundamentals of immunology for understanding immunotherapy for lymphoma. *Blood Advances, 4*, 5863–5867.

Budde, L. E., Sehn, L. H., Matasar, M., et al. (2022). Safety and efficacy of mosunetuzumab, a bispecific antibody, in patients with relapsed or refractory follicular lymphoma: A single-arm, multicentre, phase 2 study. *The Lancet Oncology, 23*, 1055–1065. https://doi.org/10.1016/S1470-2045(22)00335-7

Chaplin, D. D. (2010). Overview of the immune response. *The Journal of Allergy and Clinical Immunology, 125*, S3–S23. https://doi.org/10.1016/j.jaci.2009.12.980

Dickinson, M. J., Carlo-Stella, C., Morschhauser, F., et al. (2022). Glofitamab for relapsed or refractory diffuse large B-cell lymphoma. *The New England Journal of Medicine, 387*, 2220–2231. https://doi.org/10.1056/NEJMoa2206913

Gökbuget, N., Dombret, H., Bonifacio, M., et al. (2018). Blinatumomab for minimal residual disease in adults with B-cell precursor acute lymphoblastic leukemia. *Blood, 131*, 1522–1531. https://doi.org/10.1182/blood-2017-08-798322

Lee, D. W., Santomasso, B. D., Locke, F. L., et al. (2019). ASTCT consensus grading for cytokine release syndrome and neurologic toxicity associated with immune effector cells. *Biology of Blood and Marrow Transplantation, 25*, 625–638.

Moreau, P., Garfall, A. L., van de Donk, N. W. C. J., et al. (2022). Teclistamab in relapsed or refractory multiple myeloma. *The New England Journal of Medicine, 387*, 495–505. https://doi.org/10.1056/nejmoa2203478

Nathan, P., Hassel, J. C., Rutkowski, P., et al. (2021). Overall survival benefit with tebentafusp in metastatic uveal melanoma. *The New England Journal of Medicine, 385*, 1196–1206. https://doi.org/10.1056/nejmoa2103485

NCCN. (2023). Management of immunotherapy-related toxicities. In *Guidelines*. https://www.nccn.org/guidelines/guidelines-detail?category=3&id=1486

Santomasso, B. D., Nastoupil, L. J., Adkins, S., et al. (2021). Management of immune-related adverse events in patients treated with chimeric antigen receptor T-cell therapy: ASCO guideline. *Journal of Clinical Oncology, 39*, 3978–3992. https://doi.org/10.1200/JCO.21.01992

Shah, K., Al-Haidari, A., Sun, J., & Kazi, J. U. (2021). T cell receptor (TCR) signaling in health and disease. *Signal Transduction and Targeted Therapy, 6*, 412.

Thieblemont, C., Phillips, T., Ghesquieres, H., et al. (2023). Epcoritamab, a novel, subcutaneous CD3xCD20 bispecific T-cell-engaging antibody, in relapsed or refractory large B-cell lymphoma: Dose expansion in a phase I/II trial. *Journal of Clinical Oncology, 41*, 2238–2247. https://doi.org/10.1200/JCO.22.01725

Topp, M. S., Kufer, P., Gökbuget, N., et al. (2011). Targeted therapy with the T-cell - Engaging antibody blinatumomab of chemotherapy-refractory minimal residual disease in B-lineage acute lymphoblastic leukemia patients results in high response rate and prolonged leukemia-free survival. *Journal of Clinical Oncology, 29*, 2493–2498. https://doi.org/10.1200/JCO.2010.32.7270

van de Donk, N. W. C. J., & Zweegman, S. (2023). T-cell-engaging bispecific antibodies in cancer. *Lancet, 402*, 142–158.

Xia, A., Zhang, Y., Xu, J., et al. (2019). T cell dysfunction in cancer immunity and immunotherapy. *Frontiers in Immunology, 10*, 1719.

Chapter 4
Tumor-Infiltrating Lymphocyte (TIL) Therapy

Jeffrey E. Johnson, Velvet R. Van Ryan, and Arkadiusz Z. Dudek

Abstract Since T cells can recognize tumor-associated antigens and eliminate cancer cells, preclinical and clinical developments of therapy have been leveraging on the use of autologous tumor-infiltrating lymphocytes (TILs). Target metastatic tumor is excised from patient by trained surgeon and then transferred to laboratory, where is cut into small fragments. Lymphocytes are then enriched in culture with interleukin 2 and after several days propagated in rapid expansion phase. When TIL product is ready, patient receives lymphodepleting chemotherapy, and then TILs are infused followed by treatment with high-dose interleukin 2. Therapy with TIL has shown to be an effective treatment strategy in melanoma, even after melanoma progression following immune checkpoint inhibitor therapy with remarkable responses and improvement of progression-free survival. Recently, genetically modified TILs have been tested with a goal to further improve clinical activity.

Keywords Tumor-infiltrating lymphocytes · Interleukin 2 · Infrastructure for TIL therapy · Melanoma · Lymphodepleting therapy

Knowledge that T cells can recognize tumor-associated antigens and in turn cause elimination of melanoma cells led to the idea of tumor treatment by infusion of immunized lymphoid cells (Rosenberg et al., 1982). Success of the cancer treatment was dependent on the dose of infused sensitized to tumor cells, and therefore expansion of immune cells by interleukin-2 (IL-2) was introduced and cured of up to 93% of animals (Eberlein et al., 1982). Around the same time, the discovery that suppressive T cells will interfere with adoptive therapy led to the use of cyclophosphamide prior to infusion of immunized cells to decrease suppressive T cell population

---

J. E. Johnson · V. R. Van Ryan
Department of Surgery, Mayo Clinic, Rochester, MN, USA

A. Z. Dudek (✉)
Department of Medical Oncology, Mayo Clinic, Rochester, MN, USA
e-mail: dudek.arkadiusz@mayo.edu

(North, 1982). In 1986, Rosenberg et al. published pivotal paper demonstrating that tumor-infiltrating lymphocytes (TILs) grown from and expanded in IL-2, when injected to animals pretreated with cyclophosphamide and treated with IL-2 after infusion, were 50–100 times more effective than lymphokine-activated killer cells (Rosenberg et al., 1986). This discovery initiated the development of TIL for therapy of human patients with cancer. Optimization of culture techniques of TIL (Dudley et al., 2003) led to study of 35 patients with metastatic melanoma treated with lymphodepleting regimen of 2 days of cyclophosphamide and 5 days of fludarabine, infusion of TIL, and then high-dose IL-2. This resulted in 51% clinical response rates including three complete responses (Dudley et al., 2005). Activity of TIL therapy was confirmed in other studies (Besser et al., 2010; Radvanyi et al., 2012). With increasing number of patients treated with TIL, knowledge of best surgical techniques and metastatic sites from which to harvest TIL was gained (Goff et al., 2010).

Multi-institution phase 2 study of centrally manufactured TIL product in previously treated patients with immune checkpoint inhibitors for metastatic melanoma demonstrated that TIL can induce tumor response rate of 41% in this patient population (Sarnaik et al., 2021). With additional cohorts, pooled analysis of patients treated with TIL, lifileucel product, confirmed overall response rate of 31.4% with 41.7% of responses lasting at least 18 months (Chesney et al., 2022).

In randomized, phase 3, multicenter study outcomes of treatment of patients with unresectable or metastatic melanoma treated with TIL were compared to anti-cytotoxic T-lymphocyte antigen 4 therapy with ipilimumab. Median progression-free survival was superior inpatients receiving TIL (7.2 months) versus ipilimumab (3.1 months) (Rohaan et al., 2022).

Further research was focused on prolongation of TIL persistence (Krishna et al., 2020), increased activity (Chamberlain et al., 2022), and preservation from exhaustive phenotype (Woroniecka et al., 2020).

TIL therapy requires a multidisciplinary approach. Medical oncologists, surgeons, advanced practice providers, registered nurses, and technicians familiar with the multiple facets of TIL therapy are integral. Overall, having the lymphodepleting treatment, infusion of TIL, and high-dose IL-2 on an oncology or intensive care unit is optimal.

Appropriate patient selection is critical. Patients need to have a performance status of 0–1 with low cardiac and pulmonary comorbidities (Sarnaik et al., 2021; Rohaan et al., 2022). Cardiac stress testing and pulmonary function tests can aid in identifying acceptable respective organ function. Untreated, active brain metastases are contraindicated (Sarnaik et al., 2021; Rohaan et al., 2022).

In addition, there are a number of surgical specimen considerations that must be considered for patient's selection as well as ensuring an adequate sample for production of the cell therapy product. Multidisciplinary collaboration with surgical oncologists, other subspecialty surgeons, radiologists, and medical oncologists is needed to select patients who will tolerate anesthesia, recover quickly from surgery to allow for treatment within 3–4 weeks, and have a lesion of sufficient size, character, and accessibility to allow for surgical resection. Patient being considered for surgery will often have a range of comorbidities and diminished functional status, often related to progressive disease and receipt of multiple lines of systemic therapy prior to consideration for TIL cell therapy, which must be considered in surgical planning.

Although it depends on manufacture or clinical study criteria, generally tumor tissue measuring 1–4 cm in size is required for isolation in expansion of sufficient TILs (Goff et al., 2010; Mullinax et al., 2022). Anatomic locations that minimize morbidity and allow for outpatient surgery are favored, such as tumors involving the skin and superficial tissues or accessible lymph node basins. Tumors involving visceral organs can also be used, and minimally invasive surgery is favored to speed recovery time. Consideration for visceral surgery, for example, liver or lung resections, requires careful patient selection and discussion with surgeons experienced in performing surgery in those areas. Tumors should also have sufficient viable cellularity to allow for culture, excluding small or necrotic tumors. Additionally, tumors with a risk of bacterial contamination due to extrinsic exposure (e.g., ulceration, aerodigestive tract, genital organs) cannot be used due to risk of contamination, precluding use of the cultured cell product (Mullinax et al., 2022).

Early studies had a significant proportion of patients initiating the TIL procurement process but ultimately not receiving therapy. Since then, better patient selection, streamlined workflow, and improved production protocols have increased likelihood of completing TIL production leading to infusion to above 90% (Chesney et al., 2022; Mullinax et al., 2022). Patients may have a number of anatomic sites involved with metastatic cancer, and generally any site of disease may be used as all tissues are able to yield TILs and tumor resection site does not affect systemic efficacy of TIL therapy (Goff et al., 2010; Sarnaik et al., 2021). However, sites from secondary lymphoid organs or sites with high non-tumor reactive lymphocytes (e.g., bowel) may result in lower tumor-specific TIL yield (Goff et al., 2010).

Once a metastatic tumor has been excised, the surgeon places the tumor in the sterile field to select tumor areas avoiding necrosis or non-tumor-involved tissue and selecting well-vascularized viable tumor. It is vital that all tissue handling remain under sterile conditions to prevent contamination. Intraoperative pathology review to confirm presence of tumor and infiltrating lymphocytes may be used as needed. The prosected tissue is placed into a sealed sterile media container and transported to a Good Manufacturing (GMP) laboratory (Mullinax et al., 2022). GMP labs follow strict US Food and Drug Administration regulations to ensure products are consistently produced and controlled (Chu et al., 2023). The laboratory expands the lymphocytes ex vivo in a medium that includes IL-2 (Andersen et al., 2016; Sarnaik et al., 2021; Ernst & Giubellino, 2022). Once the cell proliferation goal has been met, the cells are cryopreserved for later use.

Upon completion of TIL expansion and transfer to treatment site, the patient can begin lymphodepletion therapy. It is important to have an oncology team of experienced physicians, advanced practice providers, and nurses to safely care for the patient and manage the ensuing side effects. The more common side effects include bone marrow suppression, electrolyte imbalances, nausea, vomiting, and diarrhea (Rohaan et al., 2022). These patients may need blood product transfusions, electrolyte replacement, and additional medical management during this time.

Within 24 h of the completion of the lymphodepletion regimen, the TIL cells are infused. The patient needs to have continuous cardiac monitoring and frequent monitoring of vital signs and be premedicated for the TIL infusion. Patients can have transient adverse effects such as chills, fever, shortness of breath, and tachycardia during and immediately following infusion (Radvanyi et al., 2012).

The first dose of IL2 is administered IV within 24 h of TIL infusion and repeated every 8 to 12 h. The side effects of IL-2 are varied, and their management can be counterintuitive. The Cytokine Working Group (CWG) recommends that centers that are naïve to the administration of IL-2 perform the first ten or so infusions in an intensive care setting (Dutcher et al., 2014). The CWG and National Cancer Institute have established best management practices for the infusion of high-dose IL-2 (Dutcher et al., 2014). Patients will need continuous cardiac monitoring, frequent monitoring of vital signs, and assessment. The CWG recommends that nurses have a low nurse-to-patient ratio to allow for frequent monitoring and management of adverse effects of IL-2 (Dutcher et al., 2014). The most common side effects are due to cytokine release syndrome and capillary leak syndrome (Dutcher et al., 2014; Rohaan et al., 2022). Function of multiple organ systems can be affected. Frequently patients develop significant hypotension and extracellular fluid overload which is better managed with inotropic therapy rather than fluid boluses. The patient should be evaluated by a provider before each infusion to ensure safety. The peak adverse effect of each dose occurs 4–6 h after the infusion. The heart rate, pulse oximetry, and blood pressure should reach or be near reaching baseline before the next infusion (Dutcher et al., 2014). If the patient needs to be moved to the intensive care unit, the experienced oncology team needs to continue care over the patient. The majority of adverse effects resolve before the patient is discharged from the hospital. Treatment-related adverse events are from lymphodepleting chemotherapy and IL-2 and include thrombocytopenia, anemia (56%), febrile neutropenia (55%), neutropenia (39%), hypophosphatemia (35%), leukopenia (35%), and lymphopenia (32%) (Sarnaik et al., 2021). No lifileucel-related serious adverse events nor recurrence of immune-related adverse events from earlier immune checkpoint inhibitor therapy were reported six months after therapy (Sarnaik et al., 2021).

In summary, TIL therapy is promising with manageable side effects and could be an effective strategy against melanoma progressing on immune checkpoint therapies (Sarnaik et al., 2021; Rohaan et al., 2022). Further improvements in TIL technology are underway with its use tested in other solid tumors (Fig. 4.1).

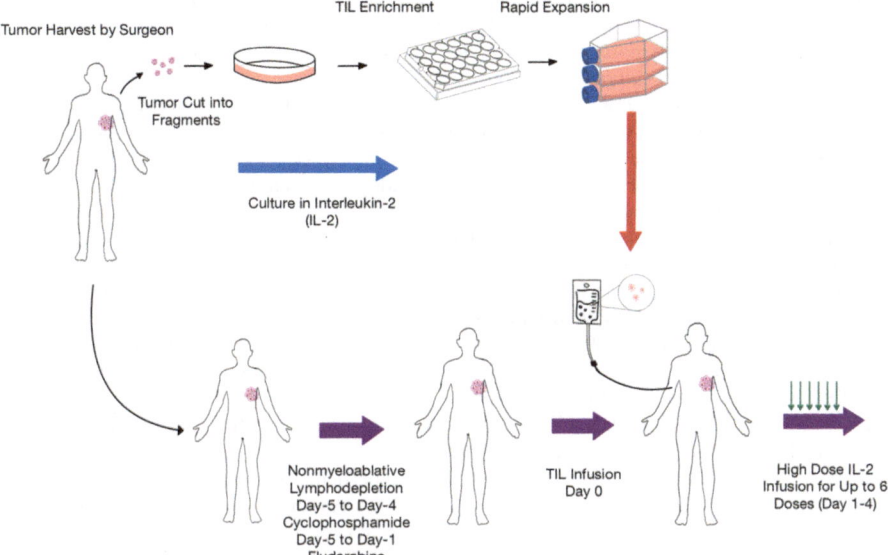

Fig. 4.1 Schematic of TIL therapy

References

Andersen, R., Donia, M., Ellebaek, E., Borch, T. H., Kongsted, P., Iversen, T. Z., Holmich, L. R., Hendel, H. W., Met, O., Andersen, M. H., Thor Straten, P., & Svane, I. M. (2016). Long-lasting complete responses in patients with metastatic melanoma after adoptive cell therapy with tumor-infiltrating lymphocytes and an attenuated IL2 regimen. *Clinical Cancer Research, 22*(15), 3734–3745.

Besser, M. J., Shapira-Frommer, R., Treves, A. J., Zippel, D., Itzhaki, O., Hershkovitz, L., Levy, D., Kubi, A., Hovav, E., Chermoshniuk, N., Shalmon, B., Hardan, I., Catane, R., Markel, G., Apter, S., Ben-Nun, A., Kuchuk, I., Shimoni, A., Nagler, A., & Schachter, J. (2010). Clinical responses in a phase II study using adoptive transfer of short-term cultured tumor infiltration lymphocytes in metastatic melanoma patients. *Clinical Cancer Research, 16*(9), 2646–2655.

Chamberlain, C. A., Bennett, E. P., Kverneland, A. H., Svane, I. M., Donia, M., & Met, O. (2022). Highly efficient PD-1-targeted CRISPR-Cas9 for tumor-infiltrating lymphocyte-based adoptive T cell therapy. *Molecular Therapy - Oncolytics, 24*, 417–428.

Chesney, J., Lewis, K. D., Kluger, H., Hamid, O., Whitman, E., Thomas, S., Wermke, M., Cusnir, M., Domingo-Musibay, E., Phan, G. Q., Kirkwood, J. M., Hassel, J. C., Orloff, M., Larkin, J., Weber, J., Furness, A. J. S., Khushalani, N. I., Medina, T., Egger, M. E., Graf Finckenstein, F., Jagasia, M., Hari, P., Sulur, G., Shi, W., Wu, X., & Sarnaik, A. (2022). Efficacy and safety of lifileucel, a one-time autologous tumor-infiltrating lymphocyte (TIL) cell therapy, in patients with advanced melanoma after progression on immune checkpoint inhibitors and targeted therapies: Pooled analysis of consecutive cohorts of the C-144-01 study. *Journal for Immunotherapy of Cancer, 10*(12).

Chu, Y., Milner, J., Lamb, M., Maryamchik, E., Rigot, O., Ayello, J., Harrison, L., Shaw, R., Behbehani, G. K., Mardis, E. R., Miller, K., Venkata, L. P. R., Chang, H., Lee, D., Rosenthal,

E., Kadauke, S., Bunin, N., Talano, J. A., Johnson, B., Wang, Y., & Cairo, M. S. (2023). Manufacture and characterization of good manufacturing practice-compliant SARS-COV-2 cytotoxic T lymphocytes. *The Journal of Infectious Diseases, 227*(6), 788–799.

Dudley, M. E., Wunderlich, J. R., Shelton, T. E., Even, J., & Rosenberg, S. A. (2003). Generation of tumor-infiltrating lymphocyte cultures for use in adoptive transfer therapy for melanoma patients. *Journal of Immunotherapy, 26*(4), 332–342.

Dudley, M. E., Wunderlich, J. R., Yang, J. C., Sherry, R. M., Topalian, S. L., Restifo, N. P., Royal, R. E., Kammula, U., White, D. E., Mavroukakis, S. A., Rogers, L. J., Gracia, G. J., Jones, S. A., Mangiameli, D. P., Pelletier, M. M., Gea-Banacloche, J., Robinson, M. R., Berman, D. M., Filie, A. C., Abati, A., & Rosenberg, S. A. (2005). Adoptive cell transfer therapy following non-myeloablative but lymphodepleting chemotherapy for the treatment of patients with refractory metastatic melanoma. *Journal of Clinical Oncology, 23*(10), 2346–2357.

Dutcher, J. P., Schwartzentruber, D. J., Kaufman, H. L., Agarwala, S. S., Tarhini, A. A., Lowder, J. N., & Atkins, M. B. (2014). High dose interleukin-2 (Aldesleukin) - expert consensus on best management practices-2014. *Journal for Immunotherapy of Cancer, 2*(1), 26.

Eberlein, T. J., Rosenstein, M., & Rosenberg, S. A. (1982). Regression of a disseminated syngeneic solid tumor by systemic transfer of lymphoid cells expanded in interleukin 2. *The Journal of Experimental Medicine, 156*(2), 385–397.

Ernst, M., & Giubellino, A. (2022). The current state of treatment and future directions in cutaneous malignant melanoma. *Biomedicine, 10*(4).

Goff, S. L., Smith, F. O., Klapper, J. A., Sherry, R., Wunderlich, J. R., Steinberg, S. M., White, D., Rosenberg, S. A., Dudley, M. E., & Yang, J. C. (2010). Tumor infiltrating lymphocyte therapy for metastatic melanoma: Analysis of tumors resected for TIL. *Journal of Immunotherapy, 33*(8), 840–847.

Krishna, S., Lowery, F. J., Copeland, A. R., Bahadiroglu, E., Mukherjee, R., Jia, L., Anibal, J. T., Sachs, A., Adebola, S. O., Gurusamy, D., Yu, Z., Hill, V., Gartner, J. J., Li, Y. F., Parkhurst, M., Paria, B., Kvistborg, P., Kelly, M. C., Goff, S. L., Altan-Bonnet, G., Robbins, P. F., & Rosenberg, S. A. (2020). Stem-like CD8 T cells mediate response of adoptive cell immunotherapy against human cancer. *Science, 370*(6522), 1328–1334.

Mullinax, J. E., Egger, M. E., McCarter, M., Monk, B. J., Toloza, E. M., Brousseau, S., Jagasia, M., & Sarnaik, A. (2022). Surgical considerations for tumor tissue procurement to obtain tumor-infiltrating lymphocytes for adoptive cell therapy. *Cancer Journal, 28*(4), 285–293.

North, R. J. (1982). Cyclophosphamide-facilitated adoptive immunotherapy of an established tumor depends on elimination of tumor-induced suppressor T cells. *The Journal of Experimental Medicine, 155*(4), 1063–1074.

Radvanyi, L. G., Bernatchez, C., Zhang, M., Fox, P. S., Miller, P., Chacon, J., Wu, R., Lizee, G., Mahoney, S., Alvarado, G., Glass, M., Johnson, V. E., McMannis, J. D., Shpall, E., Prieto, V., Papadopoulos, N., Kim, K., Homsi, J., Bedikian, A., Hwu, W. J., Patel, S., Ross, M. I., Lee, J. E., Gershenwald, J. E., Lucci, A., Royal, R., Cormier, J. N., Davies, M. A., Mansaray, R., Fulbright, O. J., Toth, C., Ramachandran, R., Wardell, S., Gonzalez, A., & Hwu, P. (2012). Specific lymphocyte subsets predict response to adoptive cell therapy using expanded autologous tumor-infiltrating lymphocytes in metastatic melanoma patients. *Clinical Cancer Research, 18*(24), 6758–6770.

Rohaan, M. W., Borch, T. H., van den Berg, J. H., Met, O., Kessels, R., Geukes Foppen, M. H., Stoltenborg Granhoj, J., Nuijen, B., Nijenhuis, C., Jedema, I., van Zon, M., Scheij, S., Beijnen, J. H., Hansen, M., Voermans, C., Noringriis, I. M., Monberg, T. J., Holmstroem, R. B., Wever, L. D. V., van Dijk, M., Grijpink-Ongering, L. G., Valkenet, L. H. M., Torres Acosta, A., Karger, M., Borgers, J. S. W., Ten Ham, R. M. T., Retel, V. P., van Harten, W. H., Lalezari, F., van Tinteren, H., van der Veldt, A. A. M., Hospers, G. A. P., Stevense-den Boer, M. A. M., Suijkerbuijk, K. P. M., Aarts, M. J. B., Piersma, D., van den Eertwegh, A. J. M., de Groot, J. B., Vreugdenhil, G., Kapiteijn, E., Boers-Sonderen, M. J., Fiets, W. E., van den Berkmortel, F., Ellebaek, E., Holmich, L. R., van Akkooi, A. C. J., van Houdt, W. J., Wouters, M., van Thienen, J. V., Blank, C. U., Meerveld-Eggink, A., Klobuch, S., Wilgenhof, S., Schumacher, T. N.,

Donia, M., Svane, I. M., & Haanen, J. (2022). Tumor-infiltrating lymphocyte therapy or ipilimumab in advanced melanoma. *The New England Journal of Medicine, 387*(23), 2113–2125.

Rosenberg, S. A., Eberlein, T. J., Grimm, E. A., Lotze, M. T., Mazumder, A., & Rosenstein, M. (1982). Development of long-term cell lines and lymphoid clones reactive against murine and human tumors: A new approach to the adoptive immunotherapy of cancer. *Surgery, 92*(2), 328–336.

Rosenberg, S. A., Spiess, P., & Lafreniere, R. (1986). A new approach to the adoptive immunotherapy of cancer with tumor-infiltrating lymphocytes. *Science, 233*(4770), 1318–1321.

Sarnaik, A. A., Hamid, O., Khushalani, N. I., Lewis, K. D., Medina, T., Kluger, H. M., Thomas, S. S., Domingo-Musibay, E., Pavlick, A. C., Whitman, E. D., Martin-Algarra, S., Corrie, P., Curti, B. D., Olah, J., Lutzky, J., Weber, J. S., Larkin, J. M. G., Shi, W., Takamura, T., Jagasia, M., Qin, H., Wu, X., Chartier, C., Graf Finckenstein, F., Fardis, M., Kirkwood, J. M., & Chesney, J. A. (2021). Lifileucel, a tumor-infiltrating lymphocyte therapy, in metastatic melanoma. *Journal of Clinical Oncology, 39*(24), 2656–2666.

Woroniecka, K. I., Rhodin, K. E., Dechant, C., Cui, X., Chongsathidkiet, P., Wilkinson, D., Waibl-Polania, J., Sanchez-Perez, L., & Fecci, P. E. (2020). 4-1BB agonism averts TIL exhaustion and licenses PD-1 blockade in glioblastoma and other intracranial cancers. *Clinical Cancer Research, 26*(6), 1349–1358.

Chapter 5
Cellular Therapies for Cancer: Chimeric Antigen Receptor T Cells (CAR-T)

Richard C. Godby, Alex Niu, and Jonas Paludo

Abstract Chimeric antigen receptor T cell (CAR-T), a novel modality of adoptive cellular therapy, is characterized by the expression of chimeric antigen receptors (CARs) engineered to bind to tumor-associated antigens while facilitating the cytotoxic activity of the CAR-T cells. CAR construct intricacies and T cell signaling play an important role in the function of CAR-T cells. Currently, various FDA-approved CAR-T products target B-cell malignancies and multiple myeloma. Despite these successes, the complex CAR-T production process, spanning collection logistics to manufacturing, coupled with the frequent occurrence of acute toxicities like cytokine release syndrome (CRS), immune effector cell-associated neurotoxicity syndrome (ICANS), cytopenias, and infections, poses a significant challenge for widespread adoption of this remarkable therapy. Ongoing developments in novel CAR-T cell generations and alternative manufacturing practices aim to address current limitations and overcome resistance mechanisms. These advancements solidify CAR-T cells' role as a revolutionary anticancer treatment.

Keywords Chimeric antigen receptors (CARs) · CAR-T cells · Cellular therapy · CAR constructs · Axicabtagene ciloleucel · Lisocabtagene maraleucel · Tisagenlecleucel · Brexucabtagene autoleucel · Idecabtagene vicleucel · Ciltacabtagene autoleucel · Cytokine release syndrome (CRS) · Immune effector cell-associated neurotoxicity syndrome (ICANS) · CAR-T manufacturing

Introduction

Chimeric antigen receptors (CARs) are engineered receptor constructs that are expressed by immune effector cells (IECs). These receptors direct the IECs to recognize a target ligand and carry out effector functions. CARs have been investigated

R. C. Godby · A. Niu · J. Paludo (✉)
Divison of Hematology, Mayo Clinic, Rochester, MN, USA
e-mail: paludo.jonas@mayo.edu

for several years, with a focus on T cells as the IEC given the pivotal roles in immunology, leading to the innovative technology of chimeric antigen receptor T cells (CAR-T) (Gross et al., 1989; Eshhar et al., 1993).

The term "chimeric" refers to the engineered protein with functionality similar to an immunoglobulin extracellularly by using single chain variable fragments (ScFvs) to recognize a target antigen and T cells intracellularly by using components of the T cell receptor (TCR) structure to carry out effector functions, such as cytotoxicity. With advancements in the understanding of immunology and T cell signaling, the incorporation of a costimulatory domain has enhanced the antitumor efficacy and in vivo persistence (Milone et al., 2009). The ongoing advancements in immunology in conjunction with emerging gene therapy technologies have formed the basis for the development of more sophisticated constructs, ultimately leading to the first clinical CAR-T product approved by the Food and Drug Administration (FDA) in 2017. Since that time, the field of cellular therapies and adoptive immunotherapies has emerged as a cornerstone in the cancer treatment landscape and is actively expanding to other domains of medicine.

T Cell Signaling and CAR Constructs

Typically, innate and adaptive arms of the immune system collaborate to achieve immunosurveillance and safeguard against harmful agents, including malignancies and microbes (Chaplin, 2010). The adaptive immune system consists of various cell types, among which T cells are particularly noteworthy as a vehicle for cancer therapeutics due to their crucial roles in both immune coordination and as IECs with inherently robust cytotoxic functionality. T cell effector functions rely on proper engagement of TCRs with antigen presentation via the major histocompatibility complex (MHC), such as that from the antigen-presenting cells (APC) or nucleated tumor cells (Fig. 5.1). TCR complexes are comprised of a diverse range of elements, encompassing both extracellular and intracellular components (Shah et al., 2021b). Additional elements and further discussion of T cell immunology can be found in Chap. 1.

T cell dysfunction has the potential to manifest in various circumstances, such as anergy from suboptimal antigen stimulation, exhaustion caused by persistent over stimulation, and senescence from repeated stimulation (Xia et al., 2019). Malignant cells often employ various mechanisms to evade immune destruction and impair the proper functioning of T cells. These include upregulation of immunosuppressive ligands (e.g., PD-L1), loss of MHC expression, and changes in the tumor microenvironment (TME) that lead to immune suppression and exhaustion (Ansell, 2020). Some of these immune escape mechanisms have been targeted by many of the most impactful advances in hematology and oncology, such as immune checkpoint inhibitors to disinhibit T cell effector functions and reverse some dysfunctional states as well as CAR-T cell technologies to provide cytotoxic activity in a directed manner independent of MHC antigen presentation. Furthermore, a number of these

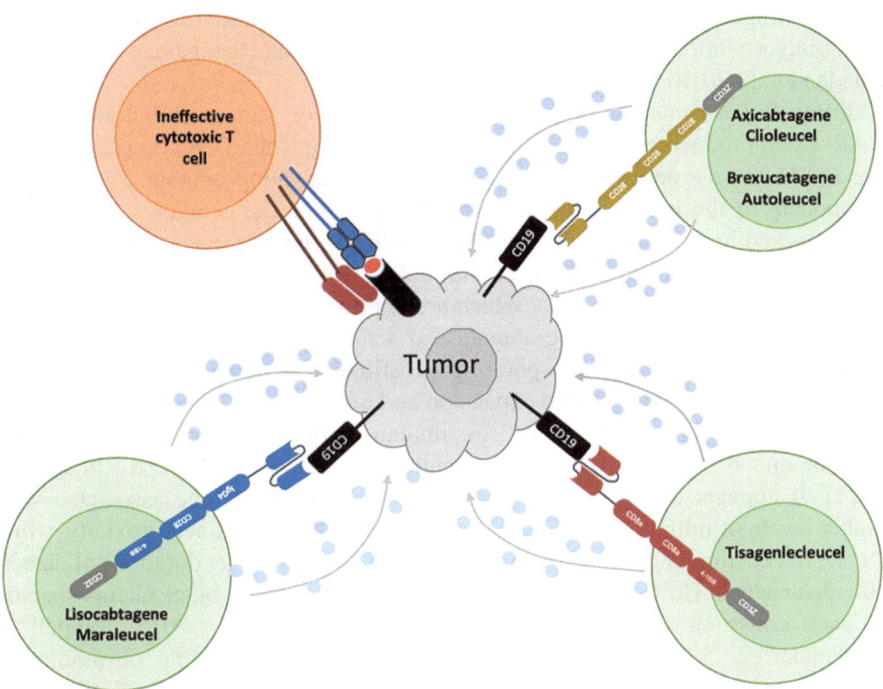

Fig. 5.1 Representation of currently FDA-approved CAR-T cell technologies, which promote effective immune cytotoxicity by the addition of a chimeric antigen receptor to autologous T cells targeting a surface tumor antigen of interest (e.g., CD19)

malignancy-associated immunoparesis phenomena may have repercussions on the collection, manufacturing, and efficacy of current cellular therapies.

CAR constructs are designed with various domains to achieve specific functions. The CAR structure typically contains an antigen binding domain, hinge region, transmembrane domain, and intracellular signaling domains with co-stimulatory and activation sub-domains (Rafiq et al., 2020).

For currently FDA-approved CAR products, the antigen binding domain is a scFv derived from antibody, allowing antigen binding independent of MHC presentation. All currently approved CAR-T cell products used in the treatment of lymphoma, tisagenlecleucel, axicabtagene ciloleucel, lisocabtagene maraleucel, and brexucabtagene autoleucel have a scFv that targets the same CD19 epitope FMC63 on the surface of B lymphocytes but with different hinge regions and intra-cellular co-signaling domains (Fig. 5.1). Both currently approved CAR-T cells used in the treatment of multiple myeloma, idecabtagene vicleucel and ciltacabtagene autoleucel, have a scFv that targets BCMA on the surface of plasma cells.

The hinge region facilitates access to the target antigen while minimizing steric hindrance with differences in design affecting binding affinity and signaling efficiency (Qin et al., 2017; Alabanza et al., 2017; Guedan et al., 2018; Zhang et al., 2021). Different products incorporate varied hinge regions, such as a CD28, CD8a, or IgG4 hinge region. The transmembrane domain anchors the CAR into the cell lipid bilayer while also influencing stability and function (Bridgeman et al., 2010; Guedan et al., 2018).

Intracellular signaling domains are composed of various sub-domains. All CAR-T cell products use the CD3ζ chain of the endogenous TCR complex containing ITAMs as the activation domain. The CD3ζ-activating domain was the only component of the intracellular signaling domain in first-generation CAR-T cells, which lacked in vivo expansion and clinical efficacy due to the absence of a second co-stimulatory signal (Kershaw et al., 2006; Tokarew et al., 2019). Second-generation CAR-T cell products, which are approved by the FDA for clinical use, contain both a CD3ζ-activating domain and a single co-stimulatory domain using either 4-1BB or CD28. By incorporating a costimulatory domain, there was a notable enhancement in both in vivo expansion and efficacy, which resulted in substantial clinical advancements. Both co-stimulatory domains are clinically active without one being clearly and consistently superior (Cappell & Kochenderfer, 2021). It appears that the CD28 costimulatory domain may be associated with higher levels of initial tumor killing, cytokine production, and neurotoxicity, while the 4-1BB costimulatory domain may be associated with longer durations of detectable persistence. However, differences may also be related to other factors specific to each construct and manufacturing process (Long et al., 2015; Cappell & Kochenderfer, 2021). Third-generation CARs combine multiple costimulatory domains, such as CD28 and 4-1BB, to maximize effector function. While third-generation CARs have demonstrated some improvements in expansion and persistence, it has not yet translated into significantly improved clinical outcomes (Ramos et al., 2018; Enblad et al., 2018).

CAR-T Production: Collection, Composition, Constructs, and Manufacturing

Collection

Currently, as an autologous, modified cellular therapy product, CAR-T cells necessitate complex coordination and logistics to manufacture in an efficient manner for a growing number of patients. From central venous access placement and scheduling leukapheresis, to post-collection processing, shipping of the cells, manufacturing the product, lymphodepletion, and infusion of the modified autologous T cells, there are many variables and teams involved in ensuring quality and safety.

There are many considerations involved in the CAR-T manufacturing process. For instance, the apheresis team must consider pre-apheresis (patient access and overall health, prior therapies, laboratory values, scheduling, etc.), peri-apheresis (total blood volume, extracorporeal volume, collection goals, efficiency, etc.), and post-apheresis (cellular composition, CAR genetic material, manufacturing techniques, manufacturing times, etc.) factors involved in optimizing collection and subsequent manufacturing (Paroder et al., 2020). CAR-T manufacturing failure has been reported in up to 20% in patients with B-cell malignancies (Bersenev, 2017). To increase manufacturing success, a minimum absolute lymphocyte count (ALC) or CD3+ count thresholds, often a minimum ALC of 100–500 cells/uL or a CD3+ count of at least 150 cells/uL, has been set by multiple centers (McGuirk et al., 2017; Ceppi et al., 2018).

Composition

Composition and fitness of the final CAR-T product depend on multiple factors that may impact both efficacy and susceptibility to resistance mechanisms. Prior therapies may influence T cell fitness by affecting the function and number of T cells, potentially limiting apheresis collection and viability. T cell fitness is also an important component for CAR-T responses and resistance. The T cell phenotype represented in the CAR-T products and different components of the CAR-construct can impact clinical efficacy and CAR-T cell persistence in vivo. Infusion of CAR-T in ratio of 1:1 CD4+ to CD8+ T cell ratio has also been associated with greater CAR-T expansion and fewer toxicities (Turtle et al., 2016a, b).

Advanced Constructs

More complex CAR constructs under development aim to use a number of approaches in overcoming antigen escape, improving effector function, overcoming on-target off-tumor toxicities, and modulating the TME (Young et al., 2022). Some of these strategies can be employed to address the problems of on-target off-tumor toxicities. Seldom does a neoplasm exhibit a sole surface antigen that is distinct and not present in healthy tissue. Instead, through the utilization of a combination of surface markers and biological logic gating, a unique array of surface signals can be leveraged to generate precise and complex actions (Rafiq et al., 2020; Hong et al., 2020). For instance, in order to initiate cytotoxic response, an engineered cellular product may require a target to possess both antigen A and antigen B, each generating part of a critical signal to proceed. On the other hand, the cellular product may be designed in a way that it necessitates a target to possess only antigen A in the absence of antigen B, with antigen A producing the critical signal to proceed while antigen B producing an overriding inhibitory signal.

Effector function can be improved and the TME can be tamed with additional intracellular signaling domains and genomic editing that alter the external, operational milieu. These approaches are collectively referred to as "armored" CARs. Strategies include activated CAR functioning to increase local levels of beneficial cytokines, cytokine receptors, surface ligands, secreted proteases, T cell engagers, monoclonal antibodies, and other components (Hong et al., 2020). These cellular systems can be designed to offer greater control and scalability, allowing for more refined and expanded capabilities. Built-in suicide switches that are druggable provide an "off-switch" if toxicities occur in excess. Alternatively, common CARs can be designed to target a specific adapter molecule linked to monoclonal antibodies such that a single CAR could work with a variety of existing therapies.

The ability to transduce these complex CAR constructs into effector cells is increasingly feasible in a variety of settings given the growingly sophisticated gene delivery (viral vectors, electroporation, nanoparticles, etc.) and gene editing (transposons, zinc finger nucleases, transcription activator-like effector nucleases, CRISPR/Cas-9, etc.) technologies (Atsavapranee et al., 2021). These technologies also make the aspiration of allogeneic CAR-T products more of a reality.

Manufacturing

The manufacturing process includes (1) isolating T cells from the apheresis collection, (2) cellular activation, (3) CAR gene transfer, (4) cell expansion, (5) formulation, (6) cryopreservation, and (7) shipping product to the care team for infusion (Wang & Rivière, 2016). As CAR-T products transition from research to commercial manufacturing, there have been efforts to simultaneously improve good manufacturing practices (GMPs) and automatization for increased reproducibility and scalability (Abou-El-Enein et al., 2021). Unfortunately, CAR-T manufacturing typically spans several weeks, posing challenges in delivering a timely product to critically ill patients. A large proportion of the manufacturing time is dedicated to quality control measures, including verification of sterility, specificity, and self-specified potency parameters that do not predict clinical efficacy (Abou-El-Enein et al., 2021).

While several enhancements to the manufacturing process are being studied and implemented, one particularly transformative concept is the generation of CAR-T cells in vivo, eliminating the need for cell collection and subsequent manufacturing obstacles. Transient generation of in vivo CAR-T cells has been demonstrated in mice using CD5-targeted lipid nanoparticles to deliver modified messenger RNA (Rurik et al., 2022). If advances in designing and optimizing in vivo CAR-T cells are studied and implemented clinically, many of the current collection and manufacturing limitations could be overcome.

Approved Products and Indications

Lymphoma

Since the first approval of CAR-T, there have been efforts to determine where and how to best deliver these novel cellular therapies within the growing field of approved treatment options. CAR-T therapy has provided new therapeutic possibilities for patients who would otherwise have had no additional effective treatments. Since tisagenlecleucel received FDA approval for the treatment of B-cell precursor acute lymphoblastic leukemia in 2017, additional CAR-T products followed with clinical trials and subsequent FDA approval; many more clinical trials are underway.

Currently, there are six commercial CAR-T products available for various hematologic malignancies (Table 5.1). Non-Hodgkin B-cell lymphomas utilize axicabtagene ciloleucel, lisocabtagene maraleucel, tisagenlecleucel, and brexucabtagene autoleucel. Multiple myeloma (MM), a plasma cell dyscrasia, utilizes idecabtagene vicleucel and ciltacabtagene autoleucel. And finally, B-precursor acute lymphoblastic leukemia enlists tisagenlecleucel and brexucabtagene autoleucel.

Axicabtagene ciloleucel initially achieved approval in 2017 for relapsed or refractory (R/R) DLBCL via the ZUMA-1 study. The study demonstrated a high level of activity in this patient population, with 82% of patients showing response, of which 54% were a complete response (CR). Most patients in the study had failed multiple lines of therapy, including an autologous stem cell transplant (ASCT) (Neelapu et al., 2017). Most recently, the ZUMA-7 study demonstrated superior benefit of axicabtagene ciloleucel to standard of care treatments for patients with large B-cell lymphoma that was primary refractory or had relapsed within 12 months after first-line chemoimmunotherapy. Results from the ZUMA-7 trial showed a 24-month event-free survival (EFS) of 41% versus 16%, an overall response (OR) of 83% versus 50%, and an estimated overall survival (OS) at 2 years of 61% versus 52%, in axicabtagene ciloleucel versus standard of care, respectively (Locke et al., 2022). And finally, the ZUMA-5 study demonstrated superior use of axicabtagene ciloleucel in R/R indolent non-Hodgkin lymphoma (of which follicular and marginal zone lymphoma were the main subsets evaluated). The study showed an OR of 92%, of which 74% had a CR (Jacobson et al., 2022). Axicabtagene ciloleucel's currently approved indications are outlined in Table 5.1.

Tisagenlecleucel was initially evaluated via the JULIET study, where adult patients with R/R large B-cell lymphomas, who were ineligible for or had disease progression after an ASCT, were treated with the CAR-T product. At a median follow-up of 40.3 months, the OR was 53% with 39% of patients having a CR as their best OR (Schuster et al., 2021). Furthermore, the ELARA study also demonstrated response with tisagenlecleucel in adults with relapsed/refractory follicular lymphoma after two or more treatment lines or who relapsed after an ASCT. A CR rate of 69.1% was observed, with an OR rate of 86.2% (Fowler et al., 2022). In addition to non-Hodgkin B-cell lymphomas, tisagenlecleucel also carries an indication for B-cell precursor acute lymphoblastic leukemia (ALL). The ELIANA study evaluated tisagenlecleucel in pediatric and young adult patients with R/R B-cell ALL. The overall remission rate within 3 months was found to be 81%, and all patients who had a response were found to be minimal residual disease negative. In addition, EFS and OS were 73% and 90% at 6 months and 50% and 76% at 12 months, respectively (Maude et al., 2018). Tisagenlecleucel's currently approved indications are outlined in Table 5.1.

Table 5.1 Approved Products and Indications

	Axicabtagene ciloleucel	Tisagenlecleucel	Lisocabtagene maraleucel	Brexucabtagene autoleucel	Idecabtagene vicleucel	Ciltacabtagene autoleucel
Relapsed/refractory follicular lymphoma ≥ 2 prior lines of therapy	x	x				
Relapsed/refractory follicular lymphoma 3B ≥ 2 prior lines of therapy			x			
Relapsed/refractory marginal zone lymphoma ≥ 2 prior lines of therapy	x		x			
Primary refractory large B-cell lymphoma	x		x			
Relapsed large B-cell lymphoma <12 months	x		x			
Relapsed/refractory large B-cell lymphoma: DLBCL (NOS) ≥ 2 prior lines of therapy	x	x	x			
Relapsed/refractory large B-cell Lymphoma: high-grade ≥ 2 prior lines of therapy	x	x	x			
Relapsed/refractory large B-cell lymphoma: primary mediastinal ≥ 2 prior lines of therapy	x		x			
Relapsed/refractory large B-cell lymphoma arising from follicular lymphoma ≥ 2 prior lines of therapy	x	x	x			
Relapsed/refractory large B-cell lymphoma arising from indolent lymphoma ≥ 2 prior lines of therapy			x			
Relapsed/refractory mantle cell lymphoma ≥ 2 prior lines of therapy (must include chemotherapy and BTKI)				x		
Adults with relapsed/refractory B-cell precursor acute lymphoblastic leukemia				x		
Age 25 or less with primary refractory or second relapse of B-cell precursor acute lymphoblastic leukemia		x				
Relapsed/refractory multiple myeloma after ≥ four prior lines of therapy, including an immunomodulatory agent, a proteasome inhibitor, and an anti-CD38 monoclonal antibody					x	x

The TRANSCEND study evaluated the use of lisocabtagene maraleucel in with R/R large B-cell lymphomas, subtypes of which included DLBCL, high-grade B-cell lymphoma with rearrangements of MYC and either BCL2, BCL6, or both ("double-hit" or "triple-hit" lymphoma), DLBCL transformed from any indolent lymphoma, primary mediastinal B-cell lymphoma, and follicular lymphoma grade 3B. OR was achieved in 73% of patients and a CR by 53% of patients (Abramson et al., 2020). Similar to axicabtagene ciloleucel and the ZUMA-7 trial, the TRANSFORM study evaluated lisocabtagene maraleucel versus standard of care in the second-line setting for primary refractory or early relapsed (≤12 months) large B-cell lymphoma. Likewise, the study found improved measures with lisocabtagene maraleucel with median EFS not reached for lisocabtagene maraleucel versus 2.4 months for standard of care. CR rate was 74% for lisocabtagene maraleucel versus 43% for standard of care, while median progression-free survival was not reached for lisocabtagene maraleucel versus 6.2 months for standard of care. Median OS was not reached for lisocabtagene maraleucel versus 29.9 months for SOC (Abramson et al., 2023). These results were reinforced in the PILOT study where patients who had R/R large B-cell lymphoma, despite receiving first-line therapy containing an anthracycline and a CD20-targeted agent, and were deemed ineligible for HSCT underwent lisocabtagene maraleucel treatment. The study found that 80% of patients had an OR and together with the TRANSFORM's study demonstrate the efficacy of lisocabtagene maraleucel in the second-line setting (Sehgal et al., 2022). Lisocabtagene maraleucel's currently approved indications are outlined in Table 5.1.

Mantle-cell lymphoma is unique among lymphoid malignancies for several reasons, among them is that the only approved CAR-T product, brexucabtagene autoleucel, is not currently used in other non-Hodgkin lymphomas. In the ZUMA-2 study, patients with R/R mantle-cell lymphoma, of which a prior therapy must have included a Bruton's tyrosine kinase inhibitor, underwent treatment with brexucabtagene autoleucel. The study revealed an OR of 93%, of which 67% of patients had a CR. In an intention-to-treat analysis involving all 74 patients, 85% had an OR while 59% had a CR. And at a median follow-up of 12.3 months, 57% of patients in the primary efficacy analysis were in CR, with the estimated PFS and OS at 61% and 83%, respectively (Wang et al., 2020). In addition to mantle-cell lymphoma, brexucabtagene autoleucel is also approved for adult patients with R/R B-precursor ALL via the ZUMA-3 study. Results showed that at the median follow-up of 16.4 months, 71% of patients had CR or CR with incomplete hematologic recovery, with 56% of patients reaching CR. Median duration of remission was 12.8 months, median relapse-free survival was 11.6 months, and median OS was 18.2 months. Among responders, the median OS was not reached, and 97% of these patients had minimal residual disease negativity (Shah et al., 2021a). Brexucabtagene autoleucel's currently approved indications are outlined in Table 5.1.

Multiple Myeloma

In addition to revolutionizing lymphoma treatment, CAR-T has also greatly impacted the treatment of MM. The two commercial products available for MM are idecabtagene vicleucel and ciltacabtagene autoleucel. Idecabtagene vicleucel demonstrated efficacy in the KarMMA-3 study, where patients with R/R MM after 2–4 prior treatments which must have included immunomodulatory agents, proteasome inhibitors, and daratumumab were treated with idecabtagene vicleucel or standard of care. Importantly, 66% of the patients had triple-class refractory disease while 95% had daratumumab-refractory disease. Results of the KarMMA-3 study showed that at a median follow-up of 18.6 months, the median PFS was 13.3 months in the idecabtagene vicleucel group versus 4.4 months in the standard of care group. An OR was seen in 71% of the idecabtagene vicleucel group and in 42% in the standard of care group, while a CR occurred in 39% and 5%, respectively (Rodriguez-Otero et al., 2023). The CARTITUDE-1 study evaluated ciltacabtagene autoleucel in patients who had received three or more prior lines of therapy, or were double-refractory to a proteasome inhibitor and an immunomodulatory drug, and similarly to KarMMA-3, had previously received a proteasome inhibitor, immunomodulatory drug, and anti-CD38 antibody. OR was seen in 97% of patients with 67% achieving CR. Neither median duration of response or PFS was reached. The 12-month PFS rate was 77%, while OS was 89% (Berdeja et al., 2021). Ciltacabtagene autoleucel's and idecabtagene vicleucel's currently approved indications are outlined Table 5.1.

Adverse Events and Limitations

Cytokine Release Syndrome (CRS)

After infusion of the CAR-T product, there is potential for rapid expansion, activation, and cytotoxic activity resulting in large amounts of cytokine release (Morris et al., 2022). Clinically, this may manifest with fevers, hypotension, and hypoxia which are used to grade the CRS and subsequently guide treatment (Lee et al., 2019; Santomasso et al., 2021; NCCN, 2023). While this may occur at any time immediately after infusion up to 2 weeks afterward, it typically occurs within the first few days after infusion and may persist up to approximately 1 week with other organ-specific toxicities (Morris et al., 2022; NCCN, 2023). Each CAR-T therapy has product-specific recommendations for management of CRS, but in addition to supportive care, the first-line treatment if clinically warranted is anti-IL6 therapy (e.g., tocilizumab) followed by dexamethasone if the CRS fails to abate, and then various additional strategies aimed at quelling the excessive immunotoxicity should it persist (Santomasso et al., 2021; NCCN, 2023; Jain et al., 2023a).

Immune Effector Cell-Associated Neurotoxicity Syndrome (ICANS)

After infusion of the CAR-T product, there is potential for rapid expansion, activation, and cytotoxic activity resulting in large amounts of cytokine release that may also disrupt the blood-brain barrier (Morris et al., 2022). Clinically, this may manifest with depressed consciousness, seizures, motor changes, and cerebral edema which are used to grade the ICANS and subsequently guide treatment (Lee et al., 2019; Santomasso et al., 2021; NCCN, 2023). If this occurs, it usually takes place relatively later than CRS typically does and lasts relatively longer, commonly occurring around 1 week after infusion and possibly persisting up to approximately 2 weeks (Santomasso et al., 2021; Morris et al., 2022; NCCN, 2023). Each CAR-T product has product-specific recommendations for management of ICANS, but in addition to supportive care, the first-line treatment if clinically warranted is high-dose steroids (e.g., dexamethasone) with the possible addition of antiepileptics; anti-IL6 therapy is usually added only for the simultaneous presence of CRS (Santomasso et al., 2021; NCCN, 2023; Jain et al., 2023a).

Cytopenias and Infections

Patients receiving cellular therapies often experience cytopenias that can arise from various etiologies. By the time patients are eligible for CAR-T products, they have already been exposed to cytotoxic chemotherapy and are reexposed to lymphodepleting therapy prior to infusion of CAR-T. While early cytopenias are often attributed to the lymphodepleting chemotherapy, there is a broad differential of diagnoses requiring etiology-specific interventions depending on the clinical course, including large granular lymphocytosis, thrombotic microangiopathies, disease relapse, hemophagocytic lymphohistiocytosis, and more (Santomasso et al., 2021; Jain et al., 2023b). Infections may also be an etiology for cytopenias but are often a consequence, requiring adequate antimicrobial prophylaxis, treatment, and vaccination (Hill et al., 2018; Hill & Seo, 2020; Santomasso et al., 2021). Another consequence of the cytopenias associated with CAR-T therapies, especially those products targeting CD19, is prolonged hypogammaglobulinemia often requiring intravenous immunoglobulin support and predisposing to additional infections complications.

Mechanisms of Resistance

Resistance to CAR-T is complex with mechanisms related to the tumor itself, T cell dysfunction, and/or the TME.

In a significant portion of patients receiving CAR-T cell therapy, antigen escape (partial or complete loss of target antigen expression by the tumor) is observed. Clinical relapse due to antigen loss was first reported with blinatumomab in MRD-positive B-ALL patients (Topp et al., 2011). Other possible mechanisms of antigen loss include CAR-T trogocytosis, lineage switching, and antigen masking. Trogocytosis is a process where the target antigen is transferred from the tumor cell to T cells which ultimately promotes T cell fratricide and exhaustion. CAR-T trogocytosis has been observed as a mechanism of resistance in preclinical models of CD19 CARs as well as CD22, BCMA, and mesothelin-directed CAR-T cells (Hamieh et al., 2019). Antigen loss may also occur when the target cell lineage switches from a lymphoid phenotype to a myeloid phenotype due to cellular reprograming and B-cell de-differentiation, which has been reported as a mechanism of antigen escape after both CD19 CAR-T and blinatumomab therapy (Dorantes-Acosta & Pelayo, 2012; Gardner et al., 2016; Wölfl et al., 2018). Antigen masking was described in the accidental transduction of a leukemic cell during CAR-T manufacturing that presumably led to masking of the CD19 epitope which led to resistance to CAR-T therapy (Ruella et al., 2018).

Another important resistance mechanism, associated with lack of early molecular response in large B-cell lymphoma cases treated with axicabtagene ciloleucel, was T cell exhaustion (Deng et al., 2020). T cell exhaustion may be an intrinsic T cell defect influenced by pretreatment factors or may be acquired via immunosuppressive ligands and immunosuppressive cells in the TME. T cell exhaustion immunophenotypes are characterized by increased expression of inhibitory receptors (PD-1, CTLA-4, TIM-3, and LAG-3), altered metabolism, decreased proliferation and cytokine production, and a distinct transcriptional signature (Long et al., 2015). Activation-induced cell death (AICD), a mechanism of peripheral tolerance resulting in T cell death rather than activation through binding of the TCR to its antigen, is another resistance mechanism (Green et al., 2003). Repetitive stimulation of the TCR is a factor that can predispose T cells to AICD and has been observed in CAR-T cells. Unlike T cell exhaustion, AICD is irreversible (Kuünkele et al., 2015).

The TME is composed of endothelial cells, extracellular matrix (ECM), myeloid-derived suppressor cells (MDSCs), tumor-associated macrophages (TAMs), regulatory T cells (Tregs), and cancer-associated fibroblasts (CAFs), which interact closely with tumor cells and contribute to tumorigenesis (Quail & Joyce, 2013). Physical barriers to tumor penetration by immune cells, upregulated checkpoint ligands, a pro-tumor stromal niche, and presence of immunosuppressive cytokines/chemokines and soluble factors are known mechanisms of TME-mediated T cell dysfunction.

Future Directions

Allogeneic CAR-T cells, manufactured from an unrelated T cell donor, are an alternative to the current autologous CAR-T products that could overcome many logistical and manufacturing related barriers to current CAR-T practices. Allogeneic

CAR-T products are an attractive "off-the-shelf" approach given the shorter wait times that patients currently experience, but they must be designed such that they avoid graft versus host disease (GVHD) and graft rejection. GVHD might occur when recipient antigens are recognized by the TCR of the allogeneic CAR-T. Additionally, the host immune system may recognize the allogeneic CAR-T cells via nonself HLAs resulting in rejection of the CAR-T product. Strategies to overcome these barriers include genome editing techniques during engineering of the CAR construct, use of alternative effector cells (e.g., NK cells), in vivo delivery of the CAR construct, and more. These cellular technologies are also being studied in various cancers, including solid tumor oncology, as well as in other fields of medicine, such as rheumatology and infectious diseases.

References

Abou-El-Enein, M., Elsallab, M., Feldman, S. A., et al. (2021). Scalable manufacturing of CAR T cells for cancer immunotherapy. *Blood Cancer Discovery, 2*, 408–422.

Abramson, J. S., Palomba, M. L., Gordon, L. I., et al. (2020). Lisocabtagene maraleucel for patients with relapsed or refractory large B-cell lymphomas (TRANSCEND NHL 001): A multicentre seamless design study. *Lancet, 396*, 839–852. https://doi.org/10.1016/S0140-6736(20)31366-0

Abramson, J. S., Solomon, S. R., Arnason, J., et al. (2023). Lisocabtagene maraleucel as second-line therapy for large B-cell lymphoma: Primary analysis of the phase 3 TRANSFORM study. *Blood, 141*, 1675–1684. https://doi.org/10.1182/blood.2022018730

Alabanza, L., Pegues, M., Geldres, C., et al. (2017). Function of novel anti-CD19 chimeric antigen receptors with human variable regions is affected by hinge and transmembrane domains. *Molecular Therapy, 25*, 2452–2465. https://doi.org/10.1016/j.ymthe.2017.07.013

Ansell, S. M. (2020). Fundamentals of immunology for understanding immunotherapy for lymphoma. *Blood Advances, 4*, 5863–5867.

Atsavapranee, E. S., Billingsley, M. M., & Mitchell, M. J. (2021). Delivery technologies for T cell gene editing: Applications in cancer immunotherapy. *eBioMedicine, 67*, 103354.

Berdeja, J. G., Madduri, D., Usmani, S. Z., et al. (2021). Ciltacabtagene autoleucel, a B-cell maturation antigen-directed chimeric antigen receptor T-cell therapy in patients with relapsed or refractory multiple myeloma (CARTITUDE-1): A phase 1b/2 open-label study. *Lancet, 398*, 314–324. https://doi.org/10.1016/S0140-6736(21)00933-8

Bersenev, A. (2017). CAR-T cell manufacturing: Time to put it in gear. *Transfusion, 57*, 1104–1106.

Bridgeman, J. S., Hawkins, R. E., Bagley, S., et al. (2010). The optimal antigen response of chimeric antigen receptors harboring the CD3ζ transmembrane domain is dependent upon incorporation of the receptor into the endogenous TCR/CD3 complex. *Journal of Immunology, 184*, 6938–6949. https://doi.org/10.4049/jimmunol.0901766

Cappell, K. M., & Kochenderfer, J. N. (2021). A comparison of chimeric antigen receptors containing CD28 versus 4-1BB costimulatory domains. *Nature Reviews. Clinical Oncology, 18*, 715–727.

Ceppi, F., Rivers, J., Annesley, C., et al. (2018). Lymphocyte apheresis for chimeric antigen receptor T-cell manufacturing in children and young adults with leukemia and neuroblastoma. *Transfusion, 58*, 1414–1420. https://doi.org/10.1111/trf.14569

Chaplin, D. D. (2010). Overview of the immune response. *The Journal of Allergy and Clinical Immunology, 125*, S3–S23. https://doi.org/10.1016/j.jaci.2009.12.980

Deng, Q., Han, G., Puebla-Osorio, N., et al. (2020). Characteristics of anti-CD19 CAR T cell infusion products associated with efficacy and toxicity in patients with large B cell lymphomas. *Nature Medicine, 26*, 1878–1887. https://doi.org/10.1038/s41591-020-1061-7

Dorantes-Acosta, E., & Pelayo, R. (2012). Lineage switching in acute leukemias: A consequence of stem cell plasticity? *Bone Marrow Research, 2012*, 1–18. https://doi.org/10.1155/2012/406796

Enblad, G., Karlsson, H., Gammelgård, G., et al. (2018). A phase I/IIa trial using CD19-targeted third-generation CAR T cells for lymphoma and leukemia. *Clinical Cancer Research, 24*, 6185–6194. https://doi.org/10.1158/1078-0432.CCR-18-0426

Eshhar, Z., Waks, T., Gross, G., & Schindler, D. G. (1993). Specific activation and targeting of cytotoxic lymphocytes through chimeric single chains consisting of antibody-binding domains and the γ or ζ subunits of the immunoglobulin and T-cell receptors. *Proceedings of the National Academy of Sciences of the United States of America, 90*, 720–724. https://doi.org/10.1073/pnas.90.2.720

Fowler, N. H., Dickinson, M., Dreyling, M., et al. (2022). Tisagenlecleucel in adult relapsed or refractory follicular lymphoma: The phase 2 ELARA trial. *Nature Medicine, 28*, 325–332. https://doi.org/10.1038/s41591-021-01622-0

Gardner, R., Wu, D., Cherian, S., et al. (2016). Acquisition of a CD19-negative myeloid phenotype allows immune escape of MLL-rearranged B-ALL from CD19 CAR-T-cell therapy. *Blood, 127*, 2406–2410. https://doi.org/10.1182/blood-2015-08-665547

Green, D. R., Droin, N., & Pinkoski, M. (2003). Activation-induced cell death in T cells. *Immunological Reviews, 193*, 70–81.

Gross, G., Waks, T., & Eshhar, Z. (1989). Expression of immunoglobulin-T-cell receptor chimeric molecules as functional receptors with antibody-type specificity. *Proceedings of the National Academy of Sciences of the United States of America, 86*, 10024–10028. https://doi.org/10.1073/pnas.86.24.10024

Guedan, S., Posey, A. D., Shaw, C., et al. (2018). Enhancing CAR T cell persistence through ICOS and 4-1BB costimulation. *JCI Insight, 3*. https://doi.org/10.1172/jci.insight.96976

Hamieh, M., Dobrin, A., Cabriolu, A., et al. (2019). CAR T cell trogocytosis and cooperative killing regulate tumour antigen escape. *Nature, 568*, 112–116. https://doi.org/10.1038/s41586-019-1054-1

Hill, J. A., & Seo, S. K. (2020). How I prevent infections in patients receiving CD19-targeted chimeric antigen receptor T cells for B-cell malignancies. *Blood, 136*, 925–935. https://doi.org/10.1182/blood.2019004000

Hill, J. A., Li, D., Hay, K. A., et al. (2018). Infectious complications of CD19-targeted chimeric antigen receptor-modified T-cell immunotherapy. *Blood, 131*, 121–130. https://doi.org/10.1182/blood-2017-07-793760

Hong, M., Clubb, J. D., & Chen, Y. Y. (2020). Engineering CAR-T cells for next-generation cancer therapy. *Cancer Cell, 38*, 473–488.

Jacobson, C. A., Chavez, J. C., Sehgal, A. R., et al. (2022). Axicabtagene ciloleucel in relapsed or refractory indolent non-Hodgkin lymphoma (ZUMA-5): A single-arm, multicentre, phase 2 trial. *The Lancet Oncology, 23*, 91–103. https://doi.org/10.1016/S1470-2045(21)00591-X

Jain, M. D., Smith, M., & Shah, N. N. (2023a). How I treat refractory CRS and ICANS after CAR T-cell therapy. *Blood, 141*, 2430–2442.

Jain, T., Olson, T. S., & Locke, F. L. (2023b). How I treat cytopenias after CAR T-cell therapy. *Blood, 141*, 2460–2469.

Kershaw, M. H., Westwood, J. A., Parker, L. L., et al. (2006). A phase I study on adoptive immunotherapy using gene-modified T cells for ovarian cancer. *Clinical Cancer Research, 12*, 6106–6115. https://doi.org/10.1158/1078-0432.CCR-06-1183

Kuünkele, A., Johnson, A. J., Rolczynski, L. S., et al. (2015). Functional tuning of CARs reveals signaling threshold above which CD8+ CTL antitumor potency is attenuated due to cell fas-FasL-Dependent AICD. *Cancer Immunology Research, 3*, 368–379. https://doi.org/10.1158/2326-6066.CIR-14-0200

Lee, D. W., Santomasso, B. D., Locke, F. L., et al. (2019). ASTCT consensus grading for cytokine release syndrome and neurologic toxicity associated with immune effector cells. *Biology of Blood and Marrow Transplantation, 25*, 625–638.

Locke, F. L., Miklos, D. B., Jacobson, C. A., et al. (2022). Axicabtagene ciloleucel as second-line therapy for large B-Cell lymphoma. *The New England Journal of Medicine, 386*, 640–654. https://doi.org/10.1056/nejmoa2116133

Long, A. H., Haso, W. M., Shern, J. F., et al. (2015). 4-1BB costimulation ameliorates T cell exhaustion induced by tonic signaling of chimeric antigen receptors. *Nature Medicine, 21*, 581–590. https://doi.org/10.1038/nm.3838

Maude, S. L., Laetsch, T. W., Buechner, J., et al. (2018). Tisagenlecleucel in children and young adults with B-Cell lymphoblastic leukemia. *The New England Journal of Medicine, 378*, 439–448. https://doi.org/10.1056/nejmoa1709866

McGuirk, J., Waller, E. K., Qayed, M., et al. (2017). Building blocks for institutional preparation of CTL019 delivery. *Cytotherapy, 19*, 1015–1024.

Milone, M. C., Fish, J. D., Carpenito, C., et al. (2009). Chimeric receptors containing CD137 signal transduction domains mediate enhanced survival of T cells and increased antileukemic efficacy in vivo. *Molecular Therapy, 17*, 1453–1464. https://doi.org/10.1038/mt.2009.83

Morris, E. C., Neelapu, S. S., Giavridis, T., & Sadelain, M. (2022). Cytokine release syndrome and associated neurotoxicity in cancer immunotherapy. *Nature Reviews. Immunology, 22*, 85–96.

NCCN. (2023). Management of immunotherapy-related toxicities. In *Guidelines*. https://www.nccn.org/guidelines/guidelines-detail?category=3&id=1486

Neelapu, S. S., Locke, F. L., Bartlett, N. L., et al. (2017). Axicabtagene ciloleucel CAR T-cell therapy in refractory large B-Cell lymphoma. *The New England Journal of Medicine, 377*, 2531–2544. https://doi.org/10.1056/nejmoa1707447

Paroder, M., Le, N., Pham, H. P., & Thibodeaux, S. R. (2020). Important aspects of T-cell collection by apheresis for manufacturing chimeric antigen receptor T cells. *Advances in Cell and Gene Therapy, 3*, e75. https://doi.org/10.1002/acg2.75

Qin, L., Lai, Y., Zhao, R., et al. (2017). Incorporation of a hinge domain improves the expansion of chimeric antigen receptor T cells. *Journal of Hematology & Oncology, 10*, 68. https://doi.org/10.1186/s13045-017-0437-8

Quail, D. F., & Joyce, J. A. (2013). Microenvironmental regulation of tumor progression and metastasis. *Nature Medicine, 19*, 1423–1437.

Rafiq, S., Hackett, C. S., & Brentjens, R. J. (2020). Engineering strategies to overcome the current roadblocks in CAR T cell therapy. *Nature Reviews. Clinical Oncology, 17*, 147–167.

Ramos, C. A., Rouce, R., Robertson, C. S., et al. (2018). In vivo fate and activity of second- versus third-generation CD19-specific CAR-T cells in B cell Non-Hodgkin's lymphomas. *Molecular Therapy, 26*, 2727–2737. https://doi.org/10.1016/j.ymthe.2018.09.009

Rodriguez-Otero, P., Ailawadhi, S., Arnulf, B., et al. (2023). Ide-cel or standard regimens in relapsed and refractory multiple myeloma. *The New England Journal of Medicine, 388*, 1002–1014. https://doi.org/10.1056/nejmoa2213614

Ruella, M., Xu, J., Barrett, D. M., et al. (2018). Induction of resistance to chimeric antigen receptor T cell therapy by transduction of a single leukemic B cell. *Nature Medicine, 24*, 1499–1503. https://doi.org/10.1038/s41591-018-0201-9

Rurik, J. G., Tombácz, I., Yadegari, A., et al. (2022). CAR T cells produced in vivo to treat cardiac injury. *Science, 375*, 91–96. https://doi.org/10.1126/science.abm0594

Santomasso, B. D., Nastoupil, L. J., Adkins, S., et al. (2021). Management of immune-related adverse events in patients treated with chimeric antigen receptor T-cell therapy: ASCO guideline. *Journal of Clinical Oncology, 39*, 3978–3992. https://doi.org/10.1200/JCO.21.01992

Schuster, S. J., Tam, C. S., Borchmann, P., et al. (2021). Long-term clinical outcomes of tisagenlecleucel in patients with relapsed or refractory aggressive B-cell lymphomas (JULIET): A multicentre, open-label, single-arm, phase 2 study. *The Lancet Oncology, 22*, 1403–1415. https://doi.org/10.1016/S1470-2045(21)00375-2

Sehgal, A., Hoda, D., Riedell, P. A., et al. (2022). Lisocabtagene maraleucel as second-line therapy in adults with relapsed or refractory large B-cell lymphoma who were not intended for haematopoietic stem cell transplantation (PILOT): An open-label, phase 2 study. *The Lancet Oncology, 23*, 1066–1077. https://doi.org/10.1016/S1470-2045(22)00339-4

Shah, B. D., Ghobadi, A., Oluwole, O. O., et al. (2021a). KTE-X19 for relapsed or refractory adult B-cell acute lymphoblastic leukaemia: Phase 2 results of the single-arm, open-label, multi-centre ZUMA-3 study. *Lancet, 398*, 491–502. https://doi.org/10.1016/S0140-6736(21)01222-8

Shah, K., Al-Haidari, A., Sun, J., & Kazi, J. U. (2021b). T cell receptor (TCR) signaling in health and disease. *Signal Transduction and Targeted Therapy, 6*, 412.

Tokarew, N., Ogonek, J., Endres, S., et al. (2019). Teaching an old dog new tricks: Next-generation CAR T cells. *British Journal of Cancer, 120*, 26–37.

Topp, M. S., Kufer, P., Gökbuget, N., et al. (2011). Targeted therapy with the T-cell - Engaging antibody blinatumomab of chemotherapy-refractory minimal residual disease in B-lineage acute lymphoblastic leukemia patients results in high response rate and prolonged leukemia-free survival. *Journal of Clinical Oncology, 29*, 2493–2498. https://doi.org/10.1200/JCO.2010.32.7270

Turtle, C. J., Hanafi, L. A., Berger, C., et al. (2016a). CD19 CAR-T cells of defined CD4+:CD8+ composition in adult B cell ALL patients. *The Journal of Clinical Investigation, 126*, 2123–2138. https://doi.org/10.1172/JCI85309

Turtle, C. J., Hanafi, L. A., Berger, C., et al. (2016b). Immunotherapy of non-Hodgkin's lymphoma with a defined ratio of CD8+ and CD4+ CD19-specific chimeric antigen receptor-modified T cells. *Science Translational Medicine, 8*, 355ra116. https://doi.org/10.1126/scitrans-lmed.aaf8621

Wang, X., & Rivière, I. (2016). Clinical manufacturing of CAR T cells: Foundation of a promising therapy. *Molecular Therapy Oncolytics, 3*, 16015.

Wang, M., Munoz, J., Goy, A., et al. (2020). KTE-X19 CAR T-Cell therapy in relapsed or refractory mantle-cell lymphoma. *The New England Journal of Medicine, 382*, 1331–1342. https://doi.org/10.1056/nejmoa1914347

Wölfl, M., Rasche, M., Eyrich, M., et al. (2018). Spontaneous reversion of a lineage switch following an initial blinatumomab-induced ALL-to-AML switch in MLL-rearranged infant ALL. *Blood Advances, 2*, 1382–1385. https://doi.org/10.1182/bloodadvances.2018018093

Xia, A., Zhang, Y., Xu, J., et al. (2019). T cell dysfunction in cancer immunity and immunotherapy. *Frontiers in Immunology, 10*, 1719.

Young, R. M., Engel, N. W., Uslu, U., et al. (2022). Next-generation CAR T-cell therapies. *Cancer Discovery, 12*, 1625–1633. https://doi.org/10.1158/2159-8290.CD-21-1683

Zhang, A., Sun, Y., Du, J., et al. (2021). Reducing hinge flexibility of CAR-T cells prolongs survival in vivo with low cytokines release. *Frontiers in Immunology, 12*, 724211. https://doi.org/10.3389/fimmu.2021.724211

Chapter 6
Viral Immunotherapy Strategies in Clinical Practice

Jeffrey Johnson and James Jakub

Abstracts Viruses are a tool that can be used to help activate the immune system against cancer. Viral genetics may be changed to make a virus less infectious or toxic to patients and more effective at combating cancer. Viruses injected into tumors help treat cancer by directly killing cancer cells as well as helping to activate the immune response in a manner similar to a vaccine. A number of viral therapies are being investigated for research. Currently, talimogene laherparepvec (T-VEC) is the only viral therapy approved for clinical use for treating recurrent melanoma. T-VEC is a genetically modified herpes simplex virus that is injected directly into recurrent melanoma lesions in the skin or lymph nodes. A number of additional viral therapies are in development to improve killing of cancer cells and activation of the immune system.

Keywords Oncolytic virus · Talimogene laherparepvec (T-VEC) · T cell · Intralesional therapy · Intralesional injection · Herpes simplex virus · Metastatic melanoma · In-transit disease

Viruses may be used as a tool for priming the immune system against cancer. Viruses are an appealing tool for treating cancer as viral genomes may be manipulated to coopt the evolutionary mechanisms the immune system has developed to combat infection. The concept that the body's response to infection may be used to prime the immune system against cancer has been studied since the late nineteenth century. Most famously, William Coley, a surgeon at the New York Hospital, published his results in using bacterial toxins injected into patients to treat inoperable sarcoma (Coley, 1910). Research using viruses, and particularly viruses developed to target

J. Johnson (✉)
Department of Surgery, Division of Breast and Melanoma Surgical Oncology, Mayo Clinic, Rochester, MN, USA
e-mail: johnson.jeffrey5@mayo.edu

J. Jakub
Department of Surgery, Division of Surgical Oncology, Mayo Clinic, Jacksonville, FL, USA

cancer, began in the middle of the twentieth century. Alice Moore, a physician researcher also working in New York, was an early pioneer in the development and characterization of viruses with oncolytic properties (Moore, 1952). However, it was not until more sophisticated techniques had been developed in the latter twentieth century, which allowed targeted genetic engineering of viruses, that therapeutic use of viruses began to be considered for clinical trials (Martuza et al., 1991). Over the last two decades, development of novel oncolytic virus therapy has expanded rapidly and has entered standard of care clinical use.

Viruses can be made to replicate nearly exclusively in cancer cells, and the viral genome can be modified to diminish its virulence and increase antitumor activity. Promoters can be added into viral genes to reduce the expression of or delete the genes that cause infection in normal cells (DeWeese et al., 2001; Brown et al., 1997). Tumor cells that are selectively infected by a virus are killed by the cancer cell rupturing secondary to viral replication, thereby releasing tumor antigens that prompt a specific antitumor immune response (Kaufman et al., 2015). Also, some oncolytic viruses can be designed to produce proteins that activate a T-cell immune response (Hu et al., 2006; Liu et al., 2003; Fukuhara et al., 2005). One challenge encountered in viral therapies is the risk of the immune system recognizing the virus and clearing it from the body before it serves its purpose. This can be overcome by methods that prevent the virus from being recognized by the host immune system, including genetically modifying the virus to inhibit immune system recognition and coating the outside of the virus so it is not recognized (Tesfay et al., 2013).

A number of viruses have been used in the development of oncolytic therapies, including herpes simplex virus, measles virus, poliovirus, adenovirus, coxsackievirus, vaccinia virus, reovirus, Newcastle disease virus, and Seneca Valley virus (Chiocca & Rabkin, 2014). While systemic administration of a virus has been considered in a model similar to vaccination, current oncolytic viral therapy is employed using targeted delivery of viruses to the site of cancer, such as direct injection in melanoma or urinary catheter-delivered irrigation in bladder cancer, to increase local antitumor effects. In addition, novel oncolytic viruses are modified to further enhance the immune response.

To date, the only FDA-approved virus for treatment of cancer is talimogene laherparepvec (T-VEC), a modified oncolytic herpes simplex virus type 1. Approval was granted in 2015 for treatment of unresectable, recurrent cutaneous melanoma. This virus has been genetically modified for tumor cell selective infection, to increase the immune system's ability to recognize it and to diminish the ability to divide in normal, nontumor cells (Liu et al., 2003). The coding sequence for granulocyte macrophage colony-stimulating factor (GM-CSF) has been inserted into its genome, which enhances the immune response and increases therapeutic efficacy (Liu et al., 2003; Toda et al., 2000).

FDA approval was granted on the results of a large, multicenter trial randomizing patients with unresectable advanced stage melanoma to intralesional injection of T-VEC or subcutaneous GM-CSF (Andtbacka et al., 2015). The study demonstrated an improved durable response rate, defined as complete or partial response lasting at least 6 months, in 16% of patients receiving T-VEC compared to 2% for those receiving GM-CSF. The overall response rate was also higher for those receiving T-VEC (26% vs. 6%). The treatment is well tolerated with the most common side effects including fever, fatigue, nausea, and reaction at the injection site (Andtbacka et al., 2015).

The indications for T-VEC remain relatively limited. It is generally used in the setting of melanoma involving the skin, subcutaneous tissue, and/or lymph nodes for which surgical removal is not advised. In-transit disease is the spread of melanoma in the lymphatics of the skin, which is the most common indication for using T-VEC. T-VEC is one of several treatment options for patients with in-transit melanoma, including regional perfusion of high-dose chemotherapy into the circulation of the limb, topical ointments that cause a local inflammatory immune response or act as a direct chemotherapy, radiation, and other injectable therapies, as well as systemic treatment with immunotherapy. The decision for which therapy to use depends on a number of clinical and institutional factors, and often these treatments are used in series (Racz et al., 2019).

A number of subsequent studies have continued to demonstrate the efficacy and tolerability of T-VEC (Louie et al., 2019, 2020). While there has been interest in combining systemic immunotherapy with T-VEC, including laboratory research suggesting a benefit, the combination has been shown in randomized clinical trials to improve response rate and local control without an improvement in overall survival or progression-free survival (Chesney et al., 2018, 2023a, b). However, T-VEC may be used after failure of immunotherapy (Carr et al., 2022).

T-VEC is delivered as an injection directly into the tumor in the office setting. T-VEC is generally contraindicated in patients with immunodeficiency, on treatment with immunosuppressive medications including high-dose steroids, and patients who are pregnant. Lesions may be injected under direct visualization or with the use of ultrasound guidance, as necessary. T-VEC dose is determined by the size of the lesion(s) with a set maximal total dose that can be administered with each cycle. Injections are generally performed every 2 weeks. Progress is followed for a minimum of 3 months, and injections may continue until there is a complete response, progression of disease, or other clinical factors requiring cessation of treatment (Collichio et al., 2018). The average time to achieve a complete response is approximately 8 months (Andtbacka et al., 2015). In some cases, additional biopsies may be required to evaluate for the presence of viable melanoma cells in pigmented skin lesions, which can persist even with complete resolution of the cancer (Park et al., 2022).

A wide number of additional oncologic viral therapies are in development and actively being tested in clinical trials, both as monotherapy and in combination with systemic therapies, including immunotherapy. The next generation of viral therapies will include additional genetic modifications to enhance tumor cell killing and the native immune response (Tripodi et al., 2023). Modifications include adding viral genes to increase tumor cell-specific viral effectiveness, antitumor activity, and immune response (Thomas et al., 2019; Kontermann et al., 2021).

References

Andtbacka, R. H., Kaufman, H. L., Collichio, F., Amatruda, T., Senzer, N., Chesney, J., et al. (2015). Talimogene laherparepvec improves durable response rate in patients with advanced melanoma. *Journal of Clinical Oncology, 33*(25), 2780–2788.

Brown, S. M., MacLean, A. R., McKie, E. A., & Harland, J. (1997). The herpes simplex virus virulence factor ICP34.5 and the cellular protein MyD116 complex with proliferating cell nuclear antigen through the 63-amino-acid domain conserved in ICP34.5, MyD116, and GADD34. *Journal of Virology, 71*(12), 9442–9449.

Carr, M. J., Sun, J., DePalo, D., Rothermel, L. D., Song, Y., Straker, R. J., et al. (2022). Talimogene Laherparepvec (T-VEC) for the treatment of advanced locoregional melanoma after failure of immunotherapy: An international multi-institutional experience. *Annals of Surgical Oncology, 29*(2), 791–801.

Chesney, J., Puzanov, I., Collichio, F., Singh, P., Milhem, M. M., Glaspy, J., et al. (2018). Randomized, open-label phase II study evaluating the efficacy and safety of talimogene laherparepvec in combination with ipilimumab versus ipilimumab alone in patients with advanced, unresectable melanoma. *Journal of Clinical Oncology, 36*(17), 1658–1667.

Chesney, J. A., Puzanov, I., Collichio, F. A., Singh, P., Milhem, M. M., Glaspy, J., et al. (2023a). Talimogene laherparepvec in combination with ipilimumab versus ipilimumab alone for advanced melanoma: 5-year final analysis of a multicenter, randomized, open-label, phase II trial. *Journal for Immunotherapy of Cancer, 11*(5).

Chesney, J. A., Ribas, A., Long, G. V., Kirkwood, J. M., Dummer, R., Puzanov, I., et al. (2023b). Randomized, double-blind, placebo-controlled, global phase III trial of talimogene laherparepvec combined with pembrolizumab for advanced melanoma. *Journal of Clinical Oncology, 41*(3), 528–540.

Chiocca, E. A., & Rabkin, S. D. (2014). Oncolytic viruses and their application to cancer immunotherapy. *Cancer Immunology Research, 2*(4), 295–300.

Coley, W. B. (1910). The treatment of inoperable sarcoma by bacterial toxins (the mixed toxins of the Streptococcus erysipelas and the Bacillus prodigiosus). *Proceedings of the Royal Society of Medicine, 3*(Surg Sect), 1–48.

Collichio, F., Burke, L., Proctor, A., Wallack, D., Collichio, A., Long, P. K., et al. (2018). Implementing a program of talimogene laherparepvec. *Annals of Surgical Oncology, 25*(7), 1828–1835.

DeWeese, T. L., van der Poel, H., Li, S., Mikhak, B., Drew, R., Goemann, M., et al. (2001). A phase I trial of CV706, a replication-competent, PSA selective oncolytic adenovirus, for the treatment of locally recurrent prostate cancer following radiation therapy. *Cancer Research, 61*(20), 7464–7472.

Fukuhara, H., Ino, Y., Kuroda, T., Martuza, R. L., & Todo, T. (2005). Triple gene-deleted oncolytic herpes simplex virus vector double-armed with interleukin 18 and soluble B7-1 constructed by bacterial artificial chromosome-mediated system. *Cancer Research, 65*(23), 10663–10668.

Hu, J. C., Coffin, R. S., Davis, C. J., Graham, N. J., Groves, N., Guest, P. J., et al. (2006). A phase I study of OncoVEXGM-CSF, a second-generation oncolytic herpes simplex virus expressing granulocyte macrophage colony-stimulating factor. *Clinical Cancer Research, 12*(22), 6737–6747.

Kaufman, H. L., Kohlhapp, F. J., & Zloza, A. (2015). Oncolytic viruses: A new class of immunotherapy drugs. *Nature Reviews. Drug Discovery, 14*(9), 642–662.

Kontermann, R. E., Ungerechts, G., & Nettelbeck, D. M. (2021). Viro-antibody therapy: Engineering oncolytic viruses for genetic delivery of diverse antibody-based biotherapeutics. *MAbs, 13*(1), 1982447.

Liu, B. L., Robinson, M., Han, Z. Q., Branston, R. H., English, C., Reay, P., et al. (2003). ICP34.5 deleted herpes simplex virus with enhanced oncolytic, immune stimulating, and anti-tumour properties. *Gene Therapy, 10*(4), 292–303.

Louie, R. J., Perez, M. C., Jajja, M. R., Sun, J., Collichio, F., Delman, K. A., et al. (2019). Real-world outcomes of talimogene laherparepvec therapy: A multi-institutional experience. *Journal of the American College of Surgeons, 228*(4), 644–649.

Louie, K. S., Banks, V., Scholz, F., Richter, H., Öhrling, K., Mohr, P., et al. (2020). Real-world use of talimogene laherparepvec in Germany: A retrospective observational study using a prescription database. *Future Oncology, 16*(8), 317–328.

Martuza, R. L., Malick, A., Markert, J. M., Ruffner, K. L., & Coen, D. M. (1991). Experimental therapy of human glioma by means of a genetically engineered virus mutant. *Science, 252*(5007), 854–856.

Moore, A. E. (1952). Viruses with oncolytic properties and their adaptation to tumors. *Annals of the New York Academy of Sciences, 54*(6), 945–952.

Park, S. Y., Green, A. R., Hadi, R., Doolittle-Amieva, C., Gardner, J., & Moshiri, A. S. (2022). Tumoral melanosis mimicking residual melanoma in the setting of talimogene laherparepvec treatment. *Journal for Immunotherapy of Cancer, 10*(10).

Racz, J. M., Block, M. S., Baum, C. L., & Jakub, J. W. (2019). Management of local or regional non-nodal disease. *Journal of Surgical Oncology, 119*(2), 187–199.

Tesfay, M. Z., Kirk, A. C., Hadac, E. M., Griesmann, G. E., Federspiel, M. J., Barber, G. N., et al. (2013). PEGylation of vesicular stomatitis virus extends virus persistence in blood circulation of passively immunized mice. *Journal of Virology, 87*(7), 3752–3759.

Thomas, S., Kuncheria, L., Roulstone, V., Kyula, J. N., Mansfield, D., Bommareddy, P. K., et al. (2019). Development of a new fusion-enhanced oncolytic immunotherapy platform based on herpes simplex virus type 1. *Journal for Immunotherapy of Cancer, 7*(1), 214.

Toda, M., Martuza, R. L., & Rabkin, S. D. (2000). Tumor growth inhibition by intratumoral inoculation of defective herpes simplex virus vectors expressing granulocyte-macrophage colony-stimulating factor. *Molecular Therapy, 2*(4), 324–329.

Tripodi, L., Sasso, E., Feola, S., Coluccino, L., Vitale, M., Leoni, G., et al. (2023). Systems biology approaches for the improvement of oncolytic virus-based immunotherapies. *Cancers (Basel), 15*(4).

Chapter 7
Chemoimmunotherapy Combination for Solid Tumors

Yiyi Yan

Abstract Novel cancer immunotherapies targeting the immunosuppressive PD-1/PD-L1 pathway result in durable clinical benefit in a subset of patients; however, primary or acquired resistance is common, affecting up to two-thirds of the patients in various tumor types. Therefore, a substantial effort is currently underway to fully elucidate the mechanisms of resistance to immune checkpoint blockade and to design more effective therapeutic strategies. Conventional anticancer treatments, including chemotherapy, radiation therapy, and targeted therapy, execute anticancer activity through direct cancer cell killing. Recent appreciations of the immune regulatory effects of these therapeutic agents have led to the exploration of their utilization in combination with immune checkpoint inhibitors, aiming to achieve synergetic effects and to improve the response and durability of immunotherapy. Here, we will provide an updated review of the immunomodulatory effects of cytotoxic chemotherapy and their impacts on reshaping modern cancer immunotherapy. The ongoing clinical trials of these combination therapies and their results will be briefly discussed here, since they will also be reviewed in other sections of this book. The combination of different immunotherapy agents, such as PD-1 antibody in combination with CTLA-4 antibody, is not a focus here; instead it is discussed in the overview and other disease-specific chapters.

Keywords Immunotherapy · Chemotherapy · Resistance · Combination therapy

Y. Yan (✉)
Division of Hematology and Medical Oncology, Mayo Clinic, Jacksonville, FL, USA
e-mail: Yan.yiyi@mayo.edu

Mechanisms of Chemotherapy
and Immunotherapy Combination

For decades, cytotoxic chemotherapies have been the mainstay of treatment for many types of advanced malignancies until the recent revolutionary advances in cancer immunotherapy. However, considering that many patients will not show a durable response to immunotherapy alone, chemotherapy is still commonly used anticancer treatment, even in malignancies where immunotherapy is approved, especially in the setting of immune checkpoint inhibitor failure.

In patients who do not respond to immune checkpoint inhibitors, additional mechanisms of immunosuppression in the tumor microenvironment (within the tumors) and derangements in systemic immune competence (homeostasis) can drive chronic tumor-promoting inflammations and therefore serve as potential barriers to treatment success (Gajewski, 2006; Gajewski et al., 2006; Nevala et al., 2009). Overcoming these dysregulations is likely to improve PD-1 blockade efficacy. The immune system, both intra-tumoral and systemic, consists of many types of immune cells orchestrating the regulation of immune surveillance that leads to tumor elimination or tumor growth that leads to cancer metastasis. While some of those cells, such as CD8+ T cells and T helper 1 cells (Th1) (Haabeth et al., 2011), are responsible for antitumor activities, others play immunosuppressive roles promoting the tumor growth and invasion. Regulatory T cells (Treg), T helper 2 cells (Th2), myeloid-derived suppressor cells (MDSCs) (Bunt et al., 2007; Gabrilovich & Nagaraj, 2009), and tumor-associated macrophages (TAM) are examples of immune cells that contribute to the suppressive immune environment favoring tumor progression. The disruption or polarization of the balance between the pro-tumorigenesis and antitumorigenic immune status can impact the outcome of the cancer immunotherapy.

Various types of chemotherapy drugs kill tumor cells through different mechanisms, such as inhibiting mitosis (a critical step in cell cycle progression) and DNA replication, as well as directly targeting cellular DNA or other key molecules that are critical for cancer cell division and survival. Interestingly, a delicate interplay between the effects of chemotherapy and one's immune system has been elucidated—the cell killing induced by chemotherapies can modulate the immune system (both inside of the tumor and systemically), while the status of the immune system can impact the effectiveness of the chemotherapy drugs.

Anticancer cytotoxic chemotherapy has been regarded historically as detrimental to immunity because of its dose-limiting myelosuppression effects. However, recent discoveries have suggested that the antitumor effect of conventional cancer chemotherapy may result in part from its ability to disrupt immune suppressive pathways in addition to direct antitumor effects. For example, studies have shown that chemotherapy-induced lymphodepletion can counterintuitively augment antitumor immunity by potentiating tumor-specific T cell responses (responsible for tumor killing) (Sampson et al., 2011; Williams et al., 2007). Possible mechanisms include depletion of Treg and regulatory B cells, promotion of Th1/Th2 polarization, and enhanced proliferation of effector T-lymphocytes (Ghiringhelli et al., 2007; Alizadeh & Larmonier, 2014).

The presence of immune-suppressing immune cells, such as MDSCs and macrophages (M2), also impairs T cell functions, resulting in a tumor microenvironment that promotes tumor growth. MDSCs are sensitive to chemotherapy drugs, including platinum drugs and 5-FU (Welters et al., 2016; Melief et al., 2020). And certain chemotherapeutic agents, such as cyclophosphamide, favor the differentiation of M1 (favoring tumor killing) than M2 (Buhtoiarov et al., 2011). These pro-immune mechanisms suggest the potential synergetic antitumor effects of chemoimmunotherapy combination.

In addition, some chemotherapeutic agents promote antitumor immunity through induction of immunogenic cell death in tumors. Debris from tumor cells killed by certain chemotherapeutic agents can be processed and then presented by APCs, triggering downstream antitumor immune responses through different proposed mechanisms (Galluzzi et al., 2020, 2017).

Given the role of chemotherapy in overcoming the immune suppression that can result in resistance to immunotherapy, it has been hypothesized that immunotherapy in addition to chemotherapy may further activate the cytotoxic T cells with improved antitumor activities. This combination strategy has been investigated in multiple recent clinical trials.

Chemoimmunotherapy in Solid Tumors

Here, we will briefly summarize the clinical applications and perspectives of chemoimmunotherapy combination in different cancers. The advance in the management of various of solid tumors in the era of modern immunotherapy will be discussed in detail in each disease-specific chapter.

Lung Cancer

Lung cancer is the most common cause of cancer morbidity and mortality worldwide. Immune checkpoint inhibitors (ICIs) represent a paradigm shift in lung cancer treatment, and the addition of chemotherapy to ICI has further improved the survival.

Non-small-Cell Lung Cancer (NSCLC)

NSCLC accounts for about 80% of all lung cancers and has poor prognosis (Siegel et al., 2023). The most success of chemotherapy in combination with immunotherapy is demonstrated in the treatment of NSCLC. For patients with non-small-cell lung cancer, initial clinical data for combinations of chemotherapy with anti-PD1 or anti-PD-L1 antibody (i.e., nivolumab and atezolizumab) have suggested that these regimens have promising antitumor activity and a manageable, nonoverlapping toxicity profile (Rizvi et al., 2016; Camidge et al., 2015).

In 2017, pembrolizumab has received accelerated approval by the FDA for the treatment of metastatic NSCLC adenocarcinomas in combination with carboplatin and pemetrexed in the first-line setting. In the clinical trial that led to this approval, KEYNOTE 021 (Langer et al., 2016), a total of 123 chemo-naïve patients who were stratified by PD-L1 tumor cell expression (<1% compared to ≥1%) were randomized to chemotherapy alone or chemotherapy with pembrolizumab. Those who received chemotherapy alone could receive maintenance pemetrexed indefinitely, and those who received the combination of chemotherapy with pembrolizumab could receive maintenance pemetrexed indefinitely and pembrolizumab for up 24 months. The response rate was significantly higher for the chemotherapy-immunotherapy (CTIO) combination group (55%) than the chemotherapy-alone group (29%). The progression-free survival was 13 months in the CTIO group versus 6 months in the chemotherapy-alone group albeit with more toxicity (39% versus 26%, respectively). Response rates of patients treated with pembrolizumab and chemotherapy combination varied by PD-L1 tumor cell expression, such that the response rate of those with <1% expression was 57%, those with ≥1% expression was 54%, those with 1–49% expression was 26%, and those with ≥50% expression was 80%. Accordingly, the expression of PD-L1 seems to enhance responses when a higher cutoff is used. This study supported CTIO as an alternative frontline therapeutic approach in non-squamous NSCLC patients who do not harbor targetable mutations and have <50% tumor PD-L1 expression, since pembrolizumab is only indicated in those with ≥50% PD-L1 expression in this setting.

The subsequent KEYNOTE-189 trial further confirmed the clinical benefit observed in KETYNOTE-021 trial. In this study, 616 patients with non-squamous advanced NSCLC were randomized in a 2:1 ratio to chemotherapy (cisplatin or carboplatin with pemetrexed) with or without pembrolizumab (Gandhi et al., 2018), unselected for PD-L1 expression status. Crossover to pembrolizumab upon progression is allowed for chemotherapy-alone group. At a median follow-up of 10.5 months, improved 12-month overall survival (OS) rates were observed in the CTIO group compared with chemotherapy-alone group (69 vs. 49%, respectively). The improvements in OS were observed in all PD-L1 categories (<1%, 1–49%, ≥50%). Similar OS benefits were seen at longer follow-up (Rodriguez-Abreu et al., 2021; Gadgeel et al., 2020) with 5-year OS rates of 19% versus 11% (Garassino et al., 2023). Patients in the CTIO-treated group had higher ORR as compared to chemotherapy-alone patients (48% vs. 19%). In addition, improvement in PFS was also observed with the addition of pembrolizumab to chemotherapy (8.8 vs. 4.9 months), across all PD-L1 subgroups, but the differences in PD-L1<1 subgroup were not statistically significant. Severe adverse events (≥grade 3) occurred in 67% of the patients in the CTIO group and in 66% of those in the chemotherapy group, with improved patient-reported quality of life (Garassino et al., 2020).

The addition of pembrolizumab to frontline platinum-based doublet chemotherapy has also shown survival benefit in NSCLC with squamous histology, without substantial additional toxicity. In the phase III KEYNOTE-407 trial, 559 patients with advanced squamous NSCLC were randomized to frontline chemotherapy (carboplatin with either paclitaxel or nabpaclitaxel) combined with either pembrolizumab or placebo. Five-year OS rates were improved in chemoimmunotherapy arm as compared to chemotherapy-alone arm (18% vs. 9.7%, respectively) (Novello et al., 2023). The ORR was 58% in the pembrolizumab-combination group and 38% in the placebo-combination group. Rates of severe adverse events ($\geq$grade 3) were similar in two groups.

Since the publication of the first edition of this book, multiple other chemoimmunotherapy regimens have also been granted regulatory approval for the frontline treatment of advanced NSCLC (lacking an epidermal growth factor receptor (*EGFR*) or anaplastic lymphoma kinase (*ALK*) mutation) based on the improved survival observed in various studies. These include (1) atezolizumab, in combination with chemotherapy, either carboplatin, paclitaxel, and bevacizumab, based on the IMpower 150 trial that randomly assigned 1202 patients with advanced non-squamous NSCLC regardless of PD-L1 status to firstline chemotherapy combined with either atezolizumab, atezolizumab plus bevacizumab, or bevacizumab (BCP) (Socinski et al., 2018); (2) atezolizumab with carboplatin and nabpaclitaxel in the IMpower 130 trial, where the addition of atezolizumab to carboplatin plus nabpaclitaxel in the frontline setting was investigated for advanced non-squamous NSCLC (West et al., 2019); (3) nivolumab plus ipilimumab in combination with platinum-based chemotherapy as studied in the CheckMate-9LA trial (Paz-Ares et al., 2021); (4) cemiplimab in combination with platinum-based chemotherapy, based on preliminary results of the randomized EMPOWER-Lung 3 trial (Gogishvili et al., 2022); (5) and tremelimumab and durvalumab in combination with platinum-based chemotherapy, based on the POSEIDON trial, where 1013 patients with *EGFR/ALK* wild-type tumors were randomly assigned to tremelimumab plus durvalumab plus chemotherapy, durvalumab plus chemotherapy, or chemotherapy alone (Johnson et al., 2023).

Chemoimmunotherapy containing pemetrexed-based regimen was studied in the IMpower 132 trial with atezolizumab (Nishio et al., 2021). The combination therapy improved median PFS in non-squamous NSCLC. However, the improvement in OS is not statistically significant. Therefore, atezolizumab in combination with pemetrexed has not yet received regulatory approval.

Small-Cell Lung Cancer (SCLC)

Extensive stage small-cell lung cancer (ES-SCLC) is a lethal disease with an estimated five-year overall survival around 7% (Siegel et al., 2023). Recent phase III studies have established the combination of chemotherapy and immunotherapy as the frontline treatment for ES-SCLC with improved overall survival.

The first treatment advance for ES-SCLC over the last 20 years was atezolizumab in combination with carboplatin and etoposide, as shown in the IMpower133 trial. In this study, 403 treatment-naïve ES-SCLC patients were randomized to carboplatin and etoposide, with or without atezolizumab for four cycles, followed by maintenance atezolizumab or placebo, accordingly to the initial randomization (Horn et al., 2018; Liu et al., 2021). The ORR was similar between groups (60.2 vs. 64.4%). However, with 23-month follow-up, improvements in median PFS (5.2 vs. 4.3 months) and median OS (12.3 and 10.3 months) were seen in patients who received atezolizumab chemotherapy combination, with no additive toxicities. Correlative studies failed to show evidence to support the use of PD-L1 or circulating tumor DNA (ctDNA) or tumor mutational burden as predictive biomarker.

The addition of the durvalumab to platinum-etoposide, in the frontline setting, has also shown improved survival outcomes compared with chemotherapy alone for ES-SCLC, as demonstrated in the phase III CASPIAN trial (Paz-Ares et al., 2019, 2022). This study randomized 537 treatment-naïve ES-SCLC patients to durvalumab plus four cycles of platinum-etoposide followed by maintenance durvalumab versus 4–6 cycles of platinum-etoposide. Updated results with median follow-up time of 25.1 months have shown that CTIO group had improved OS (12.9 vs. 10.5 months). PFS rates at 24 months were 11% for CTIO group versus 2.9% for chemotherapy group, with ORR of 68% versus 58%, respectively. Responses were durable with CTIO versus chemotherapy alone at 2 years (13.5% vs. 3.9%, respectively). Rates of grade 3 or 4 adverse events were similar in both groups, including grade 5 adverse events.

Interestingly, the addition of anti-CTLA4 antibodies, tremelimumab, to durvalumab and platinum-based chemotherapy did not further improve OS, but with increased high-grade adverse events and treatment-related death (Paz-Ares et al., 2022; Goldman et al., 2021).

The addition of pembrolizumab to platinum and etoposide was investigated in the randomized placebo-controlled KEYNOTE-604 study. Results showed improved PFS, but not OR, with the addition of pembrolizumab. In this trial, 453 treatment-naïve ES-SCLC patients received treatment with the addition of pembrolizumab or placebo to four cycles of platinum-etoposide, with continuation of pembrolizumab for up to 35 cycles in pembrolizumab group. The 12-month PFS rates were 13.6% versus 3.1%, with and without pembrolizumab (Rudin et al., 2020). Although the addition of pembrolizumab to chemotherapy numerically improved OS, it did not meet the statistical significance threshold (24-month OS rates of 23% vs. 11%, respectively). Similar to IMpower133 and CASPIAN studies, the rates of grade 3 and 4 and treated-related death are comparable in two treatment groups in KEYNOTE-604 study.

The addition of other molecules to chemoimmunotherapy combination is under investigation in several ongoing trials, aiming to further improve the outcomes for patients with ES-SCLC. These include the addition of antiangiogenic agents, which will promote T cell infiltration and reduce immunosuppression (NCT05116007, NCT04660097, etc.). Other immune checkpoint inhibitors, such as LAG3 inhibitor

(NCT05026592) and TIGIT antibody (NCT04256421), in addition to chemotherapy, are also under investigations for patients with SCLC.

Resectable Lung Cancer

In addition to its application in the non-resectable advanced stage lung cancers, chemo-immunotherapy combination has shown great success in NSCLC patients with resectable diseases in the neoadjuvant and/or adjuvant settings. For further details, please refer to the "Management of Lung Cancer" chapter in this book. These results strongly suggest the benefit of using chemoimmunotherapy in the early-stage diseases, aiming to increase chance for a cure.

Breast Cancer

HER-2-negative hormone receptor-negative (triple negative) breast cancer (TNBC) remains to be a clinical challenge with poor prognosis compared with other subtypes of breast cancer. For patients with metastatic disease, the standard of care includes chemotherapy. And chemoimmunotherapy combinations were recently investigated in this setting, yet its clinical applications in different disease stages need further clarification.

Atezolizumab was previously granted accelerated approval by the FDA in combination with nabpaclitaxel, for those with advanced TNBC with PD-L1 $\geq 1\%$ of the tumor area, based on the PFS benefit observed in the Impassion 130 study (Schmid et al., 2018). However, this approval was later withdrawn, given that the final result for OS in the intention-to-treat population was negative (Schmid et al., 2020a; Emens et al., 2020). In addition, IMpassion 131 study, a randomized phase III trial using paclitaxel with or without atezolizumab for frontline unresectable locally advanced/metastatic TNBC, showed that combining atezolizumab with paclitaxel did not improve PFS or OS versus paclitaxel alone (Miles et al., 2020).

In 2020, the FDA approved pembrolizumab in combination with chemotherapy for patients with metastatic TNBC with PD-L1 CPS ≥ 10, based on the result from KEYNOTE-355 study. In this phase III trial, 847 patients with locally recurrent, inoperable, or metastatic TNBC were randomized to chemotherapy (nabpaclitaxel, paclitaxel, or gemcitabine/carboplatin), with or without pembrolizumab (Cortes et al., 2020). In patients with CPS ≥ 10, the combination of pembrolizumab and chemotherapy significantly improved median PFS by approximately 4 months (9.7 vs. 5.6 months) compared with chemotherapy-alone group, with comparable grade 3–4 adverse events between the two groups. Multiple trials are currently ongoing to investigate the chemoimmunotherapy combination in metastatic TNBC patients.

Recently, the phase II I-SPY2 trial (Nanda et al., 2020) and the phase III KEYNOTE-522 trial (Schmid et al., 2020b) have shown that the addition of pembrolizumab to paclitaxel-based chemotherapy regimen in the neoadjuvant setting resulted in improved pathologic response rates in TNBC patients. In the phase III Impassion031 trial (Mittendorf et al., 2020), the addition of atezolizumab to chemotherapy also demonstrated benefit in pathologic complete response rates as compared with chemotherapy alone. However, the benefits in OS and PFS of chemoimmunotherapy combination from these studies are yet to be determined with longer follow-ups.

Melanoma

Before the introduction of immune checkpoint inhibitors, cytotoxic chemotherapy was the standard of care for metastatic melanoma. Prior to the FDA approval of pembrolizumab in 2014, two studies investigated ipilimumab in combination with dacarbazine compared with dacarbazine or ipilimumab alone (Robert et al., 2011; Hersh et al., 2011), respectively. Although these trials demonstrated OS benefit with chemoimmunotherapy, its clinical application was limited due to the unprecedented improvement of survival provided by the subsequently approved anti-PD1 antibody-based therapies.

Despite the success of anti-PD1 therapy, many patients with metastatic melanoma either fail to respond or experience secondary resistance with later disease progressions after initial responses. In a retrospective study from our group (Vera Aguilera et al., 2020), the clinical outcomes of patients who received chemoimmunotherapy upon disease progression on PD-1 blockade were investigated. When compared to patients who received either chemotherapy or immunotherapy alone in the post-PD1 progression setting, chemoimmunotherapy-treated patients had improved survival, with median OS of 3.5 years versus 1.8 years, with ORR of 59% versus 15%, respectively. The median event-free survival (EFS) was 7.6 months following chemoimmunotherapy versus 3.4 months following ICI or chemotherapy alone. Acceptable safety profile was also observed in the chemoimmunotherapy treatment group with no additional toxicities compared to either therapy alone. Of note, many patients included in this study have progressed after multiple lines of therapy, including ipilimumab combined with PD-1 blockade. Although it needs to be validated in prospective studies, these results provide clinical evidence supporting chemoimmunotherapy combination as an effective and safe therapeutic regimen for patients who have disease progression after anti-PD-1-based therapy, especially in those who have failed multiple lines of previous systemic treatment.

Other Cancers

Genitourinary Cancers

Before immunotherapy becoming the standard of care for renal cell carcinoma (RCC), tyrosine kinase inhibitors (TKI) used to be the first-line treatment, due to the lack of the efficacy of chemotherapy. Therefore, recent studies exploiting combination approach in RCC are mainly focused on combining ICI with antiangiogenic agents. Reader will be referred to the "GU Cancer" chapter for further details.

In contrast, platinum-based chemotherapy provides clear benefit in patients with metastatic urothelial carcinoma. However, the benefit of the addition of ICI to chemotherapy is still unclear. In a single arm phase II study, patients with chemotherapy-naïve metastatic urothelial cancer was treated with ipilimumab in combination with gemcitabine and cisplatin (Galsky et al., 2018). This study did not achieve the primary endpoint of 1-year OS. However, authors observe a significant expansion of circulating CD4 cells with the addition of ipilimumab which correlated with improved survival.

In the phase III three-arm KEYNOTE-361 trial (Powles et al., 2021), pembrolizumab in combination with chemotherapy (cisplatin or carboplatin plus gemcitabine) for patients with advanced or metastatic urothelial carcinoma in the first-line setting did not meet its pre-specified dual primary endpoints of OS or PFS, compared with standard of care chemotherapy. In the final analysis of the study, the observed improvement in OS and PFS for patients treated with chemoimmunotherapy compared to chemotherapy alone did not meet statistical significance per the pre-specified statistical plan. The pembrolizumab monotherapy arm in this study was not formally tested, since superiority was not reached for OS or PFS in the combination arm. No new safety signals were identified.

Given the lack of benefit of ICIs in metastatic castration-resistant prostate cancer, the addition of immunotherapy to chemotherapy has not been evaluated for these patients.

Head and Neck Cancers

Chemoimmunotherapy combination has shown efficacy in metastatic head and neck squamous cell carcinoma in the frontline or recurrent settings. As shown in the KEYNOTE-048 trial (Burtness et al., 2019), the addition of pembrolizumab to a platinum-based chemotherapy improved OS and PFS compared with cetuximab plus a platinum-based chemotherapy combination. For those with high PD-L1 expression (CPS $\geq$1), single-agent pembrolizumab also improved OS compared with cetuximab plus chemotherapy combination, while this benefit is mainly driven by those with a CPS $\geq$20 (Burtness et al., 2022). Based on these results, the FDA has approved the use of pembrolizumab for this indication for all patients, along with cisplatin and fluorouracil, as a single agent for those whose tumors express PD-L1 CPS $\geq$1.

The clinical benefit of chemoimmunotherapy for patients with treatment-naïve recurrent or metastatic head and neck cancer was also demonstrated in the phase IV trial KEYNOTE-B10 study (Dzienis et al., 2022), where patients were treated with up to six cycles of carboplatin plus paclitaxel in combination with pembrolizumab, followed by subsequent maintenance pembrolizumab monotherapy. In preliminary results, at median follow-up of 8 months, the ORR for the entire study population was 48%, including a complete response rate of 5%. Median PFS and OS for all patients were 6 and 12 months, respectively. Of note, the observed rate for grade ≥3 toxicity was 71%, including two deaths.

Since the majority of patients with HNSCC presented with either localized or locoregional disease, multiple ongoing studies are focused on the clinical application of chemoimmunotherapy in various perioperative settings for these patients.

Gastrointestinal Cancers

In recent years, immune checkpoint inhibitors have gained regulatory approvals in patients with microsatellite unstable metastatic colon cancer, gastric cancer, and HCC (hepatocellular carcinoma). These are discussed in detail in "GI Cancer" chapter.

For colorectal cancer, cytotoxic chemotherapy is still the first-line standard of care. The addition of ICI to chemotherapy for metastatic CRC offers future research opportunities to improve the clinical outcomes, especially in the perioperative setting, given their synergistic antitumor effects.

In patients with advanced upper GI cancers (gastric, esophageal, and GE junction cancers), multiple trials have demonstrated the OS benefits of chemoimmunotherapy combination, including CheckMate 649 (Janjigian et al., 2021; Shitara et al., 2022), KEYNOTE-859 (Rha et al., 2023), CheckMate 648 (Doki et al., 2022), and KEYNOTE-590 studies (Sun et al., 2021). For details, readers are referred to the chapter "GI Cancer." Future effort will also focus on the application of combination approach in the neoadjuvant and adjuvant settings for upper GI cancers.

For HCC and pancreatic cancer, the use of chemoimmunotherapy is yet to be explored, since chemotherapy is not used as SOC in HCC and immunotherapy with ICI has not yield any benefit for PDAC.

Antibody-Drug Conjugate

Antibody-drug conjugates (ADCs) represent another attractive approach for combination systemic therapy of metastatic cancer. ADC is an approach that aims to improve chemotherapy delivery to cancer cells by combining two classes of drugs, monoclonal antibodies and cytotoxic agents. This leverages the ability of monoclonal antibodies to selectively target tumor cells in order for cytotoxic chemotherapy to reach cancer cells more selectively, ultimately leading to improved therapeutic outcomes with less toxicity and greater antitumor efficacy (Panowski et al., 2014). Recent technologic advances have addressed some of the previous shortcomings such as unstable linkers, low antigen selectivity and high immunogenicity, and reinvigorating interest in ADC-based anticancer therapy over the last decade (Panowski et al., 2014). This is evidenced by the FDA approval of multiple immunoconjugates targeting CD33, CD30, HER2, CD22, CD79b, Nectin 4, Trop2, BCMA, CD19, tissue factor (Chia, 2022), and most recently folate receptor alpha (Moore et al., 2021). Immune checkpoint inhibitor-based ADCs are yet to be investigated in the clinical studies, but this could represent a future research direction to further improve the outcomes of currently available chemoimmunotherapy combination.

Conclusion and Future Perspectives

Despite the effectiveness demonstrated in these trials, the efficacy and safety profile of chemoimmunotherapy (CTIO) combination therapies have significant room for further improvement. In order to develop the optimum therapeutic strategy, researchers need to further elucidate the mechanisms of chemo-induced regulation on immune responses augmented by immunotherapy; to define the regimen, treatment sequence, and timing of combination therapy; and to develop the predictive and prognostic markers for patient selection and response assessment. These are all areas of focus for this recently evolving field of immunotherapy over the last few years.

Immunomodulatory Mechanisms

Chemotherapy can target proliferating cells besides cancer cells for killing, including lymphocytes. As previously mentioned, these drugs can deplete immune suppressor cells, rendering an immune environment favoring antitumor activity. However, the impact of chemotherapy drugs on the function of tumor-reactive effector T cells is largely unknown. This is of particular importance, because these types of T cells are mediators of the antitumor activity of immune checkpoint blockade. One of the research interests in our group is to identify the alterations that are caused by chemotherapy in this T cell population and the impacts of these alterations on the designs and outcomes of CTIO. We evaluated the impact of chemotherapy on these tumor-reactive T cells, taking advantage of samples from melanoma patients who failed initial PD1 blockade therapy and received subsequent salvage CTIO combination (Yan et al., 2018). We have identified a subset of circulating CD8+ T cells and CXCR1+GranzymB+CD8+ T cells, which was able to withstand the toxicity of chemotherapy with enhanced antitumor activities in melanoma patients who responded to CTIO. The adoptive transfer of this T cell subset demonstrated improved tumor control in preclinical animal models. In addition, in our clinical cohort, CXCR1+GranzymB+CD8+ T cells showed dynamic increase upon successful CITO treatment in melanoma patients who have failed previous anti-PD1 therapy. Further research focused on the interplay and modulation between chemotherapy and immunotherapy, especially the impact in the tumor microenvironment, will elucidate additional mechanisms and targets that can lead to improvement of current clinical outcomes.

Strategies for Chemoimmunotherapy Combination

The optimum sequence and timing of the CTIO therapy are still unclear. In most reported trials, chemotherapy and immunotherapy are given concurrently. However, preclinical studies have demonstrated that the timing of and the sequence of both modalities are important. For example, in metastatic melanoma patients who have failed anti-PD1 therapy, chemotherapies are commonly offered as the late-line regimen. We have showed that approximately 26% of these patients demonstrated an objective response to subsequent chemotherapy (including carboplatin and paclitaxel) compared to a lower response rate in chemotherapy-treated historic controls (Flaherty et al., 2013), suggesting increased effectiveness of cytotoxic chemotherapy even after exposure of PD-1 blockade compared to patients who have never received immunotherapy (Yan et al., 2016). Results from melanoma animal model also demonstrated that chemotherapy after immunotherapy provides better tumor control compared to concurrent CTIO (Yan et al., 2018). In contrast, a phase II study, using ipilimumab in combination with carboplatin and paclitaxel in NSCLC, showed improved PFS only in phased ipilimumab combination group (two cycles of chemotherapy followed by CTIO) but not in CTIO concurrent group (Lynch et al., 2012).

The dosing schedule of chemotherapy delivery also had a significant impact on the therapeutic effects. For example, the platinum-based chemotherapy regimen was given at an every-three-week or every-four-week regimen for NSCLC in most of the CTIO combination trials for lung cancer. However, previously studies in gynecology cancer have demonstrated differences in immunomodulatory effects of weekly versus an every 4 weeks chemotherapy. In addition, in a phase III study for patients with treatment-naïve NSCLC, weekly paclitaxel/carboplatin have shown similar efficacy to an every 3 weeks schedule. Severe neurotoxicity was significantly less frequent with the weekly schedule (4.4% vs. 9.1%), but grade 3 or 4 diarrhea was more common (4.2% vs. 1.1%) when compared with an every 3 weeks regimen (Schuette et al., 2006). Currently, the best sequence and schedule of CTIO are still inconclusive in both preclinical and clinical settings with controversial data, and the optimum combination regimens are evolving. Further studies are warranted to address and evaluate these critical questions.

Different class of chemotherapy agents exert unique immunomodulatory effects. For example, anthracyclines are capable of inducing immunogenic cell death (ICD), taxanes can selectively reduce immunosuppressive cells (Treg and MDSC) (Kodumudi et al., 2010; Li et al., 2014; Roselli et al., 2013), and 5-fluorouracil stimulates immune responses by facilitating antigen uptake (Galetto et al., 2003). Therefore, how to pair different chemotherapeutic drugs with the most appropriate immunotherapy for an ideal combination strategy remains to be elucidated in future preclinical and clinical studies. For example, a meta-analysis that included 17 randomized trials found that cisplatin, but not carboplatin-based regimens, was associated with a significantly higher survival at 1 year compared with nonplatinum regimens in lung cancer patients (Rajeswaran et al., 2008). In addition, various disease and histology types are also likely to impact the optimal agents to be combined as chemotherapy regimen in the clinical settings (Scagliotti et al., 2008; Syrigos et al., 2010). Furthermore, the dose and duration of chemotherapy used in the CTIO combination, in order to achieve maximal anticancer and immunomodulatory effects with minimal toxicities, is another crucial question that needs to be investigated in preclinical models.

Potential Biomarkers

Among the biomarkers that have been explored to predict the efficacy of ICI, PD-L1 is the most studied molecule. Despite its association with increased likelihood of response to ICI, tumor PD-L1 expression alone fails to guarantee responses in patients with high expression nor to exclude responses in those lacking PD-L1 expression. This is likely due to the intra- and inter- tumoral heterogeneity of PD-L1 as well as high rate of inadequate sampling.

PD-L1 has also been studied extensively for patients treated with chemoimmunotherapy combination. However, the values of PD-L1 as predictive and prognostic value in this setting are still inconclusive. As shown in KEYNOTE-021, KEYNOTE-35,5 and KEYNOTE-048, high PD-L1 expression is associated with higher response rates to combination therapy for NSCLC patients. However, in other disease types, such as SCLC as shown in IMpower133 study, there was no difference in the predicted OS and PFS by PD-L1 IHC subgroups. In most of the recent studies, PDL1 testing was not required for enrollment.

TMB measurement has also been deeply studied as a potential biomarker for cancer immunotherapy, where high disease responses are observed in tumors with high TMB. The FDA approved the use of pembrolizumab in any cancer type with ≥ 10 mutations/megabase who had progressed to one previous treatment line without other valid alternative treatment options. However, its clinical application is limited for chemoimmunotherapy, since TMB did not predict either OS or PFS in chemoimmunotherapy, as shown in the exploratory analysis of Impower133 trial (Horn et al., 2018). Further preclinical and clinical studies are likely to identify novel biomarkers to inform the outcomes of chemoimmunotherapy. For example, the aforementioned CX3CR1+ Granzyme B+ CD8+ T cell was associated with patients responded to CTIO treatment but not in those who did not respond to CTIO (Yan et al., 2018). In recent studies, immune profiling and immune-related gene expression appear to be involved in the prognosis and response to immunotherapy in NSCLC. These are also being investigated in the setting of chemoimmunotherapy combination.

Conclusion

Current pre-clinical and clinical research in cancer immunotherapy is focused on modulating host immune response through two main approaches—increasing the cancer killing ability of the immune system (e.g., boost the T cell function via checkpoint inhibitors) and suppressing the tumor-promoting immune process. The recent unprecedented success of immune checkpoint inhibitors in cancer treatment has rapidly reinvigorating the field of oncology and cancer research. Given the fact that they do not provide clinical benefit for many cancer patients, it is crucial to design efficacious synergic therapeutic approaches with increased response. Chemotherapy has been shown to modulate host immune system, making it more favorable for T cell antitumor activity enhanced by immune checkpoint inhibitor. Although these combinations have shown promising results with improved survival, further research is needed to elucidate the exact immune-regulatory mechanisms and the treatment strategies, such as regimens, dose, and schedule, of the combination therapy.

References

Alizadeh, D., & Larmonier, N. (2014). Chemotherapeutic targeting of cancer-induced immuno-suppressive cells. *Cancer Research, 74*, 2663–2668.

Buhtoiarov, I. N., et al. (2011). Anti-tumour synergy of cytotoxic chemotherapy and anti-CD40 plus CpG-ODN immunotherapy through repolarization of tumour-associated macrophages. *Immunology, 132*, 226–239.

Bunt, S. K., et al. (2007). Reduced inflammation in the tumor microenvironment delays the accumulation of myeloid-derived suppressor cells and limits tumor progression. *Cancer Research, 67*, 10019–10026.

Burtness, B., et al. (2019). Pembrolizumab alone or with chemotherapy versus cetuximab with chemotherapy for recurrent or metastatic squamous cell carcinoma of the head and neck (KEYNOTE-048): A randomised, open-label, phase 3 study. *Lancet, 394*, 1915–1928.

Burtness, B., et al. (2022). Pembrolizumab alone or with chemotherapy for recurrent/metastatic head and neck squamous cell carcinoma in KEYNOTE-048: Subgroup analysis by programmed death ligand-1 combined positive score. *Journal of Clinical Oncology, 40*, 2321–2332.

Camidge, R., et al. (2015). Atezolizumab (MPDL3280A) combined with platinum-based chemotherapy in Non-Small Cell Lung Cancer (NSCLC): A phase Ib safety and efficacy update. *Journal of Thoracic Oncology, 10*, S176–S177.

Chia, C. S. B. (2022). A patent review on FDA-approved antibody-drug conjugates, their linkers and drug payloads. *ChemMedChem, 17*, e202200032.

Cortes, J., et al. (2020). Pembrolizumab plus chemotherapy versus placebo plus chemotherapy for previously untreated locally recurrent inoperable or metastatic triple-negative breast cancer (KEYNOTE-355): A randomised, placebo-controlled, double-blind, phase 3 clinical trial. *Lancet, 396*, 1817–1828.

Doki, Y., et al. (2022). Nivolumab combination therapy in advanced esophageal squamous-cell carcinoma. *The New England Journal of Medicine, 386*, 449–462.

Dzienis, M. R., et al. (2022). Pembrolizumab (pembro) plus carboplatin (carbo) plus paclitaxel (pacli) as first-line (1L) therapy in recurrent/metastatic (R/M) head and neck squamous cell carcinoma (HNSCC): Phase VI KEYNOTE-B10 study. *Annals of Oncology, 33*, S839–S840.

Emens, L. A., et al. (2020). IMpassion130: Final OS analysis from the pivotal phase III study of atezolizumab plus nab-paclitaxel vs placebo plus nab-paclitaxel in previously untreated locally advanced or metastatic triple-negative breast cancer. *Annals of Oncology, 31*, S1148–S1148.

Flaherty, K. T., et al. (2013). Phase III trial of carboplatin and paclitaxel with or without sorafenib in metastatic melanoma. *Journal of Clinical Oncology, 31*, 373–379.

Gabrilovich, D. I., & Nagaraj, S. (2009). Myeloid-derived suppressor cells as regulators of the immune system. *Nature Reviews. Immunology, 9*, 162–174.

Gadgeel, S., et al. (2020). Updated analysis from KEYNOTE-189: Pembrolizumab or placebo plus pemetrexed and platinum for previously untreated metastatic nonsquamous non-small-cell lung cancer. *Journal of Clinical Oncology, 38*, 1505–1517.

Gajewski, T. F. (2006). Identifying and overcoming immune resistance mechanisms in the melanoma tumor microenvironment. *Clinical Cancer Research, 12*, 2326s–2330s.

Gajewski, T. F., et al. (2006). Immune resistance orchestrated by the tumor microenvironment. *Immunological Reviews, 213*, 131–145.

Galetto, A., et al. (2003). Drug- and cell-mediated antitumor cytotoxicities modulate cross-presentation of tumor antigens by myeloid dendritic cells. *Anti-Cancer Drugs, 14*, 833–843.

Galluzzi, L., Buque, A., Kepp, O., Zitvogel, L., & Kroemer, G. (2017). Immunogenic cell death in cancer and infectious disease. *Nature Reviews. Immunology, 17*, 97–111.

Galluzzi, L., Humeau, J., Buque, A., Zitvogel, L., & Kroemer, G. (2020). Immunostimulation with chemotherapy in the era of immune checkpoint inhibitors. *Nature Reviews. Clinical Oncology, 17*, 725–741.

Galsky, M. D., et al. (2018). Phase 2 trial of gemcitabine, cisplatin, plus ipilimumab in patients with metastatic urothelial cancer and impact of DNA damage response gene mutations on outcomes. *European Urology, 73*, 751–759.

Gandhi, L., et al. (2018). Pembrolizumab plus chemotherapy in metastatic non-small-cell lung cancer. *The New England Journal of Medicine, 378*, 2078–2092.

Garassino, M. C., et al. (2020). Patient-reported outcomes following pembrolizumab or placebo plus pemetrexed and platinum in patients with previously untreated, metastatic, non-squamous non-small-cell lung cancer (KEYNOTE-189): A multicentre, double-blind, randomised, placebo-controlled, phase 3 trial. *The Lancet Oncology, 21*, 387–397.

Garassino, M. C., et al. (2023). Pembrolizumab plus pemetrexed and platinum in nonsquamous non-small-cell lung cancer: 5-year outcomes from the phase 3 KEYNOTE-189 study. *Journal of Clinical Oncology, 41*, 1992–1998.

Ghiringhelli, F., et al. (2007). Metronomic cyclophosphamide regimen selectively depletes CD4+CD25+ regulatory T cells and restores T and NK effector functions in end stage cancer patients. *Cancer Immunology, Immunotherapy, 56*, 641–648.

Gogishvili, M., et al. (2022). Cemiplimab plus chemotherapy versus chemotherapy alone in non-small cell lung cancer: A randomized, controlled, double-blind phase 3 trial. *Nature Medicine, 28*, 2374–2380.

Goldman, J. W., et al. (2021). Durvalumab, with or without tremelimumab, plus platinum-etoposide versus platinum-etoposide alone in first-line treatment of extensive-stage small-cell lung cancer (CASPIAN): Updated results from a randomised, controlled, open-label, phase 3 trial. *The Lancet Oncology, 22*, 51–65.

Haabeth, O. A., et al. (2011). Inflammation driven by tumour-specific Th1 cells protects against B-cell cancer. *Nature Communications, 2*, 240.

Hersh, E. M., et al. (2011). A phase II multicenter study of ipilimumab with or without dacarbazine in chemotherapy-naive patients with advanced melanoma. *Investigational New Drugs, 29*, 489–498.

Horn, L., et al. (2018). First-Line atezolizumab plus chemotherapy in extensive-stage small-cell lung cancer. *The New England Journal of Medicine, 379*, 2220–2229.

Janjigian, Y. Y., et al. (2021). First-line nivolumab plus chemotherapy versus chemotherapy alone for advanced gastric, gastro-oesophageal junction, and oesophageal adenocarcinoma (CheckMate 649): A randomised, open-label, phase 3 trial. *Lancet, 398*, 27–40.

Johnson, M. L., et al. (2023). Durvalumab with or without tremelimumab in combination with chemotherapy as first-line therapy for metastatic non-small-cell lung cancer: The phase III POSEIDON study. *Journal of Clinical Oncology, 41*, 1213–1227.

Kodumudi, K. N., et al. (2010). A novel chemoimmunomodulating property of docetaxel: Suppression of myeloid-derived suppressor cells in tumor bearers. *Clinical Cancer Research, 16*, 4583–4594.

Langer, C. J., et al. (2016). Carboplatin and pemetrexed with or without pembrolizumab for advanced, non-squamous non-small-cell lung cancer: A randomised, phase 2 cohort of the open-label KEYNOTE-021 study. *The Lancet Oncology, 17*, 1497–1508.

Li, J. Y., et al. (2014). Selective depletion of regulatory T cell subsets by docetaxel treatment in patients with nonsmall cell lung cancer. *Journal of Immunology Research, 2014*, 286170.

Liu, S. V., et al. (2021). Updated overall survival and PD-L1 subgroup analysis of patients with extensive-stage small-cell lung cancer treated with atezolizumab, carboplatin, and etoposide (IMpower133). *Journal of Clinical Oncology, 39*, 619–630.

Lynch, T. J., et al. (2012). Ipilimumab in combination with paclitaxel and carboplatin as first-line treatment in stage IIIB/IV non-small-cell lung cancer: Results from a randomized, double-blind, multicenter phase II study. *Journal of Clinical Oncology, 30*, 2046–2054.

Melief, C. J. M., et al. (2020). Strong vaccine responses during chemotherapy are associated with prolonged cancer survival. *Science Translational Medicine, 12*.

Miles, D. W., et al. (2020). Primary results from IMpassion131, a double-blind placebo-controlled randomised phase III trial of first- line paclitaxel (PAC) +/− atezolizumab (atezo) for unresectable locally advanced/metastatic triple-negative breast cancer (mTNBC). *Annals of Oncology, 31*, S1147–S1148.

Mittendorf, E. A., et al. (2020). Neoadjuvant atezolizumab in combination with sequential nab-paclitaxel and anthracycline-based chemotherapy versus placebo and chemotherapy in patients with early-stage triple-negative breast cancer (IMpassion031): A randomised, double-blind, phase 3 trial. *Lancet, 396*(10257), 1090–1100. https://doi.org/10.1016/S0140-6736(20)31953-X.

Moore, K. N., et al. (2021). Phase III, randomized trial of mirvetuximab soravtansine versus chemotherapy in patients with platinum-resistant ovarian cancer: Primary analysis of FORWARD I. *Annals of Oncology, 32*, 757–765.

Nanda, R., et al. (2020). Effect of pembrolizumab plus neoadjuvant chemotherapy on pathologic complete response in women with early-stage breast cancer: An analysis of the ongoing phase 2 adaptively randomized I-SPY2 trial. *JAMA Oncology, 6*, 676–684.

Nevala, W. K., et al. (2009). Evidence of systemic Th2-driven chronic inflammation in patients with metastatic melanoma. *Clinical Cancer Research, 15*, 1931–1939.

Nishio, M., et al. (2021). IMpower132: Atezolizumab plus platinum-based chemotherapy vs chemotherapy for advanced NSCLC in Japanese patients. *Cancer Science, 112*, 1534–1544.

Novello, S., et al. (2023). Pembrolizumab plus chemotherapy in squamous non-small-cell lung cancer: 5-year update of the phase III KEYNOTE-407 study. *Journal of Clinical Oncology, 41*, 1999–2006.

Panowski, S., Bhakta, S., Raab, H., Polakis, P., & Junutula, J. R. (2014). Site-specific antibody drug conjugates for cancer therapy. *MAbs, 6*, 34–45.

Paz-Ares, L., et al. (2019). Durvalumab plus platinum-etoposide versus platinum-etoposide in first-line treatment of extensive-stage small-cell lung cancer (CASPIAN): A randomised, controlled, open-label, phase 3 trial. *Lancet, 394*, 1929–1939.

Paz-Ares, L., et al. (2021). First-line nivolumab plus ipilimumab combined with two cycles of chemotherapy in patients with non-small-cell lung cancer (CheckMate 9LA): An international, randomised, open-label, phase 3 trial. *The Lancet Oncology, 22*, 198–211.

Paz-Ares, L., et al. (2022). Durvalumab, with or without tremelimumab, plus platinum-etoposide in first-line treatment of extensive-stage small-cell lung cancer: 3-year overall survival update from CASPIAN. *ESMO Open, 7*, 100408.

Powles, T., et al. (2021). Pembrolizumab alone or combined with chemotherapy versus chemotherapy as first-line therapy for advanced urothelial carcinoma (KEYNOTE-361): A randomised, open-label, phase 3 trial. *The Lancet Oncology, 22*, 931–945.

Rajeswaran, A., Trojan, A., Burnand, B., & Giannelli, M. (2008). Efficacy and side effects of cisplatin- and carboplatin-based doublet chemotherapeutic regimens versus non-platinum-based doublet chemotherapeutic regimens as first line treatment of metastatic non-small cell lung carcinoma: A systematic review of randomized controlled trials. *Lung Cancer, 59*, 1–11.

Rha, S. Y., et al. (2023). Pembrolizumab (pembro) plus chemotherapy (chemo) as first-line therapy for advanced HER2-negative gastric or gastroesophageal junction (G/GEJ) cancer: Phase III KEYNOTE-859 study. *Annals of Oncology, 34*, 319–320.

Rizvi, N. A., et al. (2016). Nivolumab in combination with platinum-based doublet chemotherapy for first-line treatment of advanced non-small-cell lung cancer. *Journal of Clinical Oncology, 34*, 2969–2979.

Robert, C., et al. (2011). Ipilimumab plus dacarbazine for previously untreated metastatic melanoma. *The New England Journal of Medicine, 364*, 2517–2526.

Rodriguez-Abreu, D., et al. (2021). Pemetrexed plus platinum with or without pembrolizumab in patients with previously untreated metastatic nonsquamous NSCLC: Protocol-specified final analysis from KEYNOTE-189. *Annals of Oncology, 32*, 881–895.

Roselli, M., et al. (2013). Effects of conventional therapeutic interventions on the number and function of regulatory T cells. *Oncoimmunology, 2*, e27025.

Rudin, C. M., et al. (2020). Pembrolizumab or placebo plus etoposide and platinum as first-line therapy for extensive-stage small-cell lung cancer: Randomized, double-blind, phase III KEYNOTE-604 study. *Journal of Clinical Oncology, 38*, 2369–2379.

Sampson, J. H., et al. (2011). Greater chemotherapy-induced lymphopenia enhances tumor-specific immune responses that eliminate EGFRvIII-expressing tumor cells in patients with glioblastoma. *Neuro-Oncology, 13*, 324–333.

Scagliotti, G. V., et al. (2008). Phase III study comparing cisplatin plus gemcitabine with cisplatin plus pemetrexed in chemotherapy-naive patients with advanced-stage non-small-cell lung cancer. *Journal of Clinical Oncology, 26*, 3543–3551.

Schmid, P., et al. (2018). Atezolizumab and Nab-Paclitaxel in advanced triple-negative breast cancer. *The New England Journal of Medicine, 379*, 2108–2121.

Schmid, P., et al. (2020a). Atezolizumab plus nab-paclitaxel as first-line treatment for unresectable, locally advanced or metastatic triple-negative breast cancer (IMpassion130): Updated efficacy results from a randomised, double-blind, placebo-controlled, phase 3 trial. *The Lancet Oncology, 21*, 44–59.

Schmid, P., et al. (2020b). Pembrolizumab for early triple-negative breast cancer. *The New England Journal of Medicine, 382*, 810–821.

Schuette, W., et al. (2006). Multicenter randomized trial for stage IIIB/IV non-small-cell lung cancer using every-3-week versus weekly paclitaxel/carboplatin. *Clinical Lung Cancer, 7*, 338–343.

Shitara, K., et al. (2022). Nivolumab plus chemotherapy or ipilimumab in gastro-oesophageal cancer. *Nature, 603*, 942–948.

Siegel, R. L., Miller, K. D., Wagle, N. S., & Jemal, A. (2023). Cancer statistics, 2023. *CA: a Cancer Journal for Clinicians, 73*, 17–48.

Socinski, M. A., et al. (2018). Atezolizumab for first-line treatment of metastatic nonsquamous NSCLC. *The New England Journal of Medicine, 378*, 2288–2301.

Sun, J. M., et al. (2021). Pembrolizumab plus chemotherapy versus chemotherapy alone for first-line treatment of advanced oesophageal cancer (KEYNOTE-590): A randomised, placebo-controlled, phase 3 study. *Lancet, 398*, 759–771.

Syrigos, K. N., et al. (2010). Prognostic and predictive factors in a randomized phase III trial comparing cisplatin-pemetrexed versus cisplatin-gemcitabine in advanced non-small-cell lung cancer. *Annals of Oncology, 21*, 556–561.

Vera Aguilera, J., et al. (2020). Chemo-immunotherapy combination after PD-1 inhibitor failure improves clinical outcomes in metastatic melanoma patients. *Melanoma Research, 30,* 364–375.

Welters, M. J., et al. (2016). Vaccination during myeloid cell depletion by cancer chemotherapy fosters robust T cell responses. *Science Translational Medicine, 8,* 334ra352.

West, H., et al. (2019). Atezolizumab in combination with carboplatin plus nab-paclitaxel chemotherapy compared with chemotherapy alone as first-line treatment for metastatic non-squamous non-small-cell lung cancer (IMpower130): A multicentre, randomised, open-label, phase 3 trial. *The Lancet Oncology, 20,* 924–937.

Williams, K. M., Hakim, F. T., & Gress, R. E. (2007). T cell immune reconstitution following lymphodepletion. *Seminars in Immunology, 19,* 318–330.

Yan, Y., et al. (2016). The Mayo Clinic experience in patients with metastatic melanoma who have failed previous pembrolizumab treatment. *ASCO Meeting Abstracts, 34,* e21014.

Yan, Y., et al. (2018). CX3CR1 identifies PD-1 therapy-responsive CD8+ T cells that withstand chemotherapy during cancer chemoimmunotherapy. *JCI Insight, 3.*

Chapter 8
Melanoma Immunotherapy

Erica L. Andres and Matthew S. Block

Abstract Melanoma is considered a highly immunogenic tumor due to its high level of somatic mutations and frequent expression of type I interferons. As such, investigators have tested many immunotherapies in patients with metastatic and resected melanoma. Although earlier forms of immunotherapy such as interleukin-2 and interferon alpha had modest efficacy, immune checkpoint inhibitors, including ipilimumab, pembrolizumab, nivolumab, and relatlimab, have demonstrated significant benefit and have transformed the care of melanoma patients. Combinations of immune checkpoint inhibitors (ipilimumab and nivolumab or nivolumab with relatlimab) have become standard first-line therapy for patients with metastatic melanoma, while anti-PD-1 monotherapy (pembrolizumab or nivolumab) is routinely used to treat high-risk resected melanoma. Neoadjuvant immunotherapy is emerging as a promising treatment approach for resectable melanoma at high risk for recurrence. Other forms of immunotherapy include oncolytic viruses such as talimogene laherparepvec, and bispecific T-cell engagers such as tebentafusp have also demonstrated benefit to certain populations of melanoma patients. Finally, newer immunotherapy approaches, including tumor-infiltrating lymphocytes (TILs), vaccines targeting melanoma neoantigens, and antibodies to novel immune checkpoints like T-cell immunoreceptor with immunoglobulin (Ig) and immunoreceptor tyrosine-based inhibitory motif domains (TIGIT) are showing promise in recently reported and ongoing clinical trials. In summary, immunotherapies have transformed and now dominate systemic therapy for melanoma patients.

Keywords Melanoma · Ipilimumab · Nivolumab · Pembrolizumab · Relatlimab · Adjuvant · Neoadjuvant · Metastatic · Talimogene laherparepvec · Tebentafusp · Tumor-infiltrating lymphocyte · Vaccine · TIGIT

E. L. Andres · M. S. Block (✉)
Department of Oncology, Mayo Clinic, Rochester, MN, USA
e-mail: block.matthew@mayo.edu

© The Author(s), under exclusive license to Springer Nature Switzerland AG 2024
H. Dong, S. N. Markovic (eds.), *The Basics of Cancer Immunotherapy*,
https://doi.org/10.1007/978-3-031-59475-5_8

Part 1: Melanoma and the Immune System

Melanoma has long been considered one of the most "immunogenic" tumors. Early evidence suggesting that the host immune response that could eradicate cancer came from observations that melanomas, including disseminated melanomas, would occasionally regress without therapy (Baker, 1964; Everson, 1967; Nathanson, 1976). Although the mechanisms involved in spontaneous regression of melanoma were not initially known, many investigators felt that the host immune system was responsible. As the components of the cellular immune response were identified, a relationship was observed between tumor-infiltrating lymphocytes (TILs) and outcome in melanoma (Clark Jr. et al., 1969; Poppema et al., 1983; Strohal et al., 1994), and investigators noted a correlation between TILs and spontaneous melanoma regression (Mackensen et al., 1994). The demonstration that cloned TILs could recognize and lyse autologous melanoma cells provided an important proof of the concept of tumor immunotherapy (Topalian et al., 1989; Itoh et al., 1988; Sensi et al., 1993). This was further substantiated by the recognition that vitiligo (the loss of pigment in the skin due to destruction of benign melanocytes), which is seen in higher frequency in melanoma patients, is mediated by the immune system (Bystryn, 1989). Because of the early recognition of the immunogenicity of melanomas (as well as the relative futility of cytotoxic chemotherapy and radiotherapy approaches to metastatic melanoma), melanoma has been the cancer in which immunotherapy has been most studied and has also shown remarkable efficacy in treating even patients with widely metastatic disease. Thus, to describe the rationale for various immunotherapies for melanoma, we will first discuss the means by which melanomas both stimulate as well as suppress and evade the host antitumor immune response.

Inherent Immunogenicity of Melanoma

Once it became clear that the immune system was capable of recognizing melanomas, investigators sought to determine the antigens responsible for immune recognition. Melanoma antigens have been classified into cancer-testis antigens, overexpression antigens, melanocyte differentiation antigens, and neoantigens. Cancer-testis antigens are germline-encoded antigens with no expression or minimal expression by most tissues of the body but are expressed in the testis (which normally has no HLA class I expression) and by a subset of melanoma cells. The prototypic cancer-testis antigens are the melanoma antigen-encoding (MAGE) proteins (van der Bruggen et al., 1991; Chomez et al., 2001). Overexpression antigens are normally expressed at low levels but are expressed at higher levels by tumors; these include the proteins, survivin (Schmitz et al., 2000), melanoma antigen preferentially expressed in tumors (PRAME) (Ikeda et al., 1997), and telomerase (Vonderheide et al., 1999). Melanocyte differentiation antigens have shared expression by melanoma cells and normal melanocytes. While the presence of differentiation antigens on nonmalignant melanocytes suggests that self-tolerance may be a key concern, tumor-infiltrating lymphocytes recognizing the differentiation antigens Melan A (MART-1) (Kawakami et al., 1994), glycoprotein 100 (gp100) (Bakker et al., 1994), and tyrosinase (Brichard et al., 1993) have been described.

The advent of next-generation sequencing and algorithms capable of predicting the binding of peptide antigens to HLA molecules has allowed for recognition of new antigens, called neoantigens, comprised of mutated proteins unique to each tumor and expressed in tumor cells only (Overwijk et al., 2013). These neoantigens are generated through mutations in the genomic DNA or in alterations in the posttranscriptional or posttranslational steps. Cutaneous melanomas harbor a relatively high number of non-synonymous mutations and have, on average, the highest number of neoantigens of any tumor type (Schumacher & Schreiber, 2015). These neoantigens are presented on the surface of tumor cells or via an antigen-presenting cells and can be recognized by activated T-cells. The number of mutations per megabase (muts/Mb) harbored by a tumor is known as tumor mutation burden (TMB). Increased TMB has been shown to correlate with increased response to immune checkpoint inhibitor therapy by allowing for improved recognition and then elimination of tumor cells by the immune system (Darvin et al., 2018).

Within melanoma, anatomic location of the primary site has been shown to directly correlate with the TMB and response to immunotherapy. Cutaneous melanomas in chronically sun-exposed sites have the highest TMB, with mucosal, acral, and uveal melanomas having a lower TMB. Exposure to ultraviolet rays causes pyrimidine-pyrimidine photodimers leading to mutagenesis. The intraocular space in which uveal melanoma develops is completely protected from the sun and therefore has the lowest TMB (Dousset et al., 2021). As will be discussed below, many forms of immunotherapy are more frequently effective in sun-exposed cutaneous melanomas versus acral, mucosal, and uveal melanomas.

In addition to being the tumor most capable of stimulating the adaptive immune response with a very high mutational burden, melanoma stimulates the innate immune system via a variety of mechanisms. Gene expression profiling of melanoma metastases has demonstrated significant expression of type I interferons (Harlin et al., 2009), which are produced by innate immune cells in response to a variety of stimuli. Type I interferons are typically produced in response to the binding of innate immune receptors, including the Toll-like receptors (TLRs), nod-like receptors (NLRs), C-type lectin receptors, and the STING receptor (Gajewski et al., 2012). Melanomas have also been reported to express high levels of many damage-associated molecular patterns (DAMPs) capable of stimulating type I interferon production. The significant expression of type I interferon by these mechanisms contributes to the inherent immunogenicity of melanoma.

Mechanisms of Immune Evasion and Immunosuppression Employed by Melanoma

Despite containing a relatively high number of antigens and innate immune stimuli, most advanced melanomas are not eradicated by the host immune response. This is due in part to immune editing (selection of subclones of melanoma cells that do not express dominant antigens) but is also due to melanoma-induced immunosuppression. Insights into the immune escape mechanisms used by melanoma and other tumors has led to the development of multiple immunotherapy agents that have transformed the care of melanoma patients.

Initial research focused on melanoma immune escape mechanisms involving alterations in the tumor microenvironment (TME). One key means of melanoma immune evasion is the loss of HLA class I molecules, leading to a lack of antigen presentation (Ferrone & Marincola, 1995). Loss of class I molecules would be expected to lead to increased sensitivity to natural killer (NK) cell recognition and killing, but melanomas often downregulate NK cell ligands as well.

More recently, research has shifted to focus on co-inhibitory ligands and receptors that help regulate tumor immunity. These ligand and receptor pairs are known as immune checkpoints and can be targeted to enhance the antitumor activity of the immune system. The first immune checkpoint to be successfully targeted in melanoma immunotherapy was cytotoxic T-lymphocyte-associated protein 4 (CTLA-4). CTLA-4 is a co-inhibitory receptor expressed on activated T-cells. CTLA4 and CD28 are both expressed on the surface of T-cells and bind to the CD80 and CD86 ligands on antigen-presenting cells. However, while CD28 serves to amplify the immune response, CTLA-4 serves to keep the immune response in check by downregulating the amplitude of early stages of T-cell activation. Blocking CTLA-4 leads to increased amplitude of T-cell activation and thereby an increased antitumor response by the T-cells (Chikuma, 2017; Rowshanravan et al., 2018).

Perhaps the most well-known immunosuppressive factor produced by melanoma is programmed death ligand 1 (PD-L1). By binding to the co-inhibitory T-cell receptor programmed death 1 (PD-1), PD-L1 activates tyrosine-protein phosphatase non-receptor type 11 (PTPN11, also known as Shp2) and decreases signaling through CD28 and the T-cell receptor. In most melanomas, PD-L1 is not constitutively expressed but is rather induced in response to one of several stimuli. Classically, PD-L1 expression is induced by IFNγ, which is expressed by TILs (Spranger et al., 2013). In this way, PD-L1 limits the degree of immune damage done to melanomas via upregulation in the context of Th1-mediated immune responses. Additionally, PD-L1 is upregulated in response to BRAF inhibition (Jiang et al., 2013) and thus can subvert the clinical efficacy of targeted therapy. While most investigators have focused on the immunosuppressive properties of membrane-bound PD-L1, a subset of melanomas also secrete a soluble splice variant of PD-L1 (Zhou et al., 2017); expression of soluble PD-L1 is a poor prognostic marker in melanoma. The key role played by PD-L1 in melanoma-mediated immunosuppression is perhaps best demonstrated by the clinical efficacy of antibodies that disrupt the interaction between PD-L1 and PD-1, as discussed below.

However, some tumors are resistant or become resistant to PD-1 blockade, and thus focus has turned to other immune checkpoints that may work individually or synergistically with PD-1. One such checkpoint is lymphocyte activation gene-3 (LAG-3). LAG-3 is a type 1 transmembrane protein with an extracellular component that is structurally similar to CD4 and binds MHC class II among other ligands. It is expressed on exhausted CD4+ and CD8+ tumor-infiltrating T-cells; once bound, LAG-3 inhibits T-cell activation (Maruhashi et al., 2020). Immune cells that are chronically activated eventually become exhausted; this normally plays an important role in the prevention of autoimmunity. However, in malignancy, T-cell exhaustion leads to decreased numbers and functionality of T-cells which leads to the negative effects of decreased antitumor activity. Blocking the LAG-3 checkpoint has been shown to both increase the numbers of T-cells as well as inflammatory cytokines (Graydon et al., 2020).

T-cell immunoreceptor with immunoglobulin and immunoreceptor tyrosine-based inhibition motif domain (TIGIT) is another co-inhibitory receptor in the immunoglobulin superfamily, and it binds to the ligands CD155 and CD112 that are expressed on tumor and dendritic cells. TIGIT inhibits both innate and adaptive immunities through the inhibition of T-cells and NK cells and by enhancing the immunosuppressive effects of Tregs. TIGIT has been shown to be upregulated in over 30 cancer types including melanoma (Wen et al., 2021) and like LAG-3 also helps promote T-cell exhaustion and subsequently the progressive loss of T-cell function and proliferation (Tang et al., 2023).

While the immunosuppressive mediators described above primarily work within the melanoma TME, melanomas have also been demonstrated to cause regional and systemic alterations in immunity, which can also lead to suppression of anti-melanoma immune responses. Sentinel lymph nodes from resected early-stage melanoma patients demonstrate evidence of Th2 polarization, including a decrease in CD8+ T-cells and an increase in VEGF (Grotz et al., 2015). Once melanoma has metastasized, many patients demonstrate systemic Th2 polarization, as demonstrated by Th1 cell dysfunction and high levels of Th2 cytokines circulating in plasma (Nevala et al., 2009). Patients with metastatic melanoma also exhibit decreased circulating dendritic cells (DCs) and altered monocyte function (Chavan et al., 2014). While the mechanisms behind the systemic shift from Th1- to Th2-dominated immunity are not completely clear, one cause may be galectin 9, which is commonly found in plasma of metastatic melanoma patients and which converts immune responses from Th1 to Th2 (Enninga et al., 2016). The presence of regional and systemic immune dysregulation has the potential to impact the efficacy of melanoma immunotherapies.

Part 2: Current Immunotherapy Treatments for Melanoma

Whereas the majority of resected solid organ cancers can be treated effectively with cytotoxic chemotherapy, this approach has not proven beneficial for melanoma. However, building on the early discoveries of melanoma's intricate relationship with the immune system, there are now multiple effective systemic therapies to treat melanoma by using strategies that take advantage of the inherent immunogenicity of melanoma as well as its mechanisms of immune evasion and suppression. We will discuss immunotherapies for both unresectable and resectable melanomas below.

Part 2a: Unresectable Melanoma

Interleukin 2 (IL-2) and Tumor-Infiltrating Lymphocyte (TIL) Therapy

The first immune-based therapy approved for unresectable melanoma involved giving high-dose interleukin 2 (IL-2), a cytokine produced by activated T-cells. IL-2 serves as a growth factor for both T-cells and natural killer (NK) cells. Upon binding to its receptor, IL-2 activates multiple pathways within T and NK cells to drive cell proliferation and prevent apoptotic cell death. It was hypothesized that IL-2 drives expansion of melanoma-specific T-cells and allows them to infiltrate tumors. However, while highly effective for a small percentage of patients, the overall response rate to IL-2 was poor, and the therapy was associated with significant toxicity. Due to adverse events such as respiratory distress and capillary leak syndrome, IL-2 was often administered in the intensive care unit. A case record-based analysis of 631 patients treated on multiple clinical trials demonstrated a single-agent response rate of 14.9%, a response rate to IL-2 plus chemotherapy of 20.8%, a response rate to IL-2 plus IFNγ of 23.0%, and a response rate to IL-2 plus IFNγ plus chemotherapy (known as biochemotherapy) of 44.9% (Keilholz et al., 1998). The median overall survival for the entire cohort was 10.5 months.

Investigators also tried combining IL-2 with tumor-infiltrating lymphocyte (TIL) therapy. TIL therapy attempted to passively immunize patients with melanoma-specific activated T-cells by harvesting T-cells from tumors (so-called tumor-infiltrating lymphocytes or TILs), expanding them in vitro using cytokines, and then reinfusing them into patients. Initial trials of TILs alone rarely resulted in durable clinical benefit, as the TILs often failed to persist for more than a few days after adoptive transfer. However, the added steps of preconditioning patients with high doses of chemotherapy and infusing IL-2 after TIL therapy did lead to improved TIL persistence and a higher frequency of objective responses, albeit at a cost of increased toxicity. Future directions in TIL therapy will be discussed in Part 3 of this chapter.

While IL-2 is highly toxic and has proved only marginally effective, a new strategy targeting co-inhibitory ligands and receptors that help regulate tumor immunity has developed. Immune checkpoint inhibitors are not only more effective but also less toxic, can be given in outpatient infusion centers at local oncology practices, and do not require the single-patient manufacturing requirements of high-dose IL-2 and TIL therapies. The FDA approval of the first immune checkpoint inhibitor, ipilimumab, and its widespread adoption into clinical practice in 2011 ushered cancer immunotherapeutics into mainstream oncology practice.

Ipilimumab

As discussed in Part 1, the discovery that the inducible T-cell surface protein cytotoxic T lymphocyte antigen 4 (CTLA-4) functions as a coinhibitory receptor led rapidly to the finding that targeting of CTLA-4 with monoclonal antibodies can lead to the enhancement of antitumor immune responses (Leach et al., 1996). This led to the testing and subsequent FDA approval of the CTLA-4-binding monoclonal antibody ipilimumab in the setting of metastatic melanoma. Ipilimumab binds to CTLA-4 and prevents it from binding to its ligands B7-1 and B7-2, thus preventing CTLA-4-driven coinhibitory signaling. As such, CTLA-4 blockade leads to increased expansion of activated T-cells.

Ipilimumab was approved for use in metastatic melanoma on the basis of two randomized clinical trials. The first trial employed a 1:1:3 randomization of HLA-A2-positive previously treated metastatic melanoma patients to ipilimumab 3 mg/kg, a vaccine targeting gp100, or ipilimumab plus vaccine (Hodi et al., 2010). Although median progression-free survival was similar between the three groups, median overall survival was improved from 6.4 months in the vaccine only arm to 10.1 and 10.0 months in the ipilimumab only and ipilimumab plus vaccine arms, respectively. Importantly, the overall survival rates at 24 months were 23.5% and 21.6% for ipilimumab alone and ipilimumab plus vaccine, versus 13.7% for vaccine alone. The second trial randomized untreated metastatic melanoma patients to receive the cytotoxic chemotherapy drug dacarbazine (DTIC) plus placebo versus DTIC plus ipilimumab dosed at 10 mg/kg (Robert et al., 2011). Median overall survival was 9.1 months in the DTIC plus placebo arm and 11.2 months in the DTIC plus ipilimumab arm.

Toxicities observed with ipilimumab were primarily immune-mediated adverse events including colitis, dermatitis, and hepatitis. Grade 3 and 4 adverse events occurred in 45.8%, 45.5%, and 56.3% of patients treated with ipilimumab alone, ipilimumab plus vaccine, and ipilimumab plus DTIC, respectively. Of the patients allocated to ipilimumab treatment, 52% discontinued therapy due to adverse events. Ultimately, the 3 mg/kg dose of ipilimumab was approved for use in metastatic melanoma.

Pembrolizumab and Nivolumab

Just as CTLA-4 is expressed on activated T-cells as a co-inhibitory receptor to the B7-1 and B7-2 ligands, programmed death 1 (PD-1) is expressed by activated T-cells and triggers T-cell death and anergy when bound by one of its ligands:

PD-L1 (B7-H1) or PD-L2 (Dong & Chen, 2003). PD-L1 is expressed by many tumors and tumor-infiltrating leukocytes; most often, PD-L1 expression is induced by IFNγ (Dong et al., 2002). In this way, expression of PD-L1 is a means for tumors to attenuate productive antitumor-immune responses.

Monoclonal antibodies that bind to PD-1 or PD-L1 can block the interaction between receptor and ligand and can prevent the resultant T-cell inhibition. In this way, anti-PD-1 antibodies allow for increased persistence of activated TILs in tumors that express PD-L1. The first PD-1-targeting monoclonal antibodies to be tested in clinical trials were pembrolizumab (initially known as lambrolizumab) and nivolumab.

The first report of pembrolizumab in melanoma was in 2013 by Dr. Hamid and colleagues (Hamid et al., 2013). Patients with advanced melanoma were treated with one of three dosing schedules: 10 mg/kg every 2 weeks, 10 mg/kg every 3 weeks, or 2 mg/kg every 3 weeks. Confirmed tumor responses were seen in 38% of patients, and response rates were similar in patients who were naïve to ipilimumab or had received prior ipilimumab. On this basis, pembrolizumab at 2 mg/kg every 3 weeks was approved by the FDA for use in metastatic melanoma in patients who had previously been treated with ipilimumab.

Pembrolizumab was then compared with ipilimumab, which had emerged as a standard for first-line therapy of metastatic melanoma. Patients were randomized to receive either ipilimumab or pembrolizumab at 10 mg/kg every 2 weeks or pembrolizumab at 10 mg/kg every 3 weeks (Robert et al., 2015a). Median progression-free survival times were 5.5 months, 4.1 months, and 2.8 months for pembrolizumab every 2 weeks, pembrolizumab every 33 weeks, and ipilimumab, respectively. Although median overall survival was not reached at the time of the trial report, the 12-month survival rates were 74.1%, 68.4%, and 58.2%, while the objective response rates were 33.7%, 32.9%, and 11.9% for pembrolizumab every 2 weeks, pembrolizumab every 3 weeks, and ipilimumab, respectively. On this basis, pembrolizumab monotherapy was approved as first-line therapy for melanoma.

Similar to pembrolizumab, nivolumab is a monoclonal antibody that binds to PD-1 and disrupts the ability of PD-1 to bind to ligands and drive T-cell death and anergy. Nivolumab was developed in parallel as a single-agent therapy and in combination with ipilimumab. As a single agent, nivolumab was compared to DTIC in a placebo-controlled randomized phase III trial (CheckMate 066) in untreated patients with metastatic melanoma without a BRAF mutation (Robert et al., 2015b). Here, nivolumab was given at 3 mg/kg every 2 weeks. Nivolumab therapy led to objective responses in 40.0% of patients, versus 13.9% of patients with DTIC. Median progression-free survival was 5.1 months with nivolumab versus 2.2 months with DTIC. The 1 year overall survival benefit was significantly improved with at 79.2% for nivolumab versus 42.1% for DTIC. Based on a significant improvement over DTIC, nivolumab was approved as monotherapy for metastatic melanoma.

The toxicities associated with single-agent pembrolizumab and single-agent nivolumab are similar both to each other and to those associated with ipilimumab. However, the frequency of severe adverse events was considerably lower for either anti-PD-1 therapy than for ipilimumab. Grade 3 or higher adverse events were seen in 34.8% of patients receiving pembrolizumab (Hamid et al., 2013) (31.8% of patients treated with 2 mg/kg every 3 weeks) and in 34% of patients treated with nivolumab (Robert et al., 2015b) (recall that 45.8% of patients treated with ipilimumab (Hodi et al., 2010) had grade 3 or higher adverse events). Thus, the PD-1-targeting drugs are associated with both higher objective response rates and lower toxicity as single agents than ipilimumab, which targets CTLA-4.

Combined Ipilimumab and Nivolumab

Given that CTLA-4 and PD-1 send distinct negative regulatory signals to T-cells, and given that they are frequently engaged at different times and locations in the body, investigators hypothesized that combined targeting of CTLA-4 and PD-1 might lead to better control of melanoma than either agent alone. As such, the combination of ipilimumab (at 3 mg/kg every 3 weeks for four cycles) and nivolumab (1 mg/kg every 3 weeks for four cycles, followed by 3 mg/kg every 2 weeks) was compared against either agent alone in patients with untreated metastatic melanoma (Larkin et al., 2015). This led to statistical improvements in multiple oncologic outcomes over ipilimumab monotherapy, as well as numeric increases in multiple oncologic measures over nivolumab monotherapy. However, this improvement came at a cost of increased toxicity compared with either single agent. Nonetheless, the impressive rate of melanoma control by combined therapy with ipilimumab and nivolumab led to FDA approval of the combination in 2015. A summary of the outcomes of this phase III trial is shown in Table 8.1.

Nivolumab/Retlatinib Combination Therapy

Unfortunately, not all patients initially respond to immune checkpoint inhibitor therapy, and some who do respond eventually stop responding. With the success of combining multiple immunotherapies that target complimentary but distinct immune checkpoints as seen in nivolumab/ipilimumab, investigators sought to identify other immune checkpoint inhibitor combinations. One such combination is

Table 8.1 Comparison of outcomes in phase III randomized clinical trial with combined ipilimumab and nivolumab, single-agent nivolumab, and single-agent ipilimumab in patients with metastatic melanoma

Regimen	Ipilimumab + nivolumab	Nivolumab	Ipilimumab
Objective response rate	57.6%	43.7%	19.0%
Median progression-free survival (months)	11.5	6.9	2.9
Grade 3+ adverse events	68.7%	43.5%	55.6%
Grade 3+ treatment-related adverse events	55.0%	16.3%	27.3%

nivolumab/retlatinib. Retlatinib is a lymphocyte-activation gene 3 (LAG-3) monoclonal antibody that like the PD-1 antibody, nivolumab, prevents T-cell exhaustion.
LAG-3 has been found to be co-expressed with PD-1 on TILs in mouse models. By
blocking both LAG-3 and PD-1, investigators hoped to achieve a better overall
response rate with prolonged progression-free survival.

In order to study this, the investigators used a unique double-blind phase II trial
that then bled into a phase III trial. The RELATIVITY-047 trial compared the combination nivolumab/relatlimab with single-agent nivolumab in patients with previously untreated metastatic or unresectable melanoma (Tawbi et al., 2022). They
excluded patients with uveal melanoma and patients with untreated brain metastases. Participants were randomized 1:1 to either 160 mg of relatlimab with fixed dose
of 480 mg of nivolumab or 480 mg of nivolumab monotherapy given every 4 weeks.
The primary endpoint of progression-free survival was met with PFS of 10.1 months
for patients receiving nivolumab/relatlimab compared to 4.6 months with nivolumab.
The secondary endpoint of overall response rate was also significantly improved
with 43.1% of patients responding in the relatlimab-nivolumab group compared to
32.65 in the single-agent nivolumab group. Overall survival however was not statistically significant between the groups. (Tawbi et al., 2022) Grade 3 or 4 treatment-
related adverse events were 18.9% in the combination group and 9.7% in the
nivolumab monotherapy group. Importantly, benefit of relatlimab-nivolumab over
single-agent nivolumab was seen regardless of LAG-3 expression status. The results
from the trial are listed in Table 8.2.

Comparison of CTLA-4 Monotherapy, PD-1 Monotherapy, and Combination CTLA-4/PD-1 Therapy for Metastatic Melanoma

There are now multiple effective immune checkpoint inhibitors approved as first-
line therapy for metastatic melanoma with the optimal approach for each patient
dependent on a number of considerations and at discretion of the treating oncologist. In young, otherwise healthy patients or patients with aggressive disease or
high-risk biology such as patients with acral or mucosal tumors, combination ICI

Table 8.2 Comparison of outcomes in phase II–III randomized clinical trial with combined
relatlimab-nivolumab compared to single-agent nivolumab in patients with metastatic melanoma

Regimen	Relatlimab + nivolumab	Nivolumab
Objective response rate	43.1%	32.6%
Median progression-free survival (months)	10.1	4.6
Progression-free survival at 12 months	47.7%	36.0%
Grade 3+ treatment-related adverse events	18.9%	9.7%

therapy with ipilimumab-nivolumab is often given as first-line therapy. It has been demonstrated to have an improved response rate (57.6% vs. 43.7%) over PD-1 monotherapy with nivolumab but carries with it an increased risk of grade 3 and 4 adverse events (55.0% vs. 16.3%). Additionally, both nivolumab and ipilimumab-nivolumab regimens have shown efficacy in the treatment of brain metastases and are therefore the preferred regimens in this setting (Combination nivolumab and ipilimumab or nivolumab alone in melanoma brain metastases: a multicentre randomised phase 2 study - The Lancet Oncology). In patients who are frail, monotherapy with nivolumab or pembrolizumab, which have shown similar efficacy and tolerability to each other, is typically considered first line due to the decreased rate of adverse events. The more recent success of nivolumab-relatlimab as an effective ICI doublet therapy with efficacy and tolerability similar to ipilimumab-nivolumab makes it an attractive emerging option for patients who are healthy and/or have aggressive disease (Table 8.3).

Talimogene Laherparepvec (T-VEC)

Another FDA-approved immunotherapy for patients with unresectable, metastatic melanoma is the oncolytic virus therapy, talimogene laherparepvec (T-VEC). T-VEC is a genetically modified herpes virus that has been engineered to target, infect, and then lyse cancer cells and causes infected cells to secrete granulocyte-macrophage colony-stimulating factor (GM-CSF). In the phase III randomized clinical trial, OPTiM, patients were assigned to receive either intralesional T-VEC every 2 weeks or daily GM-CSF injections for 14 days of a 28-day cycle (Andtbacka et al., 2015). T-VEC was directly injected into the sites of cutaneous, subcutaneous, or nodal metastases. The trial's primary endpoint of durable response rate (DRR) defined as an objective response lasting greater than sixth months was reached with patients in the T-VEC group achieving a DRR of 16.3% compared to 2.1% in the GM-CSF group. The secondary endpoint of median overall survival was not statistically significant but showed a median OS of 23.3 months in the T-VEC group compared to 18.9 months in the GM-CSF group ($P = 0.051$). The results of the OPTiM trial led to the FDA approval of T-VEC in 2015.

The efficacy of T-VEC is thought to be due to both direct effects from the virus through lysis of the cancer cell as well as through the enhancement of the antitumor immune response. The latter has led to multiple clinical trials looking for a synergistic effect between oncolytic viruses and immune checkpoint inhibitors. T-VEC was recently trialed in combination with pembrolizumab in a phase III clinical trial where patients with stage IIIB-IVM1c unresectable melanoma were given either T-VEC and pembrolizumab or placebo and pembrolizumab (Chesney et al., 2023). Unfortunately the study did not achieve either of its primary endpoints as the addition of T-VEC to pembrolizumab did not significantly improve PFS or OS.

Table 8.3 Comparison of phase III clinical trial results for immune checkpoint inhibitor therapies in patients with unresectable melanoma

	Checkmate-067			Keynote-006		Relativity-047	
	Ipilimumab 3 mg/kg	Nivolumab 1 mg/kg	Ipilimumab 3 mg/kg + nivolumab 1 mg/kg	Pembrolizumab 10/kg	Ipilimumab 3 mg/kg	Nivolumab 480 mg	Nivolumab 480 mg + relatlimab 160 mg
Objective response rate	19.0%	43.7%	57.6%	33.2%	11.9%	32.6%	43.1%
Median progression free survival	2.9 months	6.9 months	11.5 months	8.4 months	3.4 months	4.6 months	10.1 months
Median overall survival	19.9 months	37.6 months	Not reached	32.7 months	15.9 months	33.2 months	Not reached
≥ Grade 3 adverse treatment events	27.3%	16.3%	55.0%	17%	20%	9.7%	18.9%

Tebentafusp for Uveal Melanoma

A unique immunotherapy for metastatic or unresectable uveal melanoma was approved in January 2022. While uveal melanoma arises from melanocytes, it has a very different tumor microenvironment and genetic signature compared to cutaneous melanoma. It is often metastatic at presentation with over 50% of patients having metastatic disease to the liver. Uveal melanoma has a low TMB and low PD-L1 expression compared to cutaneous melanoma and therefore, as expected, has not had the same robust response to immune checkpoint inhibitors that is seen in cutaneous melanoma. Uveal melanoma is also considered a "cold" tumor, with infiltration of very few CD8+ T-cells. However, uveal melanomas do display the pigment-associated antigen glycoprotein 100 (gp1000) which is recognized by T-cells (Carvajal et al., 2022). Tebentafusp is a bispecific protein that was developed to help T-cells engage the gp100 peptide and kill gp100-expressing melanoma cells. It was approved for use in patients who are positive for HLA-A*02:01, as the bispecific protein consists of a HLA-A*02:01-restricted T-cell receptor (TCR) that is specific for the gp100 peptide.

In a phase III randomized clinical trial comparing previously untreated HLA-A-*02:01-positive patients with metastatic uveal melanoma to either tebentafusp versus investigator's choice with single-agent pembrolizumab, ipilimumab, or dacarbazine, the overall survival at 1 year was 73% in the tebentafusp group and 59% in the control group (Nathan et al., 2021). While cytokine-mediated adverse events due to T-cell activation were noted in over 90% of patients, only 2% of patients discontinued trial treatment. Despite only modest benefit compared to that of immune checkpoint inhibitor therapy for cutaneous melanoma, Tebentafusp pioneered multiple firsts and became not only the first FDA treatment approved for metastatic uveal melanoma but also the first T-cell engager to demonstrate overall survival benefit in any solid tumor.

Part 2b: Resectable Melanoma

Adjuvant Immunotherapy in Resectable Melanoma

Once a primary melanoma has been resected, the risk for recurrence depends on the site of the primary tumor, the depth of invasion, and the presence or absence of regional lymph node metastasis. For a thin cutaneous melanoma with no lymph node metastasis, the risk for distant melanoma metastasis is minimal, and no systemic therapy is recommended. However, for non-cutaneous melanomas, thick primary cutaneous melanomas, and melanomas with lymph node metastasis, the risk for recurrence after definitive surgery is relatively high.

Patients with high-risk resectable cutaneous melanoma, defined as those with stage IIB to stage IIID melanoma, have also shown significant improvements in both progression-free and overall survival with immunotherapy. Patients with stage

IIB and stage IIC melanoma have thick and/or ulcerated melanomas, while patients with stage III disease have lymph node involvement. At these stages, the primary cutaneous tumors and their lymph node metastases can often be surgically resected with a margin of healthy tissue which ideally helps to eradicate any microscopic cancerous cells in the surrounding tissue and prevent further spread of the melanoma. However, there may still be some cancerous cells outside this area that go undetected, allowing for future tumor growth and metastasis. Systemic therapies are given in the postoperative or adjuvant setting in an attempt to kill these remaining cells and decrease the rates of tumor recurrence and metastasis.

Prior to the approval of the first immune checkpoint inhibitor, the standard of care for patients with high-risk resectable cutaneous melanoma was adjuvant interferon alfa. Interferons are proteins produced naturally by the body in response to several pathogens, most notably viruses. Interferon alpha (IFNγ) is secreted by leukocytes of the innate immune system and stimulates a number of host immune functions, including increased expression of MHC class I molecules (Schiavoni et al., 2013), increased T-cell co-stimulation, (Snell et al., 2017) and direct impairment of tumor cell growth (Balmer, 1985). A 2017 meta-analysis combining results from trials testing several different forms and dosing schedules of interferon alpha showed that the use of adjuvant interferon alpha was associated with only marginal improvement in event-free survival and overall survival. The absolute 10-year event-free survival benefit was 2.5% with an overall survival benefit of 2.6% (Ives et al., 2017). The use of adjuvant interferon was also associated with considerable toxicity in a majority of patients including fatigue, depression, liver test abnormalities, pyrexia, headache, and myalgia. The success of immune checkpoint therapy in unresectable melanoma paved the way for immunotherapy to replace interferon therapy for patients with high-risk resectable melanoma.

It is important to note that the initial adjuvant trials for stage III melanoma were undertaken before the January 1, 2018, implementation of the American Joint Committee on Cancer (AJCC) eighth edition staging guidelines. Both the seventh and eighth edition staging systems classified patients with any nodal disease but no distant metastatic spread as stage III. However, in the seventh edition guidelines, stage IIIA melanomas included patients with T1–T4a melanomas, but the eighth edition limited stage IIIA disease to patients with T1–T2a tumors. This is key as some patients who had deep tumors but only micrometastatic foci in their lymph nodes (<1 mm) and were therefore staged at IIIA per the seventh AJCC guidelines were excluded from the initial adjuvant clinical trials. Some of these patients would now be classified as stage IIIB due to the size of their tumor (Gershenwald et al., 2017).

Ipilimumab

Given the success of adjuvant ipilimumab in the metastatic setting, investigators queried whether ipilimumab could provide benefit to patients with resected stage III melanoma. To that end, a trial was conducted comparing adjuvant ipilimumab dosed at 10 mg/kg with a placebo in patients with resected stage III cutaneous melanoma (with the caveat that for patients with stage IIIA melanoma which included T1-T4a, the metastatic nodal focus must be greater than 1 mm in maximal diameter) (Eggermont et al., 2015). Adjuvant ipilimumab was associated with improved recurrence-free survival (HR 0.75, median RFS 26.1 months vs. 17.1 months) and was approved by the FDA in 2015 on this basis. It was later demonstrated that ipilimumab was also associated with an improvement in overall survival when compared with placebo (HR 0.72, 5-year OS 65.4% vs. 54.4%) (Eggermont et al., 2016). A trial directly comparing ipilimumab at 3 mg/kg and the previous standard of care of high-dose IFNγ demonstrated a statistically significant 5 year overall survival benefit with ipilimumab compared to high-dose IFNγ (HR 0.78; OS 72% vs. 67%) with a significantly lower rate of grade 3 and 4 adverse events (38.6% vs. 78.8%) (Tarhini et al., 2020).

Pembrolizumab and Nivolumab

The development of the PD-1 checkpoint inhibitors, pembrolizumab and nivolumab, further revolutionized the standard of care for patients not only with unresectable melanoma as noted previously but also as an adjuvant therapy for those with high-risk resectable melanoma. Checkmate 238 was a phase III randomized clinical trial that enrolled 906 patients across 130 academic centers in 25 countries (https://www. thelancet.com/article/S1470-2045(20)30494-0/fulltext). Patients with resected stage IIIB-C or resected oligometastatic stage IV melanoma were randomized 1:1 to receive nivolumab 3 mg/kg every 2 weeks or ipilimumab 10 mg/kg every 3 weeks for 4 doses and then every 12 weeks for up to 1 year of treatment. The 4 year recurrence-free survival was statistically significant at 51.7% in the nivolumab group versus 41.2% in the ipilimumab group. The 4 year overall survival was not statistically significant between the two groups at 77.9% for nivolumab and 76.6% for ipilimumab. However, given the improved RFS with better tolerability of nivolumab compared to ipilimumab, single-agent nivolumab and not ipilimumab is now recommended as first-line adjuvant therapy for patients with stage IIIB or IIIC melanoma.

Pembrolizumab was then successfully trialed in the adjuvant setting for patients with stage III melanoma. The landmark KEYNOTE-054 trial was conducted at 123 academic centers and community hospitals across 23 countries. The trial randomized patients 1:1 with resected stage III cutaneous melanoma with metastatic nodal focus >1 mm and without in-transit metastasis to receive either pembrolizumab 200 mg or placebo every 3 weeks for up to 18 doses. At the initial time of follow-up at 42 months, the distant metastasis-free survival was significantly longer in the pembrolizumab group than in the placebo group (HR 0.60; 65.3% vs. 49.4%) with the benefit similar between patients with PD-L1-positive and PD-L1-negative tumor marker status (Eggermont et al., 2021). At 5 years, the distant metastasis-free survival was still significantly improved over placebo (HR 0.62; 60.6% vs. 44.5%) as was recurrence-free survival (HR 0.61; 55.4% vs. 38.3%) (https://evidence.nejm.

org/doi/full/10.1056/EVIDoa2200214). Pembrolizumab was therefore approved by the FDA for use in patients with resected stage III melanoma regardless of PD-L1 tumor status in 2019.

Attention was then turned to patients that have high-risk disease but do not have evidence of lymph node involvement at time of sentinel lymph node biopsy, patients with stage IIB and stage IIC cutaneous melanoma. Patients with stage IIB-C cutaneous melanomas with deep or ulcerated tumors at T3b-T4b actually have a higher risk of recurrence than patients with stage IIIA disease who have micrometastases to the lymph nodes but have shallower T1a-T2a tumors which ultimately led to a change in the AJCC staging system for melanoma as noted above (Yushak et al., 2019).

Pembrolizumab became the first immunotherapy to be approved for patients with stage II melanoma in the adjuvant setting. In the KEYNOTE-716 phase III trial, patients aged 12 years and older with stage IIB or IIC melanoma were randomized 1:1 to receive either pembrolizumab at a fixed dose of 200 mg in adults (or 2 mg/kg in pediatric patients) or placebo every 3 weeks for up to 17 cycles. At 21 months, 15% of patients in the pembrolizumab compared with 24% of patients in the placebo group had a first recurrence or died which was a statistically significant improvement (https://www.thelancet.com/journals/lancet/article/PIIS0140-6736(22)00562-1/fulltext). Median recurrence-free survival was not met in either group. However, this still led to the FDA approval of pembrolizumab for patients with stage IIB and stage IIC melanoma in 2021.

Nivolumab is currently undergoing review by the FDA for potential approval for treatment of patients with completely resected stage IIB or IIC melanoma. The phase III CheckMate 76K trial randomly assigned patients 1:1 to receive either 480 mg of nivolumab or placebo every 4 weeks for up to 12 months. The 12-month recurrence-free survival rates were statistically significant compared to placebo for patients with stage IIB disease (93% vs. 84%) and stage IIC disease (84% vs. 72%) (https://www.thelancet.com/journals/lanonc/article/PIIS1470-2045(22)00559-9/fulltext). Toxicities were similar to those previously observed with grade 3 and 4 adverse events in 10% of patients receiving nivolumab and 2% patients receiving placebo.

Of note, while we see benefit of using dual immune checkpoint therapy known as "ICI doublet" therapy in the metastatic setting, this has not yet been proven to be beneficial in patients with high-risk resectable melanoma. The phase III trial CheckMate 915 enrolled 1844 patients and compared nivolumab monotherapy to ipilimumab-nivolumab combination therapy in patients with completely resected stage III and IV diseases. ICI doublet therapy did not show a statistically significant benefit over ICI monotherapy in a 2 year recurrence-free survival (Weber et al., 2023).

Neoadjuvant Immunotherapy in Resectable Melanoma

In certain solid tumors responsive to cytotoxic chemotherapy, chemotherapy before surgery, known as neoadjuvant therapy, has shown multiple benefits. Neoadjuvant therapy is typically given to reduce tumor burden to help facilitate surgical resection as well as eradicate micrometastases. Patients also often have a better performance status prior to surgery and are able to withstand higher doses of chemotherapy with fewer dose reductions and interruptions in treatment. These principles apply to neo-adjuvant immunotherapy as well, but there are also some unique advantages to giving immunotherapies in the neoadjuvant setting. By giving immunotherapy before surgery when tumors are intact, it allows for the immune system to be activated against a broader array of antigens and enhance tumor-antigen presentation in the lymph nodes (Bilusic & Gulley, 2021). It also avoids the negative effects of surgery-mediated immunosuppression seen in the postoperative period when adjuvant therapies are given. While neoadjuvant immunotherapy is standard of care for certain lung and breast cancers, there have been no completed phase III trials for neoadjuvant immunotherapy in patients with melanoma. We will however discuss the results of some promising phase II studies below.

Pembrolizumab

Neoadjuvant pembrolizumab was studied in the phase II SWOG S1801 study. A total of 159 patients with resectable clinically stage IIIB–IV melanomas were randomized 1:1 to receive either 3 doses of neoadjuvant pembrolizumab at 200 mg before surgery followed by an additional 15 doses or adjuvant pembrolizumab at 200 mg for 18 doses. At 14.7 months, patients who received neoadjuvant pembrolizumab had a significantly improved event-free survival (EFS) compared to those in the adjuvant arm (HR 0.58; 72% vs. 49%) with similar incidence of treatment-related adverse events between the groups (Patel et al., 2023). While no phase III data is available yet, these results are significant, and the current NCCN guidelines now include a recommendation to consider neoadjuvant therapy as part of a clinical trial for patients who have clinically stage III melanoma versus considering therapeutic lymph node dissection.

Ipilimumab-Nivolumab

The two initial phase I clinical trials of dual ICI therapy in the neoadjuvant study were associated with high rates of toxicity. The phase IB OpACIN study randomized 20 patients 1:1 to receive either 6 weeks of adjuvant therapy with ipilimumab 3 mg/kg plus nivolumab 1mk/kg or 6 weeks of neoadjuvant therapy plus 6 weeks of adjuvant therapy with ipilimumab 3 mg/kg and nivolumab 1 mg/kg. In each arm, nine of the ten patients experienced a grade 3 or 4 toxicity (Blank et al., 2018). However, at 4 years, nine of the ten patients in the neoadjuvant arm and seven of the ten patients in the adjuvant arm were still alive (Rozeman et al., 2021).

This led to the follow-up phase IIb trial, OpACIN-neo, to try and determine an optimal dosing regimen that would decrease toxicity without sacrificing effectiveness. A total of 86 patients with macroscopic stage III melanoma were randomized to one of three treatment arms with the regimens, and results are listed in Table 8.4.

Table 8.4 Summary of dosing schedule, adverse events, and results from the phase IIb OpACIN-neo trial

Group	Dosing schedule	Grade 3/grade 4 adverse events after 12 weeks	Radiographic response rate	Pathologic response rate
A	Ipilimumab 3 mg/kg + nivolumab 1 mg/kg every 3 weeks for two cycles	12/30 (40%)	19/30 (63%)	24/30 (80%)
B	Ipilimumab 1 mg/kg + nivolumab 3 mg/kg every 3 weeks for two cycles	6/30 (20%)	17/30 (57%)	23/30 (77%)
C	Ipilimumab 3 mg/kg every 3 weeks for 2 cycles and then nivolumab 3 mg/kg every 3 weeks for two cycles	13/26 (50%)	9/26 (35%)	17/26 (65%)

Overall, these results indicated that the two cycles of ipilimumab 1 mg/kg plus nivolumab 3 mg/kg provided the most benefit with the fewest grade 3 and 4 adverse events (Rozeman et al., 2019).

Nivolumab-Relatlimab

Investigators have also done some early work in evaluating the doublet ICI regimen nivolumab-relatlimab in the neoadjuvant setting for patients with resectable stage III or IV melanoma. This regimen has been previously shown to improve progression-free survival over nivolumab monotherapy in patients with unresectable melanoma (Tawbi et al., 2022). Relatlimab inhibits the immune checkpoint LAG-3 which is distinct from the PD-1 checkpoint inhibitor, nivolumab, but both help prevent T-cell exhaustion. A total of 30 patients were enrolled at two centers and received two neoadjuvant doses of nivolumab 480 mg and relatlimab 160 mg every 4 weeks for two doses and then proceeded to surgery. After surgery, they completed an additional ten doses of treatment. Twenty-nine of the thirty patients proceeded to surgery. The primary end point was pathologic complete response (pCR) rate. The combination resulted in a 57% pCR rate and 70% overall pathologic response rate (Amaria et al., 2022). The 2 year recurrence-free survival rate was 92% for patients with any pathologic response compared to 55% for patients who did not have a pathologic response.

Unanswered Questions

Many unanswered questions remain. These neoadjuvant regimens have not been compared head to head in the neoadjuvant setting nor have there been any phase III clinical trials comparing neoadjuvant to adjuvant immunotherapy. Therefore, the efficacy, broad applicability, and optimal first-line regimen, and dosing schedule is not known. It is also important to remember that neoadjuvant therapy delays definitive surgery in patients who may be cured with surgery alone and there is as of yet no model to predict which patients will respond to and benefit from immunotherapy. This delay in potentially curable surgery also comes with the possibility the tumor may progress and become inoperable during the neoadjuvant treatment period. The rates of grade 3 and 4 adverse events were also high in the phase I and II trials as well which is especially notable for patients who may have otherwise been cured.

Additional questions to consider include if patients do have a pathologic response to neoadjuvant therapy in the index lymph node, can this be used to tailor further therapy? If an index node subsequently shows a complete pathologic response rate, can a therapeutic lymph node dissection and its associated morbidities be avoided? These are just some of the many questions that remain to be answered.

Summary

In summary, perhaps no other solid organ cancer setting has experienced a more dramatic clinical impact from immunotherapy than that of melanoma. While there is a long-standing history of the use of high-dose interleukin 2 and tumor-infiltrating lymphocytes in metastatic melanoma patients, the advent of immune checkpoint-inhibiting monoclonal antibodies has allowed immunotherapy to emerge as a standard of care for first-line therapy for both resectable and unresectable melanomas. Whereas prior to the advent of immune checkpoint inhibitor therapy, the median overall survival of patients with metastatic melanoma was 6.2 months (Korn et al., 2008); many current clinical trials in metastatic melanoma demonstrate median survivals in excess of 2 years. While other drugs (viz., small molecule inhibitors of BRAF and MEK) have undoubtedly contributed to this increase in patients with BRAF-mutated melanoma, immunotherapies have been responsible for the majority of this improvement in clinical outcomes.

Part 3: New Treatments on the Horizon

There are additional promising new immunotherapies on the horizon with potential for further impact on survival rates for patients with advanced melanoma. These include other immune checkpoint inhibitors, immunostimulatory monoclonal antibodies, vaccines, oncolytic viruses, and small molecule inhibitors of proteins involved in modulating the nature of the immune response, as well as combinations of the above and combinations of immunotherapies with other treatments. It is beyond the scope of this book to discuss all of the ongoing clinical research efforts in the field of melanoma immunotherapy. However, we will discuss a few of the most promising therapies currently undergoing clinical testing.

TIL Therapy

Another type of immunotherapy that has been utilized in patients long before immune checkpoint therapy is adoptive cell therapy (ACT). In ACT, a patient's immune cells are removed, manipulated in the lab, and then infused back into the patient. Tumor-infiltrating lymphocyte (TIL) therapy and chimeric antigen receptor T-cell (CAR-T) therapy are both forms of adoptive cell therapy. In TIL therapy, lymphocytes are harvested from a patient's surgically resected tumor and expanded in the laboratory. Patients then receive chemotherapy to eradicate their existing lymphocyte population before the expanded tumor-specific lymphocytes are infused back into the patient. In order to allow the newly infused cells to persist in a more durable fashion, patients are then given the growth factor IL-2.

The first studies of TIL therapies in melanoma were published over 30 years ago. In 1988, the National Cancer Institute (NCI) published a study describing the response of a 20 patient cohort to TIL therapy. The patients were given a single dose of intravenous cyclophosphamide followed by transfer of TILs and administration of IL-2. The overall response rate was 55% (Rosenberg et al., 1988).

Over the past three decades, the therapy has been continually fine-tuned and expanded. Initially, while the therapy had a high overall response rate, it was also associated with a large number of adverse effects and was time, labor, and cost intensive. Only a few academic medical centers had the technology and expertise to harvest and expand the TILs in the laboratory, and it was given to only a small number of patients, often in the intensive care unit.

However, in 2022, the first phase III, multicenter, open-label trial was completed. In the trial, 168 patients with stage IIIC or IV melanoma refractory to PD-1 therapy were randomly assigned 1:1 to receive TIL therapy or the CTLA-4 immune checkpoint inhibitor, ipilimumab. In the intention to treat population, the median PFS was 7.2 months in the TIL group and 3.1 months in the ipilimumab group (Rohaan et al., 2022). Median overall survival was 25.8 months in the TIL group and 18.9 months in the ipilimumab group. Of the patients who received TIL therapy, 100% experienced at least one grade 3 or higher adverse event while in the ipilimumab group the rate was 57%. In the TIL group, 30% of patients experienced capillary leak syndrome secondary to IL-2. The toxicity in the group who received IL-2 was expected based on the initial trials using high-dose IL-2 monotherapy, but unlike IL-2 monotherapy where the response rate was just 14.9%, the response rate with the addition of IL-2 to TILs was 49%.

The subsequent SITC C-144-01 multicohort phase II trial studied the TIL therapy, Lifileucel. The trial pooled results from multiple consecutive patient cohorts totaling 153 patients with metastatic melanoma refractory to ICI therapy (and BRAF/MEK therapy if BRAF V600 mutation is positive) and who had received a median of 3.0 lines of prior therapies. The overall response rate was 31.4% with 8 complete responses and 40 partial responses. At greater than 18 months of follow-up, 41.7% of responses were maintained (Chesney et al., 2022). Medial overall survival was 13.9 months. Based on these results, Lifileucel is currently enrolling for a phase III clinical trial and is awaiting expedited approval for its biologics license application which was submitted to the FDA in March 2023.

Vaccines

Cancer vaccines have long been studied with the hope that they would induce an effective immune response against a tumor. However, these efforts have been met with two major challenges (D'Alise & Scarselli, 2023). The first challenge is the immune suppressive environment created by the tumor as described in Part 1 of this chapter. The second is the selection of the cancer antigens used in the vaccines. The first attempted cancer vaccines used shared tumor-associated antigens (TAAs), which are self-antigens overexpressed on tumors but are not tumor specific. Vaccines targeting these antigens were not successful due to immune tolerance of these self-antigens and often led to vaccine-induced autoimmune toxicities. The advent of next-generation sequencing made possible the identification of neoantigens which revolutionized the field of cancer vaccines.

Neoantigens are comprised of mutated proteins unique to each tumor and expressed in tumor cells only (Overwijk et al., 2013). Melanomas harbor a relatively high number of non-synonymous mutations and have, on average, the highest number of neoantigens of any tumor type (Schumacher & Schreiber, 2015). Advances in bioinformatics have allowed for the identification of neoantigens with the highest probability of inducing a T-cell response and therefore the best candidates for vaccines.

There are several different types of neoantigen vaccines that have been studied including those that make use of dendritic cells, viral vectors, mRNA, and long peptides. Platforms that allow for the use of multiple neoantigens are being developed, as it is estimated that only about 1–2% of neoantigens spontaneously elicit T-cell responses (Karpanen & Olweus, 2017). To date, melanoma vaccines are still largely being evaluated in phase I trials with one phase II trial currently recruiting. However, there are several promising vaccine candidates.

NeoVax is a neoantigen-long peptide vaccine that was studied in six patients with high-risk surgically resected melanoma. The vaccine targeted approximately 20 neoantigens per patient (Ott et al., 2017). At median follow-up of 25 months, the four patients with stage IIIB/stage C melanoma remained free of disease. The two patients with stage IV disease (due to lung metastases) both had progression noted on their first restaging scans after their last vaccination. However, both patients were then treated with pembrolizumab, and both achieved complete radiographic response after 4 months and also remain disease free. At median follow-up of 55 months after initial surgical resection, all six patients were still alive (Hu et al., 2021).

Many of the current early phase clinical trials are combining vaccines with immune checkpoint inhibitors. Vaccines work to enhance the activation and infiltration of immune cells into the tumor microenvironment. However, tumors also express molecules that quickly lead to T-cell exhaustion. By combining immune checkpoint inhibitor therapy which works to reinvigorate T-cells with vaccines, these therapies can work synergistically to enhance the anti-tumor response (Oladejo et al., 2023).

There are currently multiple phase I and II studies underway to study mRNA vaccines, most of which are being done in combination with immune checkpoint inhibitors. The largest of these is the phase IIb trial, KEYNOTE-942. The trial randomized patients 2:1 with resected stage IIIB-IV melanoma to receive either an intramuscular mRNA vaccine with up to 34 personalized neoantigens in combination with pembrolizumab or pembrolizumab alone. In data presented at the American Association for Cancer Research Annual Meeting in April 2023, at 2 years, disease recurrence or death occurred in 22.4% of patients receiving the vaccine and pembrolizumab and 40% of those receiving pembrolizumab monotherapy. Notably, the combination therapy was well tolerated compared with some other immunotherapies with grade 3 adverse events occurring in 25% of patients receiving the vaccine.

Khattak A, Carlino M, Meniawy T et al. A personalized cancer vaccine, mRNA-4157, combined with pembrolizumab versus pembrolizumab in patients with resected high-risk melanoma: efficacy and safety results from the randomized, open-label phase II mRNA-4157-P201/Keynote-942 trial. Abstract presented at the American Association for Cancer Research Annual Meeting; April 14–19, 2023; Orlando, FL. Abstract CT001.

TIGIT

A new immune checkpoint inhibitor therapy that has demonstrated mixed benefit in non-small-cell lung cancer (NSCLC) is being evaluated for a potential role in the treatment of melanoma and many other solid tumors. T-cell immunoreceptor with immunoglobulin (Ig) and immunoreceptor tyrosine-based inhibitory motif domains (TIGIT) is a co-inhibitory receptor in the immunoglobulin superfamily that inhibits both innate and adaptive immunities through the inhibition of T-cells and NK cells and by enhancing the immunosuppression effects of Tregs (Tang et al., 2023).

In the phase II CITYSCAPE trial, 135 patients with recurrent or metastatic NSCLC with tumors positive for PD-L1 at >1% were randomized 1:1 to receive the anti-TIGIT antibody tiragolumab plus anti-PD-1 therapy, atezolizumab, or atezolizumab alone. After a median follow-up of 5.9 months, median progression-free survival was 5.4 months in the combination group versus 3.6 months in the monotherapy group (Cho et al., 2022). Rates of grade 3 or worse treatment-related adverse events were similar between the groups. TIGIT is currently being trialed in five phase III trials in patients with NSCLC.

The TIGIT inhibitor, vibostolimab, is also being studied in a phase III trial in patients with stage IIB–IV melanoma. The KEYVIBE-010 trial started enrolling patients in January 2023 and will be randomizing patients 1:1 to receive either adjuvant vibostolimab plus pembrolizumab or pembrolizumab monotherapy (NCT05665595) with the primary endpoint of recurrence-free survival.

Summary

In summary, melanomas tend to be quite immunogenic but employ many mechanisms to evade or subvert anti-melanoma immune responses. At present, immunotherapy is considered a standard of care as adjuvant or neoadjuvant therapy for patients with resected stage IIB–IV melanoma. For most patients with overt metastatic melanoma, combination immune checkpoint inhibitor therapy, typically with antibodies to PD-1 and either CTLA-4 or LAG3, is the preferred first-line approach. Additional immunotherapies are being studied in ongoing clinical research, and it is likely that there will be additional immunotherapy options for melanoma in the near future.

References

Amaria, R. N., Postow, M., Burton, E. M., et al. (2022). Neoadjuvant relatlimab and nivolumab in resectable melanoma. *Nature, 611*(7934), 155–160. https://doi.org/10.1038/s41586-022-05368-8

Andtbacka, R. H., Kaufman, H. L., Collichio, F., et al. (2015). Talimogene laherparepvec improves durable response rate in patients with advanced melanoma. *Journal of Clinical Oncology, 33*(25), 2780–2788. https://doi.org/10.1200/JCO.2014.58.3377

Baker, H. W. (1964). Spontaneous regression of malignant melanoma. *The American Surgeon, 30*, 825–829.

Bakker, A. B., Schreurs, M. W., de Boer, A. J., et al. (1994). Melanocyte lineage-specific antigen gp100 is recognized by melanoma-derived tumor-infiltrating lymphocytes. *Journal of Experimental Medicine, 179*(3), 1005–1009.

Balmer, C. M. (1985). The new alpha interferons. *Drug Intelligence & Clinical Pharmacy, 19*(12), 887–893.

Bilusic, M., & Gulley, J. L. (2021). Neoadjuvant immunotherapy: An evolving paradigm shift? *Journal of the National Cancer Institute, 113*(7), 799–800. https://doi.org/10.1093/jnci/djaa217

Blank, C. U., Rozeman, E. A., Fanchi, L. F., et al. (2018). Neoadjuvant versus adjuvant ipilimumab plus nivolumab in macroscopic stage III melanoma. *Nature Medicine, 24*(11), 1655–1661. https://doi.org/10.1038/s41591-018-0198-0

Brichard, V., Van Pel, A., Wolfel, T., et al. (1993). The tyrosinase gene codes for an antigen recognized by autologous cytolytic T lymphocytes on HLA-A2 melanomas. *The Journal of Experimental Medicine, 178*(2), 489–495.

Bystryn, J. C. (1989). Immune mechanisms in vitiligo. *Immunology Series, 46*, 447–473.

Carvajal, R. D., Nathan, P., Sacco, J. J., et al. (2022). Phase I study of safety, tolerability, and efficacy of tebentafusp using a step-up dosing regimen and expansion in patients with metastatic uveal melanoma. *Journal of Clinical Oncology, 40*(17), 1939–1948. https://doi.org/10.1200/JCO.21.01805

Chavan, R., Salvador, D., Gustafson, M. P., Dietz, A. B., Nevala, W., & Markovic, S. N. (2014). Untreated stage IV melanoma patients exhibit abnormal monocyte phenotypes and decreased functional capacity. *Cancer Immunology Research, 2*(3), 241–248. https://doi. org/10.1158/2326-6066.CIR-13-0094

Chesney, J., Lewis, K. D., Kluger, H., et al. (2022). Efficacy and safety of lifileucel, a one-time autologous tumor-infiltrating lymphocyte (TIL) cell therapy, in patients with advanced melanoma after progression on immune checkpoint inhibitors and targeted therapies: Pooled analysis of consecutive cohorts of the C-144-01 study. *Journal for Immunotherapy of Cancer, 10*(12). https://doi.org/10.1136/jitc-2022-005755

Chesney, J. A., Ribas, A., Long, G. V., et al. (2023). Randomized, double-blind, placebo-controlled, global phase III trial of talimogene laherparepvec combined with pembrolizumab for advanced melanoma. *Journal of Clinical Oncology, 41*(3), 528–540. https://doi. org/10.1200/JCO.22.00343

Chikuma, S. (2017). CTLA-4, an essential immune-checkpoint for T-cell activation. *Current Topics in Microbiology and Immunology, 410*, 99–126.

Cho, B. C., Abreu, D. R., Hussein, M., et al. (2022). Tiragolumab plus atezolizumab versus placebo plus atezolizumab as a first-line treatment for PD-L1-selected non-small-cell lung cancer (CITYSCAPE): Primary and follow-up analyses of a randomised, double-blind, phase 2 study. *The Lancet Oncology, 23*(6), 781–792. https://doi.org/10.1016/S1470-2045(22)00226-1

Chomez, P., De Backer, O., Bertrand, M., De Plaen, E., Boon, T., & Lucas, S. (2001). An overview of the MAGE gene family with the identification of all human members of the family. *Cancer Research, 61*(14), 5544–5551.

Clark, W. H., Jr., From, L., Bernardino, E. A., & Mihm, M. C. (1969). The histogenesis and biologic behavior of primary human malignant melanomas of the skin. *Cancer Research, 29*(3), 705–727.

D'Alise, A. M., & Scarselli, E. (2023). Getting personal in metastatic melanoma: Neoantigen-based vaccines as a new therapeutic strategy. *Current Opinion in Oncology, 35*(2), 94–99. https://doi.org/10.1097/CCO.0000000000000923

Darvin, P., Toor, S. M., Nair, V. S., & Elkord, E. (2018). Immune checkpoint inhibitors: Recent progress and potential biomarkers. *Experimental & Molecular Medicine, 50*(12), 165.

Dong, H., & Chen, L. (2003). B7-H1 pathway and its role in the evasion of tumor immunity. *Journal of Molecular Medicine (Berlin, Germany), 81*(5), 281–287. https://doi.org/10.1007/s00109-003-0430-2

Dong, H., Strome, S. E., Salomao, D. R., et al. (2002). Tumor-associated B7-H1 promotes T-cell apoptosis: A potential mechanism of immune evasion. *Nature Medicine, 8*(8), 793–800. https://doi.org/10.1038/nm730

Dousset, L., Poizeau, F., Robert, C., Mansard, S., Mortier, L., & Caumont, C. (2021). Positive association between location of melanoma, ultraviolet signature, tumor mutational burden, and response to anti-PD-1 therapy. *JCO Precision Oncologia, 5*. https://doi.org/10.1200/PO.21.00084

Eggermont, A. M., Chiarion-Sileni, V., Grob, J. J., et al. (2015). Adjuvant ipilimumab versus placebo after complete resection of high-risk stage III melanoma (EORTC 18071): A randomised, double-blind, phase 3 trial. *The Lancet Oncology, 16*(5), 522–530. https://doi.org/10.1016/S1470-2045(15)70122-1

Eggermont, A. M., Chiarion-Sileni, V., Grob, J. J., et al. (2016). Prolonged survival in stage III melanoma with ipilimumab adjuvant therapy. *The New England Journal of Medicine, 375*(19), 1845–1855. https://doi.org/10.1056/NEJMoa1611299

Eggermont, A. M. M., Blank, C. U., Mandala, M., et al. (2021). Adjuvant pembrolizumab versus placebo in resected stage III melanoma (EORTC 1325-MG/KEYNOTE-054): Distant metastasis-free survival results from a double-blind, randomised, controlled, phase 3 trial. *The Lancet Oncology, 22*(5), 643–654. https://doi.org/10.1016/S1470-2045(21)00065-6

Enninga, E. A., Nevala, W. K., Holtan, S. G., Leontovich, A. A., & Markovic, S. N. (2016). Galectin-9 modulates immunity by promoting Th2/M2 differentiation and impacts survival in patients with metastatic melanoma. *Melanoma Research, 26*(5), 429–441. https://doi. org/10.1097/CMR.0000000000000281

Everson, T. C. (1967). Spontaneous regression of cancer. *Progress in Clinical Cancer, 3*, 79–95.

Ferrone, S., & Marincola, F. M. (1995). Loss of HLA class I antigens by melanoma cells: Molecular mechanisms, functional significance and clinical relevance. *Immunology Today, 16*(10), 487–494.

Gajewski, T. F., Fuertes, M. B., & Woo, S. R. (2012). Innate immune sensing of cancer: Clues from an identified role for type I IFNs. *Cancer Immunology, Immunotherapy, 61*(8), 1343–1347. https://doi.org/10.1007/s00262-012-1305-6

Gershenwald, J. E., Scolyer, R. A., Hess, K. R., et al. (2017). Melanoma staging: Evidence-based changes in the American joint committee on cancer eighth edition cancer staging manual. *CA: a Cancer Journal for Clinicians, 67*(6), 472–492. https://doi.org/10.3322/caac.21409

Graydon, C. G., Mohideen, S., & Fowke, K. (2020). LAG3's enigmatic mechanism of action. *Frontiers in Immunology, 11*, 615317.

Grotz, T. E., Jakub, J. W., Mansfield, A. S., et al. (2015). Evidence of Th2 polarization of the sentinel lymph node (SLN) in melanoma. *Oncoimmunology, 4*(8), e1026504. https://doi.org/10.1080/2162402X.2015.1026504

Hamid, O., Robert, C., Daud, A., et al. (2013). Safety and tumor responses with lambrolizumab (anti-PD-1) in melanoma. *The New England Journal of Medicine, 369*(2), 134–144. https://doi.org/10.1056/NEJMoa1305133

Harlin, H., Meng, Y., Peterson, A. C., et al. (2009). Chemokine expression in melanoma metastases associated with CD8+ T-cell recruitment. *Cancer Research, 69*(7), 3077–3085. https://doi.org/10.1158/0008-5472.CAN-08-2281

Hodi, F. S., O'Day, S. J., McDermott, D. F., et al. (2010). Improved survival with ipilimumab in patients with metastatic melanoma. *The New England Journal of Medicine, 363*(8), 711–723. https://doi.org/10.1056/NEJMoa1003466

Hu, Z., Leet, D. E., Allesoe, R. L., et al. (2021). Personal neoantigen vaccines induce persistent memory T cell responses and epitope spreading in patients with melanoma. *Nature Medicine, 27*(3), 515–525. https://doi.org/10.1038/s41591-020-01206-4

Ikeda, H., Lethe, B., Lehmann, F., et al. (1997). Characterization of an antigen that is recognized on a melanoma showing partial HLA loss by CTL expressing an NK inhibitory receptor. *Immunity, 6*(2), 199–208.

Itoh, K., Platsoucas, C. D., & Balch, C. M. (1988). Autologous tumor-specific cytotoxic T lymphocytes in the infiltrate of human metastatic melanomas. Activation by interleukin 2 and autologous tumor cells, and involvement of the T cell receptor. *The Journal of Experimental Medicine, 168*(4), 1419–1441.

Ives, N. J., Suciu, S., Eggermont, A. M. M., et al. (2017). Adjuvant interferon-alpha for the treatment of high-risk melanoma: An individual patient data meta-analysis. *European Journal of Cancer, 82*, 171–183. https://doi.org/10.1016/j.ejca.2017.06.006

Jiang, X., Zhou, J., Giobbie-Hurder, A., Wargo, J., & Hodi, F. S. (2013). The activation of MAPK in melanoma cells resistant to BRAF inhibition promotes PD-L1 expression that is reversible by MEK and PI3K inhibition. *Clinical Cancer Research, 19*(3), 598–609. https://doi.org/10.1158/1078-0432.CCR-12-2731

Karpanen, T., & Olweus, J. (2017). The potential of donor T-cell repertoires in neoantigen-targeted cancer immunotherapy. *Frontiers in Immunology, 8*, 1718. https://doi.org/10.3389/fimmu.2017.01718

Kawakami, Y., Eliyahu, S., Sakaguchi, K., et al. (1994). Identification of the immunodominant peptides of the MART-1 human melanoma antigen recognized by the majority of HLA-A2-restricted tumor infiltrating lymphocytes. *The Journal of Experimental Medicine, 180*(1), 347–352.

Keilholz, U., Conradt, C., Legha, S. S., et al. (1998). Results of interleukin-2-based treatment in advanced melanoma: A case record-based analysis of 631 patients. *Journal of Clinical Oncology, 16*(9), 2921–2929. https://doi.org/10.1200/JCO.1998.16.9.2921

Korn, E. L., Liu, P. Y., Lee, S. J., et al. (2008). Meta-analysis of phase II cooperative group trials in metastatic stage IV melanoma to determine progression-free and overall survival benchmarks for future phase II trials. *J Clin Oncol, 26*(4), 527–534. https://doi.org/10.1200/JCO.2007.12.7837

Larkin, J., Chiarion-Sileni, V., Gonzalez, R., et al. (2015). Combined nivolumab and ipilimumab or monotherapy in untreated melanoma. *The New England Journal of Medicine, 373*(1), 23–34. https://doi.org/10.1056/NEJMoa1504030

Leach, D. R., Krummel, M. F., & Allison, J. P. (1996). Enhancement of antitumor immunity by CTLA-4 blockade. *Science, 271*(5256), 1734–1736.

Mackensen, A., Carcelain, G., Viel, S., et al. (1994). Direct evidence to support the immunosurveillance concept in a human regressive melanoma. *The Journal of Clinical Investigation, 93*(4), 1397–1402. https://doi.org/10.1172/JCI117116

Maruhashi, T., Sugiura, D., Okazaki, I.-M., & Okazaki, T. (2020). LAG-3: From molecular functions to clinical applications. *Journal for ImmunoTherapy of Cancer, 8*, e001014.

Nathan, P., Hassel, J. C., Rutkowski, P., et al. (2021). Overall survival benefit with tebentafusp in metastatic uveal melanoma. *The New England Journal of Medicine, 385*(13), 1196–1206. https://doi.org/10.1056/NEJMoa2103485

Nathanson. (1976). Spontaneous regression of malignant melanoma: A review of the literature on incidence, clinical features, and possible mechanisms. *National Cancer Institute Monograph, 44*, 67–76.

Nevala, W. K., Vachon, C. M., Leontovich, A. A., et al. (2009). Evidence of systemic Th2-driven chronic inflammation in patients with metastatic melanoma. *Clin Cancer Res, 15*(6), 1931–1939. https://doi.org/10.1158/1078-0432.CCR-08-1980

Oladejo, M., Paulishak, W., & Wood, L. (2023). Synergistic potential of immune checkpoint inhibitors and therapeutic cancer vaccines. *Seminars in Cancer Biology, 88*, 81–95. https://doi.org/10.1016/j.semcancer.2022.12.003

Ott, P. A., Hu, Z., Keskin, D. B., et al. (2017). An immunogenic personal neoantigen vaccine for patients with melanoma. *Nature, 547*(7662), 217–221. https://doi.org/10.1038/nature22991

Overwijk, W. W., Wang, E., Marincola, F. M., Rammensee, H. G., & Restifo, N. P. (2013). Mining the mutanome: Developing highly personalized immunotherapies based on mutational analysis of tumors. *Journal for Immunotherapy of Cancer, 1*, 11. https://doi.org/10.1186/2051-1426-1-11

Patel, S. P., Othus, M., Chen, Y., et al. (2023). Neoadjuvant-adjuvant or adjuvant-only pembrolizumab in advanced melanoma. *The New England Journal of Medicine, 388*(9), 813–823. https://doi.org/10.1056/NEJMoa2211437

Poppema, S., Brocker, E. B., de Leij, L., et al. (1983). In situ analysis of the mononuclear cell infiltrate in primary malignant melanoma of the skin. *Clinical and Experimental Immunology, 51*(1), 77–82.

Robert, C., Thomas, L., Bondarenko, I., et al. (2011). Ipilimumab plus dacarbazine for previously untreated metastatic melanoma. *The New England Journal of Medicine, 364*(26), 2517–2526. https://doi.org/10.1056/NEJMoa1104621

Robert, C., Schachter, J., Long, G. V., et al. (2015a). Pembrolizumab versus Ipilimumab in Advanced Melanoma. *The New England Journal of Medicine, 372*(26), 2521–2532. https://doi.org/10.1056/NEJMoa1503093

Robert, C., Long, G. V., Brady, B., et al. (2015b). Nivolumab in previously untreated melanoma without BRAF mutation. *The New England Journal of Medicine, 372*(4), 320–330. https://doi.org/10.1056/NEJMoa1412082

Rohaan, M. W., Borch, T. H., van den Berg, J. H., et al. (2022). Tumor-infiltrating lymphocyte therapy or ipilimumab in advanced melanoma. *New England Journal of Medicine, 387*(23), 2113–2125. https://doi.org/10.1056/NEJMoa2210233

Rosenberg, S. A., Packard, B. S., Aebersold, P. M., et al. (1988). Use of tumor-infiltrating lymphocytes and interleukin-2 in the immunotherapy of patients with metastatic melanoma. *New England Journal of Medicine, 319*(25), 1676–1680. https://doi.org/10.1056/nejm198812223192527

Rowshanravan, B., Halliday, N., & Sansom, D. (2018). CTLA-4: A moving target in immunotherapy. *Blood, 131*(1), 58–67.

Rozeman, E. A., Menzies, A. M., van Akkooi, A. C. J., et al. (2019). Identification of the optimal combination dosing schedule of neoadjuvant ipilimumab plus nivolumab in macroscopic stage III melanoma (OpACIN-neo): A multicentre, phase 2, randomised, controlled trial. *The Lancet Oncology, 20*(7), 948–960. https://doi.org/10.1016/S1470-2045(19)30151-2

Rozeman, E. A., Hoefsmit, E. P., Reijers, I. L. M., et al. (2021). Survival and biomarker analyses from the OpACIN-neo and OpACIN neoadjuvant immunotherapy trials in stage III melanoma. *Nature Medicine, 27*(2), 256–263. https://doi.org/10.1038/s41591-020-01211-7

Schiavoni, G., Mattei, F., & Gabriele, L. (2013). Type I interferons as stimulators of DC-mediated cross-priming: Impact on anti-tumor response. *Frontiers in Immunology, 4*, 483. https://doi.org/10.3389/fimmu.2013.00483

Schmitz, M., Diestelkoetter, P., Weigle, B., et al. (2000). Generation of survivin-specific CD8+ T effector cells by dendritic cells pulsed with protein or selected peptides. *Cancer Research, 60*(17), 4845–4849.

Schumacher, T. N., & Schreiber, R. D. (2015). Neoantigens in cancer immunotherapy. *Science, 348*(6230), 69–74. https://doi.org/10.1126/science.aaa4971

Sensi, M., Salvi, S., Castelli, C., et al. (1993). T cell receptor (TCR) structure of autologous melanoma-reactive cytotoxic T lymphocyte (CTL) clones: Tumor-infiltrating lymphocytes overexpress in vivo the TCR beta chain sequence used by an HLA-A2-restricted and melanocyte-lineage-specific CTL clone. *The Journal of Experimental Medicine, 178*(4), 1231–1246.

Snell, L. M., McGaha, T. L., & Brooks, D. G. (2017). Type I interferon in chronic virus infection and cancer. *Trends in Immunology, 38*(8), 542–557. https://doi.org/10.1016/j.it.2017.05.005

Spranger, S., Spaapen, R. M., Zha, Y., et al. (2013). Up-regulation of PD-L1, IDO, and T(regs) in the melanoma tumor microenvironment is driven by CD8(+) T cells. *Science Translational Medicine, 5*(200), 200ra116. https://doi.org/10.1126/scitranslmed.3006504

Strohal, R., Marberger, K., Pehamberger, H., & Stingl, G. (1994). Immunohistological analysis of anti-melanoma host responses. *Archives of Dermatological Research, 287*(1), 28–35.

Tang, W., Chen, J., Ji, T., & Cong, X. (2023). TIGIT, a novel immune checkpoint therapy for melanoma. *Cell Death & Disease, 14*, 466. https://doi.org/10.1038/s41419-023-05961-3

Tarhini, A. A., Lee, S. J., Hodi, F. S., et al. (2020). Phase III study of adjuvant ipilimumab (3 or 10 mg/kg) versus high-dose interferon Alfa-2b for resected high-risk melanoma: North American intergroup E1609. *Journal of Clinical Oncology, 38*(6), 567–575. https://doi.org/10.1200/JCO.19.01381

Tawbi, H. A., Schadendorf, D., Lipson, E. J., et al. (2022). Relatlimab and nivolumab versus nivolumab in untreated advanced melanoma. *The New England Journal of Medicine, 386*(1), 24–34. https://doi.org/10.1056/NEJMoa2109970

Topalian, S. L., Solomon, D., & Rosenberg, S. A. (1989). Tumor-specific cytolysis by lymphocytes infiltrating human melanomas. *Journal of Immunology, 142*(10), 3714–3725.

van der Bruggen, P., Traversari, C., Chomez, P., et al. (1991). A gene encoding an antigen recognized by cytolytic T lymphocytes on a human melanoma. *Science, 254*(5038), 1643–1647.

Vonderheide, R. H., Hahn, W. C., Schultze, J. L., & Nadler, L. M. (1999). The telomerase catalytic subunit is a widely expressed tumor-associated antigen recognized by cytotoxic T lymphocytes. *Immunity, 10*(6), 673–679.

Weber, J. S., Schadendorf, D., Del Vecchio, M., et al. (2023). Adjuvant therapy of nivolumab combined with ipilimumab versus nivolumab alone in patients with resected stage IIIB-D or stage IV melanoma (CheckMate 915). *Journal of Clinical Oncology, 41*(3), 517–527. https://doi.org/10.1200/JCO.22.00533

Wen, J., Mao, X., Cheng, Q., Liu, Z., & Liu, F. (2021). A pan-cancer analysis revealing the role of TIGIG in tumor microenvironment. *Scientific Reports, 11*, 22502.

Yushak, M., Mehnert, J., Luke, J., & Poklepovic, A. (2019). Approaches to high-risk resected stage II and III melanoma. *American Society of Clinical Oncology Educational Book, 39*, e207–e211. https://doi.org/10.1200/EDBK_239283

Zhou, J., Mahoney, K. M., Giobbie-Hurder, A., et al. (2017). Soluble PD-L1 as a biomarker in malignant melanoma treated with checkpoint blockade. *Cancer Immunology Research, 5*(6), 480–492. https://doi.org/10.1158/2326-6066.CIR-16-0329

Chapter 9
Significance of Immune Checkpoints in Lung Cancer

Anastasios Dimou and Konstantinos Leventakos

Abstract Lung cancer is the second most common cancer in both men and women and is associated with the highest number of cancer-related deaths among all cancer diagnoses. The major types of lung cancer include non-small-cell lung cancer (NSCLC) and small-cell lung cancer (SCLC). Systemic therapy is part of treatment for patients with earlier-stage NSCLC, when the goal is to cure, and in patients with later stage, where the goal is to prevent cancer-related complications. In addition to chemotherapy and targeted therapy, systemic therapy also includes immunotherapy in the form of immune checkpoint inhibitors. These drugs block either PD-1, PD-L1, or CTLA4 and are used either alone or in combination with chemotherapy. Inhibitors of PD-L1 also improve outcomes for patients with extensive stage SCLC, where the goal of treatment is palliation. Their use in patients with limited stage SCLC, where the goal of treatment is cure, is currently being explored. PD-L1 expression and tumor mutation burden are generally predictive of benefit from immunotherapy in NSCLC but not in SCLC. There is active ongoing research for additional immunotherapy targets and biomarkers to better select patients with lung cancer who might benefit from immunotherapy agents.

Keywords NSCLC · SCLC · PD-L1 TPS · CTLA4 · Chemoimmunotherapy · Chemoradiation · Lung adenocarcinoma · Lung squamous cell carcinoma · Extensive stage · Limited stage · Immune escape · Neoadjuvant · Adjuvant · Lung cancer

A. Dimou · K. Leventakos (✉)
Division of Medical Oncology, Mayo Clinic, Rochester, MN, USA
e-mail: Leventakos.Konstantinos@mayo.edu

Introduction

Lung cancer is the most common cause of cancer-related mortality in the USA (Siegel et al., 2017) and worldwide (Ferlay et al., 2015). As such, lung cancer represents a major global disease burden. Over the last few years, there have been major advances in the treatment of lung cancer with the development of drugs that can target specific molecular abnormalities and with the advent of immunotherapy.

Lung cancer is not a single disease, but it represents many types of cancers that can arise within the lungs. Lung cancer is classified primarily in the small-cell lung cancer (SCLC) or non-small-cell lung cancer (NSCLC) types. There are multiple types of NSCLC, but the two most common are adenocarcinoma and squamous cell carcinoma, of which adenocarcinoma is the most common. Sadly, many cases of lung cancer are due to tobacco exposure, but a large proportion of these patients are never smokers. Other risk factors include radiation, asbestos, radon, air, and other environmental pollutants.

Staging and Treatments

Lung cancer stage is very important because it determines treatment options and influences survival. Although both NSCLC and SCLC are staged by the same TNM system, clinical decisions for SCLC are based on the Veterans Administration (VA) staging system. For NSCLCs that are localized to the lung, and whose removal would not significantly compromise breathing, surgical removal of the tumor is considered. Sometimes because of comorbidities such as heart or lung disease, patients cannot undergo surgery, and ablation or radiotherapy may be considered instead. In patients with NSCLC that has spread to the lymph nodes, consideration is given to a combination of therapies that might include cytotoxic chemotherapy, radiation therapy, surgery, and immunotherapy. Once the disease has spread beyond the lung(s) and chest lymph nodes, or if radiation therapy cannot be safely administered, systemic therapies with palliative intent are considered. Systemic treatment options can include cytotoxic chemotherapy, immunotherapy, or targeted therapy. The selection of targeted therapy depends on the detection of a mutation in *EGFR*, *ALK*, *ROS1*, HER2, RET, NTRK, MET, KRAS, or *BRAF*.

The treatment of SCLC is different to that of NSCLC. Surgery is rarely considered for the former type. More commonly, patients with SCLC will receive the combination of chemotherapy with radiation therapy if the disease is limited to a field of radiation (called limited stage). Prophylactic radiation to the brain to prevent brain metastases can be considered in some cases with limited disease. If the disease is more widespread (called extensive stage), treatment with the combination of chemotherapy with immunotherapy is preferred. In select patients with extensive disease and significant improvement after initial therapy with chemotherapy and immunotherapy, radiation to the chest might be offered.

Immunotherapy

The treatment landscape of NSCLC and SCLC is rapidly changing. The discovery of programmed cell death ligand 1 (PD-L1, aka B7-H1 and CD274) at the Mayo Clinic (Dong et al., 1999), the detection of PD-L1 on lung cancer tumor cells (Boland et al., 2013; Velcheti et al., 2014), and the negative regulation of T-cell proliferation through apoptosis of tumor-specific T-cells following engagement of PD-L1 with its receptor programmed cell death protein 1 (PD-1) (Dong et al., 2002) suggest that blocking the PD-L1/PD-1 axis in lung cancer is a reasonable therapeutic strategy for this malignancy (Pardoll, 2012). As of 2023, five drugs that block this axis have been approved by the FDA for patients with NSCLC, and others are far along in development (Leventakos & Mansfield, 2014; Leventakos & Mansfield, 2016). Additionally, two drugs that block the PD-1/PD-L1 axis are approved by the FDA for use in patients with SCLC.

Additionally, cytotoxic T-lymphocyte-associated protein 4 (CTLA4) has emerged as another target for patients with NSCLC. There are currently two drugs that block CTLA4 which are approved by the FDA in combination with anti-PD1 or anti-PDL1 drugs. The PD-1/PD-L1 axis and CTLA4 are collectively known as immune checkpoints because their physiologic function is to block excessive immune reactions in the body. A number of drugs targeting immune checkpoints other than PD-1/PD-L1 and CTLA4 are currently under investigation.

Immunotherapy in Perioperative Treatment

Perioperative systemic therapy improves outcomes for patients with NSCLC who receive surgical resection of their tumors. For a long time, this has taken the form of four cycles of chemotherapy with platinum (carboplatin or cisplatin) in combination with a second cytotoxic agent, administered before (neoadjuvant) or after (adjuvant) surgery. In recent years, the addition of immune checkpoint inhibitors in perioperative treatment extends the time of survival without lung cancer recurrence.

Neoadjuvant Therapy

Four independent large phase III randomized studies established the role of anti-PD-1 or anti-PD-L1 agents in addition to chemotherapy as neoadjuvant therapy for patients with NSCLC who have resectable disease at diagnosis. In the first study (CheckMate 816), patients with resectable NSCLC received three cycles of platinum-based chemotherapy and nivolumab (an anti-PD-1 immunotherapy drug) or platinum-based chemotherapy alone (Forde et al., 2022). Both groups of patients were evaluated for resection of their tumors. In the second study (AEGEAN),

patients with resectable NSCLC received either four cycles of platinum-based chemotherapy and durvalumab (an anti-PD-L1 immunotherapy drug) or four cycles of
platinum-based chemotherapy and placebo (Heymach et al., 2022; Heymach et al.,
2023). Both groups of patients were evaluated for surgical resection. After surgery,
patients in the first group received durvalumab for a year, and patients in the second
group received placebo for a year. In the third study (KEYNOTE 671), patients with
resectable NSCLC received either four cycles of cisplatin-based chemotherapy and
pembrolizumab (an anti-PD-1 immunotherapy drug) or four cycles of cisplatin-
based chemotherapy and placebo (Wakelee et al., 2023). Both groups of patients
were evaluated for surgical resection. After surgery, patients in the first group
received pembrolizumab for a year, and patients in the second group received placebo for a year. Finally, the Neotorch study, conducted in China, randomized
patients with resectable NSCLC to a group treated with three cycles of platinum-
based chemotherapy plus toripalimab, a PD-1 inhibitor, and a group that received
three cycles of platinum-based chemotherapy and placebo (10.1200/
JCO.2023.41.36_suppl.425126). Patients in both groups were taken to surgery.
Subsequently, patients in the experimental group received adjuvant therapy with
one cycle of chemotherapy and toripalimab followed by toripalimab to complete a
year of treatment, whereas patients in the placebo group received one cycle of chemotherapy and placebo followed by placebo.

Despite their differences, all four studies produced similar results: first, there was
improvement in the rate of complete eradication of the cancer with adding immunotherapy to neoadjuvant chemotherapy. Complete eradication, formally known as
complete pathologic response, is a term that describes the state of no viable tumor
upon microscopic evaluation of the surgical specimen and is a predictor of cure after
surgery. A similar endpoint, major pathologic response referring to the condition
where very little viable tumor remains in the resected tumor after neoadjuvant therapy was also improved with the addition of immunotherapy. Second, the complexity
of surgery was similar in patients who received prior immunotherapy and those who
were treated with chemotherapy alone. Third, patients who received preoperative
chemotherapy and immunotherapy survived without cancer recurrence for longer
time following surgery compared to patients who received chemotherapy alone. The
rates of patients who were able to have a complete resection of their tumors (about
80–90%) as well as the rates of patients who had their surgery delayed (about 3–5%)
or cancelled (about 1%) because of side effects from neoadjuvant therapy were
similar for patients in the chemoimmunotherapy- and chemotherapy-alone groups.

Adjuvant Therapy

The use of anti PD-1 or anti-PD-L1 agents as adjuvant therapy for patients with
resected NSCLC extends survival without relapse. Two drugs have been approved
by the FDA in this space, the anti-PD-L1 agent atezolizumab and the anti-PD1
agent pembrolizumab. Treatment with atezolizumab for a year was compared to no

treatment following surgical resection and adjuvant chemotherapy in the IMpower 010 study (Felip et al., 2021)(PMID: 34555333). Patients with tumors staining for positive PD-L1 in the atezolizumab group had a longer relapse-free survival. On the basis of these results, atezolizumab was approved for PD-L1-positive tumors only. On the other major study in this field, pembrolizumab for a year was compared to placebo following surgical resection and adjuvant chemotherapy in the PEARLS/Keynote 091 study (O'Brien et al., 2022). Patients in the pembrolizumab group had prolonged relapse-free survival regardless of the PD-L1 status of the tumor, and on the basis of these results, pembrolizumab was approved by the FDA as adjuvant therapy for patients with PD-L1-negative as well as patients with PD-L1-positive tumors.

Patients with Stage III Disease Receiving Concurrent Chemotherapy and Radiation

For a long time, chemoradiation has been the standard of care for patients with unresectable stage III NSCLC. Concurrent use of chemotherapy with chest radiation is superior to sequential treatment. Further efforts to improve outcomes with induction chemotherapy prior to chemoradiation or consolidation chemotherapy after chemoradiation failed to show benefit (Gadgeel, 2011). With this background, consolidation immunotherapy in the form of durvalumab, an anti-PD-L1 inhibitor, was the first intervention to improve outcomes in this space. In the PACIFIC study, patients with unresectable stage III NSCLC were randomized to receive a year of durvalumab or placebo following completion of definitive dose chest radiation with concurrent chemotherapy (Spigel et al., 2022). Patients in the experimental group had superior progression-free survival and overall survival compared to patients who received placebo. This led to regulatory approval of durvalumab as consolidation therapy following chemoradiation for patient with unresectable stage III lung cancer. The approval by the FDA involves patients regardless of PD-L1 status; however, patients with no PD-L1 expression in their tumors did not have improved outcomes with durvalumab versus placebo in an ad hoc analysis.

Patients with Advanced or Metastatic Disease

Immune checkpoint inhibitors provide durable responses to patients with NSCLC who receive treatment with palliative intent. Long-term survival at five years increased from 5% to 15–20% with the adoption of immunotherapy and targeted therapy in the treatment algorithm for this population. In the original studies that led to approval of the anti-PD-1 inhibitors nivolumab and pembrolizumab in both squamous and non-squamous NSCLC, those drugs compared favorably to standard chemotherapy when used as single agents for patients progressing in the first-line treatment (Borghaei et al., 2015; Brahmer et al., 2015; Herbst et al., 2021). Since then, more agents have received regulatory approvals, and immunotherapy is preferably administered as the first treatment for patients who are diagnosed with noncurable but treatable NSCLC with or without chemotherapy. Additionally, CTLA4 inhibitors ipilimumab and tremelimumab may be used in combination with anti-PD-1 or anti-PD-L1 inhibitors.

PD-1 and PD-L1 Inhibitors as Single Agents in Treatment-Naïve Patients

Inhibition of the PD-1/PD-L1 axis induces durable responses in cases where there is high expression of PD-L1 in the tumor. Three immune checkpoint inhibitors have received regulatory approval by the FDA for use as first treatment for patients with advanced NSCLC and high PD-L1 expression (more than 50% of tumor cells) on the basis of independent phase III clinical trials in treatment-naïve patients with high PD-L1-expressing tumors. Pembrolizumab was approved for this population on the basis of the Keynote 024 study which randomized patients to pembrolizumab or chemotherapy in the form of standard platinum doublet (Reck et al., 2021a). The IMpower110 randomized patients to atezolizumab or chemotherapy (Jassem et al., 2021), and finally in EMPOWER-Lung-01, patients were treated with cemiplimab or chemotherapy (Sezer et al., 2021). Median overall survival ranged between 20 and 30 months for patients treated with immunotherapy, while it was only 11–14.2 months for patients treated with chemotherapy in those studies. In landmark analyses, a significant proportion of patients was alive with ongoing follow-up in patients who received immunotherapy, quite unprecedented outcomes compared to chemotherapy alone and what is historically known for patients with advanced NSCLC. For example, up to 30% of the patients in the pembrolizumab group in the Keynote024 trial were alive at five years (Reck et al., 2021a).

PD-1 or PD-L1 Inhibitors in Combination with Chemotherapy

Addition of PD-1 or PD-L1 to platinum doublet-based chemotherapy improves the response rate, the progression-free survival, and the overall survival for patients with advanced NSCLC regardless of PD-L1 expression. Three agents, pembrolizumab, atezolizumab, and cemiplimab, have received approval by the FDA for palliative use in patients with advanced treatment-naïve NSCLC in combination with chemotherapy. Regulatory approval followed positive results from phase III randomized clinical trials. In the Keynote 189 study, patients with non-squamous NSCLC were randomized to receive pembrolizumab or placebo in addition to chemotherapy with carboplatin and pemetrexed (Garassino et al., 2023). The Keynote 407 study randomized patients with squamous NSCLC into pembrolizumab or placebo in addition to carboplatin and paclitaxel or nab paclitaxel (Novello et al., 2023). Atezolizumab was studied in combination with carboplatin- or cisplatin-based chemotherapy in the same setting in the IMpower 130 (patients with non-squamous histology, platinum combined with pemetrexed), IMpower 132 (patients with non-squamous histology, platinum combined with nab-paclitaxel), IMpower 150 (patients with non-squamous histology, platinum combined with paclitaxel or nab-paclitaxel and bevacizumab), and the IMpower 131 (patients with squamous histology, platinum combined with nab-paclitaxel) (Jotte et al., 2020; Nishio et al., 2021; Socinski et al., 2018; West et al., 2019). Finally, cemiplimab was studied in the EMPOWER-Lung 03 in combination with histology-specific platinum-based chemotherapy (Zhao et al., 2023).

A number of alternative anti PD-1 immune checkpoint inhibitors have shown similar benefit when added to platinum-based chemotherapy for patients with NSCLC in studies performed in China. Sintilimab, camrelizumab, and tislelizumab are all inhibitors of PD-1 in this space (Lu et al., 2021; Ren et al., 2022; Wang et al., 2021; Yang et al., 2020; Zhou et al., 2021, 2023). These agents are not approved by the FDA yet, as they were studied in Asian populations only.

It is an open question whether the combination of chemotherapy and immunotherapy or immunotherapy alone as first treatment followed by chemotherapy at progression should be preferred for cases with high PD-L1 expression (more than 50% of the tumor cells). In two retrospective real-world cohorts, overall survival was similar with either approach (Perol et al., 2022; Pons-Tostivint et al., 2023). Generally, patients with high disease burden and disease-associated symptoms who are candidates for chemotherapy, the combination is favored as it is more likely to induce a response. On the other hand, treatment with either pembrolizumab, atezolizumab, or cemiplimab alone is a very reasonable choice for high PD-L1 expressers and when the window for treatment is larger.

Combination of Anti-PD-1 and Anti-CTLA-4 Agents

Inhibition of CTLA4 in addition to anti-PD-1 or anti-PD-L1 may be more effective than anti-PD-1 or anti-PD-L1 alone for certain subgroups of patients with NSCLC. In the CheckMate 227 trial, treatment-naïve patients with stage IV or recurrent NSCLC were randomized to receive the combination of ipilimumab, an anti-CTLA4 inhibiting monoclonal antibody, in combination with nivolumab, nivolumab without (for tumors with PD-L1 $\geq$ 1%) or with platinum doublet chemotherapy (PD-L1 < 1%), or platinum doublet alone (PMID: 31562796). The study met its primary endpoint for superior overall survival in the ipilimumab plus nivolumab arm over chemotherapy for cases with PD-L1 $\geq$ 1%. In CheckMate 9LA, patients with treatment-naïve, stage IV, or recurrent NSCLC were randomized to receive the combination of ipilimumab and nivolumab with two cycles of histology appropriate platinum doublet chemotherapy for two cycles or chemotherapy alone (Reck et al., 2021b). The study showed improvement in overall survival for patients receiving the immunotherapy combination regardless of PD-L1 status. Finally, in the POSEIDON phase III study, patients with stage IV NSCLC were randomized to receive the combination of durvalumab with tremelimumab, an anti-CTLA4 inhibitory antibody, and platinum doublet chemotherapy, the combination of durvalumab with platinum doublet chemotherapy or platinum doublet chemotherapy alone. Overall survival and progression-free survival were prolonged in the durvalumab plus tremelimumab plus chemotherapy arm compared to chemotherapy-alone arm (Johnson et al., 2023). Progression-free survival but not overall survival was prolonged for the durvalumab plus chemotherapy versus chemotherapy arms. In another phase III study (Lung-MAP S1400I), addition of ipilimumab to nivolumab did not show a benefit in overall survival over nivolumab alone for patients with advanced squamous NSCLC, after progression on chemotherapy (Gettinger et al., 2021).

Overall, the combinations of chemotherapy with ipilimumab and nivolumab or tremelimumab and durvalumab were approved by the FDA and are available options for patients with metastatic NSCLC receiving treatment with palliative intent. Additionally, the combination of ipilimumab and nivolumab is approved for patients with positive PD-L1 status (PD-L1 $\geq$ 1%). These combinations are not approved for patients with EGFR or ALK mutations, as patients with those molecular abnormalities were not involved in the study populations. Adding CTLA4 inhibition with ipilimumab or tremelimumab to frontline therapy for patients with NSCLC increases the rates of significant immune-related toxicity over anti-PD1 or anti-PD-L1 alone. Additionally, it is not clear whether the outcomes are superior to the combination of chemotherapy plus anti-PD1 without anti-CTLA4. At the time of this writing, identification of patient subgroups who might benefit from adding anti-CTLA4 drugs to the frontline regimen is an area of active investigation.

Immunotherapy for Patients with EGFR and ALK Mutations

Early preclinical studies linked PD-L1 expression to downstream effects of mutated EGFR leading to the hypothesis that EGFR mutated tumors might respond to immune checkpoint inhibitors (Chen et al., 2015). However, it was quickly realized that the use of single-agent anti-PD-1 or anti-PD-L1 inhibitors when used as single agents is less effective for patients with EGFR or ALK mutated NSCLC. In a meta-analysis of four studies with single-agent nivolumab, pembrolizumab, or atezolizumab versus docetaxel for second-line treatment of patients with NSCLC, there was no difference in overall survival between immunotherapy and docetaxel for patients with EGFR mutated tumors (Yang et al., 2022). In the subgroup of patients with EGFR mutated tumors in the PACIFIC trial, durvalumab did not prolong overall survival over placebo (Naidoo et al., 2023). In a study of pembrolizumab for patients with treatment-naïve EGFR mutated tumors, no objective responses were reported, and the study was terminated early (Lisberg et al., 2018). Additionally, there were no responses to single-agent anti-PD-1 or anti-PD-L1 for patients with ALK fusions in the IMMUNOTARGET registry. Responses were observed in 12% of patients with EGFR mutations in the same retrospective multi-institution cohort.

Later studies of immune checkpoint inhibitors in combination with chemotherapy in patients with NSCLC largely excluded patients with EGFR or ALK mutations. In the few studies where patients with EGFR mutations were included, the effectiveness signal for immunotherapy is mixed. Patients with EGFR mutated tumors in the IMpower150 study had the same benefit from adding atezolizumab to the backbone of carboplatin, paclitaxel or nab-paclitaxel, and bevacizumab as the patients with no EGFR or ALK mutations (Nogami et al., 2022). Additionally, in the ORIENT-31 clinical trial that was performed in China, patients with EGFR mutated advanced or metastatic non-squamous NSCLC who have progressed on EGFR-directed therapies were randomized to receive chemotherapy with or without sintilimab, an anti-PD1 inhibitory antibody. There was an additional arm of patients who received the bevacizumab biosimilar IBI305 in addition to chemotherapy and sintilimab. Patients who received sintilimab had superior progression-free and overall survival compared to the patients who received chemotherapy only (Lu et al., 2023). Finally, in the global Keynote 789 study, patients with EGFR mutated metastatic non-squamous NSCLC who have progressed on EGFR tyrosine kinase inhibitors were randomized to receive pembrolizumab and platinum doublet chemotherapy or platinum-based chemotherapy alone (10.1200/JCO.2023.41.17_suppl.LBA9000). Enrollment was delayed amidst the COVID-19 pandemic, and the study was underpowered to show a difference at the time the data were reported. Nevertheless, the study did not show a benefit from pembrolizumab in this population.

Finally, patients with EGFR or ALK mutations were included in some studies that tested the role of perioperative immunotherapy in NSCLC with mixed results. Specifically, patients with EGFR mutated tumors did not benefit from adjuvant therapy with atezolizumab in the subgroup analysis of the IMpower010; however, there was benefit for patients with EGFR mutations and positive PD-L1 status. Patients with ALK mutations did not have benefit from atezolizumab in this study regardless of PD-L1 expression (Felip et al., 2021). Benefit from adjuvant pembrolizumab was seen in the subgroup of patients with EGFR mutations in the PEARLS/Keynote-091 study (O'Brien et al., 2022). At this time, there is no reliable biomarker to select patients with EGFR or Alk mutated NSCLC who might benefit from treatment with immune checkpoint inhibitors, and further research is required.

Immune Checkpoint Inhibitors in Later Lines of Treatment

In the current therapeutic algorithm of NSCLC, the majority of patients with advanced disease will receive treatment with immunotherapy as frontline treatment. There is no standard use of immune checkpoint inhibitors after resistance to anti-PD1, anti-PD-L1 inhibitors, either alone or in combination with anti-CTLA4. A number of approaches are worth mentioning in this space. Patients with NSCLC who progressed on previous treatment with immune checkpoint inhibitors and chemotherapy and received the combination of pembrolizumab with ramucirumab, an inhibitory antibody for vascular endothelial growth factor receptor-2, had superior overall survival compared to patients who received standard treatment in the phase II Lung-MAP-S1800A clinical trial (Reckamp et al., 2022). Results were more pronounced for patients with squamous compared to patients with non-squamous histology. In another phase II study, patients with advanced NSCLC who had progressed to prior anti-PD1 or anti-PD-L1 agents received treatment with the combination of durvalumab and tremelilumab (Garon et al., 2023). There were rare responses among patients with disease that was refractory to prior anti-PD-(L)1 treatment and no responses among patients with disease that had relapsed after initial response to prior immunotherapy. In addition to PD-1 and CTLA4, a large number of additional immune checkpoints are being examined as targets for therapy in NSCLC, and the landscape of immunotherapy in this disease is evolving.

Small-Cell Lung Cancer

A number of earlier clinical trials provided proof of concept that immune checkpoint inhibitors are effective for patients with SCLC. Finally, in 2023, there are two immunotherapy regimens approved for first-line treatment of extensive stage SCLC. The Impower 133 trial (Horn et al., 2018) led to atezolizumab being approved for this indication, and the Caspian trial (Paz-Ares et al., 2022) led to the FDA approval of durvalumab. Even though there are some differences in the design of these trials, we believe that these two regimens are practically similar and the final decision on which they can be used in each patient has to come by discussion between the treating physician and the patient. In general, the use of immunotherapy in small-cell lung cancer has increased the overall survival and the progression-free survival of patients with some patients surviving more than previously. We usually cite that now with immunotherapy three times, more patients will be long-term survivors which is exciting for this disease.

Regarding limited-stage SCLC, there are not FDA-approved immunotherapies, but many clinical trials are actively looking into the incorporation of immunotherapy in the treatment plan after the concurrent chemotherapy and radiation. One of the largest is NRG LU005 (NCT03811002) in which patients are randomly assigned in a 1:1 ratio to standard chemotherapy with concurrent radiation (45 Gy BID or 66 Gy QD) with or without atezolizumab beginning concurrently with radiation and continues every 3 weeks for up to 12 months. The thoracic oncology community is eagerly awaiting the results of these trials.

With the incorporation of immunotherapy in the first line of treatment, it is still unclear what is the role of immunotherapy at the time of progression. Clinical trials are either looking into adding immunotherapy in the second-line approved treatments. For example, at the Mayo Clinic, the clinical trial MC1923 is adding durvalumab on second-line lurbinectedin (NCT04607954).

In contrast with NSCLC, where PD-L1 and TMB can be used as a biomarker to refine the immunotherapy strategy, these biomarkers have not been validated clinically for SCLC. Thus, all patients today will receive immunotherapy independent of their PD-L1 or TMB status. Recent advances in the description of SCLC subtypes (Gay et al., 2021) have led to subtype characterization of patients based on their subtype, but the use of immunotherapy should be offered to all patients. More research is needed to identify novel ways where immunotherapy can be used more efficiently for patients with SCLC who relapse.

PD-L1 Assessment and Companion Assays

Since immunotherapy causes immune-related side effects that are occasionally serious only to benefit a fraction of patients, development of biomarkers to guide benefit to risk discussions is necessary. Further, an important decision in the therapeutic algorithm of patients with NSCLC is whether to select treatment with immunotherapy alone or the combination of chemotherapy and immunotherapy. Among the plausible companion diagnostics, PD-L1 expression in cancer cells has emerged as the most relevant biomarker for patients with NSCLC to determine response to anti-PD1 or anti-PDL1 treatment. PD-L1 tumor proportion score (TPS) is assessed as the proportion of tumor cells that have membranous expression of PD-L1. Patients with metastatic NSCLC and PD-L1 TPS $\geq$ 50% may be treated with pembrolizumab, cemiplimab, or atezolizumab alone (Akinboro et al., 2022; Pai-Scherf et al., 2017). Additionally, patients with PD-L1 TPS $\geq$ 1% and early-stage disease could receive atezolizumab as adjuvant therapy (Mathieu et al., 2023). Third, benefit from immunotherapy is increasing with higher PD-L1 TPS in patients who receive the combination of immunotherapy and chemotherapy. Benefit is present even for patients with PD-L1 TPS 0% (Garassino et al., 2023; Novello et al., 2023).

PD-L1 TPS predicts response to anti-PD1 or anti-PD-L1 treatment as a continuous variable, and it is difficult to select a cut point that will separate NSCLC patients who will, from those who will not, benefit from immunotherapy. Rather than being the sole determinant, PD-L1 TPS is one of the factors along with clinical judgment to determine whether immunotherapy could be given alone or in combination with chemotherapy to patients with advanced or metastatic NSCLC. Interestingly, PD-L1 TPS does not predict benefit from immunotherapy among patients with small-cell lung cancer (Liu et al., 2021).

A number of other biomarkers to select patients who will benefit from immunotherapy are worth mentioning. Tumor mutation burden (TMB) reflects the number of mutations in a given cancer. The cutpoint of ten mutations/MB is widely used to separate the TMB high from the TMB low groups. Pembrolizumab is approved by the FDA for solid tumors including lung cancer regardless of histology with TMB $\geq$ 10 mutations/MB on the basis of clinical trial data (Marabelle et al., 2020). TMB but not PD-L1 TPS emerged as a predictor for long-term benefit from treatment with immune checkpoint inhibitors among patients with NSCLC

(Thummalapalli et al., 2023). Additionally, a growing body of literature supports the use of biomarkers based on human leukocyte antigen (HLA) typing (Jiang et al., 2023; Naranbhai et al., 2022).

Conclusion

Immunotherapy in the form of PD1, PD-L1, and CTLA4 immune checkpoint inhibitors is standard of care for patients with early-stage, regional, and advanced stage NSCLC, also for patients with extensive stage SCLC. Intensive research is focused to discover new modes of immunotherapy, better select patients who benefit from existing immunotherapy, and address resistance.

References

Akinboro, O., et al. (2022). FDA approval summary: Pembrolizumab, atezolizumab, and Cemiplimab-rwlc as single agents for first-line treatment of advanced/metastatic PD-L1-high NSCLC. *Clinical Cancer Research, 28*, 2221–2228.

Boland, J. M., et al. (2013). Tumor B7-H1 and B7-H3 expression in squamous cell carcinoma of the lung. *Clinical Lung Cancer, 14*, 157–163.

Borghaei, H., et al. (2015). Nivolumab versus docetaxel in advanced nonsquamous non-small-cell lung cancer. *The New England Journal of Medicine, 373*, 1627–1639.

Brahmer, J., et al. (2015). Nivolumab versus docetaxel in advanced squamous-cell non-small-cell lung cancer. *The New England Journal of Medicine, 373*, 123–135.

Chen, N., et al. (2015). Upregulation of PD-L1 by EGFR activation mediates the immune escape in EGFR-driven NSCLC: Implication for optional immune targeted therapy for NSCLC patients with EGFR mutation. *Journal of Thoracic Oncology, 10*, 910–923.

Dong, H., Zhu, G., Tamada, K., & Chen, L. (1999). B7-H1, a third member of the B7 family, co-stimulates T-cell proliferation and interleukin-10 secretion. *Nature Medicine, 5*, 1365–1369.

Dong, H., et al. (2002). Tumor-associated B7-H1 promotes T-cell apoptosis: A potential mechanism of immune evasion. *Nature Medicine, 8*, 793–800.

Felip, E., et al. (2021). Adjuvant atezolizumab after adjuvant chemotherapy in resected stage IB-IIIA non-small-cell lung cancer (IMpower010): A randomised, multicentre, open-label, phase 3 trial. *Lancet, 398*, 1344–1357.

Ferlay, J., et al. (2015). Cancer incidence and mortality worldwide: Sources, methods and major patterns in GLOBOCAN 2012. *International Journal of Cancer, 136*, E359–E386.

Forde, P. M., et al. (2022). Neoadjuvant nivolumab plus chemotherapy in Resectable lung cancer. *The New England Journal of Medicine, 386*, 1973–1985.

Gadgeel, S. M. (2011). The optimal chemotherapy for stage III non-small cell lung cancer patients. *Current Oncology Reports, 13*, 272–279.

Garassino, M. C., et al. (2023). Pembrolizumab plus pemetrexed and platinum in nonsquamous non-small-cell lung cancer: 5-year outcomes from the phase 3 KEYNOTE-189 study. *Journal of Clinical Oncology, 41*, 1992–1998.

Garon, E. B., et al. (2023). Brief report: Safety and antitumor activity of durvalumab plus tremelimumab in programmed cell death-(ligand)1-monotherapy pretreated, advanced NSCLC: Results from a phase 1b clinical trial. *Journal of Thoracic Oncology, 18*, 1094–1102.

Gay, C. M., et al. (2021). Patterns of transcription factor programs and immune pathway activation define four major subtypes of SCLC with distinct therapeutic vulnerabilities. *Cancer Cell, 39*, 346–360 e347.

Gettinger, S. N., et al. (2021). Nivolumab plus ipilimumab vs nivolumab for previously treated patients with stage IV squamous cell lung cancer: The lung-MAP S1400I phase 3 randomized clinical trial. *JAMA Oncology, 7*, 1368–1377.

Herbst, R. S., et al. (2021). Five year survival update from KEYNOTE-010: Pembrolizumab versus docetaxel for previously treated, programmed death-ligand 1-positive advanced NSCLC. *Journal of Thoracic Oncology, 16*, 1718–1732.

Heymach, J. V., et al. (2022). Design and Rationale for a phase III, double-blind, placebo-controlled study of neoadjuvant durvalumab + chemotherapy followed by adjuvant durvalumab for the treatment of patients with Resectable stages II and III non-small-cell lung cancer: The AEGEAN trial. *Clinical Lung Cancer, 23*, e247–e251.

Heymach, J. V. H. D., Mitsudomi, T., Taube, J. M., Galffy, G., Hochmair, M., Winder, T., Zukov, R., Garbaos, G., Gao, S., Kuroda, H., You, J., Lee, K. Y., Antonuzzo, L., Aperghis, M., Doherty, G. J., Mann, H., Fouad, T. M., & Reck, M. (2023). AEGEAN: A phase 3 trial of neoadjuvant durvalumab + chemotherapy followed by adjuvant durvalumab in patients with resectable NSCLC. In *AACR annual meeting* (Vol. 83).

Horn, L., et al. (2018). First-line atezolizumab plus chemotherapy in extensive-stage small-cell lung cancer. *The New England Journal of Medicine, 379*, 2220–2229.

Jassem, J., et al. (2021). Updated overall survival analysis from IMpower110: Atezolizumab versus platinum-based chemotherapy in treatment-naive programmed death-ligand 1-selected NSCLC. *Journal of Thoracic Oncology, 16*, 1872–1882.

Jiang, T., et al. (2023). HLA-I evolutionary divergence confers response to PD-1 blockade plus chemotherapy in untreated advanced non-small-cell lung cancer. *Clinical Cancer Research, 29*(23), 4830–4843.

Johnson, M. L., et al. (2023). Durvalumab with or without tremelimumab in combination with chemotherapy as first-line therapy for metastatic non-small-cell lung cancer: The phase III POSEIDON study. *Journal of Clinical Oncology, 41*, 1213–1227.

Jotte, R., et al. (2020). Atezolizumab in combination with carboplatin and nab-paclitaxel in advanced squamous NSCLC (IMpower131): Results from a randomized phase III trial. *Journal of Thoracic Oncology, 15*, 1351–1360.

Leventakos, K., & Mansfield, A. S. (2014). Reflections on immune checkpoint inhibition in non-small cell lung cancer. *Translational Lung Cancer Research, 3*, 411–413.

Leventakos, K., & Mansfield, A. S. (2016). Advances in the treatment of non-small cell lung cancer: Focus on nivolumab, pembrolizumab, and atezolizumab. *BioDrugs, 30*, 397–405.

Lisberg, A., et al. (2018). A phase II study of pembrolizumab in EGFR-mutant, PD-L1+, tyrosine kinase inhibitor naive patients with advanced NSCLC. *Journal of Thoracic Oncology, 13*, 1138–1145.

Liu, S. V., et al. (2021). Updated overall survival and PD-L1 subgroup analysis of patients with extensive-stage small-cell lung cancer treated with atezolizumab, carboplatin, and etoposide (IMpower133). *Journal of Clinical Oncology, 39*, 619–630.

Lu, S., et al. (2021). Tislelizumab plus chemotherapy as first-line treatment for locally advanced or metastatic nonsquamous NSCLC (RATIONALE 304): A randomized phase 3 trial. *Journal of Thoracic Oncology, 16*, 1512–1522.

Lu, S., et al. (2023). Sintilimab plus chemotherapy for patients with EGFR-mutated non-squamous non-small-cell lung cancer with disease progression after EGFR tyrosine-kinase inhibitor therapy (ORIENT-31): Second interim analysis from a double-blind, randomised, placebo-controlled, phase 3 trial. *The Lancet Respiratory Medicine, 11*, 624–636.

Marabelle, A., et al. (2020). Association of tumour mutational burden with outcomes in patients with advanced solid tumours treated with pembrolizumab: Prospective biomarker analysis of the multicohort, open-label, phase 2 KEYNOTE-158 study. *The Lancet Oncology, 21*, 1353–1365.

Mathieu, L. N., et al. (2023). FDA approval summary: Atezolizumab as adjuvant treatment following surgical resection and platinum-based chemotherapy for stage II to IIIA NSCLC. *Clinical Cancer Research, 29,* 2973–2978.

Naidoo, J., et al. (2023). Brief report: Durvalumab after chemoradiotherapy in unresectable stage III EGFR-mutant NSCLC: A post Hoc subgroup analysis from PACIFIC. *Journal of Thoracic Oncology, 18,* 657–663.

Naranbhai, V., et al. (2022). HLA-A*03 and response to immune checkpoint blockade in cancer: An epidemiological biomarker study. *The Lancet Oncology, 23,* 172–184.

Nishio, M., et al. (2021). Atezolizumab plus chemotherapy for first-line treatment of nonsquamous NSCLC: Results from the randomized phase 3 IMpower132 trial. *Journal of Thoracic Oncology, 16,* 653–664.

Nogami, N., et al. (2022). IMpower150 final exploratory analyses for atezolizumab plus bevacizumab and chemotherapy in key NSCLC patient subgroups with EGFR mutations or metastases in the liver or brain. *Journal of Thoracic Oncology, 17,* 309–323.

Novello, S., et al. (2023). Pembrolizumab plus chemotherapy in squamous non-small-cell lung cancer: 5-year update of the phase III KEYNOTE-407 study. *Journal of Clinical Oncology, 41,* 1999–2006.

O'Brien, M., et al. (2022). Pembrolizumab versus placebo as adjuvant therapy for completely resected stage IB-IIIA non-small-cell lung cancer (PEARLS/KEYNOTE-091): An interim analysis of a randomised, triple-blind, phase 3 trial. *The Lancet Oncology, 23,* 1274–1286.

Pai-Scherf, L., et al. (2017). FDA approval summary: Pembrolizumab for treatment of metastatic non-small cell lung cancer: First-line therapy and beyond. *The Oncologist, 22,* 1392–1399.

Pardoll, D. M. (2012). The blockade of immune checkpoints in cancer immunotherapy. *Nature Reviews. Cancer, 12,* 252–264.

Paz-Ares, L., et al. (2022). Durvalumab, with or without tremelimumab, plus platinum-etoposide in first-line treatment of extensive-stage small-cell lung cancer: 3-year overall survival update from CASPIAN. *ESMO Open, 7,* 100408.

Perol, M., et al. (2022). Effectiveness of PD-(L)1 inhibitors alone or in combination with platinum-doublet chemotherapy in first-line (1L) non-squamous non-small-cell lung cancer (Nsq-NSCLC) with PD-L1-high expression using real-world data. *Annals of Oncology, 33,* 511–521.

Pons-Tostivint, E., et al. (2023). Real-world multicentre cohort of first-line pembrolizumab alone or in combination with platinum-based chemotherapy in non-small cell lung cancer PD-L1 >/= 50. *Cancer Immunology, Immunotherapy, 72,* 1881–1890.

Reck, M., et al. (2021a). Five-year outcomes with pembrolizumab versus chemotherapy for metastatic non-small-cell lung cancer with PD-L1 tumor proportion score >/= 50. *Journal of Clinical Oncology, 39,* 2339–2349.

Reck, M., et al. (2021b). First-line nivolumab plus ipilimumab with two cycles of chemotherapy versus chemotherapy alone (four cycles) in advanced non-small-cell lung cancer: CheckMate 9LA 2-year update. *ESMO Open, 6,* 100273.

Reckamp, K. L., et al. (2022). Phase II randomized study of ramucirumab and pembrolizumab versus standard of care in advanced non-small-cell lung cancer previously treated with immunotherapy-lung-MAP S1800A. *Journal of Clinical Oncology, 40,* 2295–2306.

Ren, S., et al. (2022). Camrelizumab plus carboplatin and paclitaxel as first-line treatment for advanced squamous NSCLC (CameL-Sq): A phase 3 trial. *Journal of Thoracic Oncology, 17,* 544–557.

Sezer, A., et al. (2021). Cemiplimab monotherapy for first-line treatment of advanced non-small-cell lung cancer with PD-L1 of at least 50%: A multicentre, open-label, global, phase 3, randomised, controlled trial. *Lancet, 397,* 592–604.

Siegel, R. L., Miller, K. D., & Jemal, A. (2017). Cancer statistics, 2017. *CA: a Cancer Journal for Clinicians, 67,* 7–30.

Socinski, M. A., et al. (2018). Atezolizumab for first-line treatment of metastatic nonsquamous NSCLC. *The New England Journal of Medicine, 378,* 2288–2301.

Spigel, D. R., et al. (2022). Five-year survival outcomes from the PACIFIC trial: Durvalumab after chemoradiotherapy in stage III non-small-cell lung cancer. *Journal of Clinical Oncology, 40*, 1301–1311.

Thummalapalli, R., et al. (2023). Clinical and molecular features of long-term response to immune checkpoint inhibitors in patients with advanced non-small cell lung cancer. *Clinical Cancer Research, 29*(21), 4408–4418.

Velcheti, V., et al. (2014). Programmed death ligand-1 expression in non-small cell lung cancer. *Laboratory Investigation, 94*, 107–116.

Wakelee, H., et al. (2023). Perioperative pembrolizumab for early-stage non-small-cell lung cancer. *The New England Journal of Medicine, 389*, 491–503.

Wang, J., et al. (2021). Tislelizumab plus chemotherapy vs chemotherapy alone as first-line treatment for advanced squamous non-small-cell lung cancer: A phase 3 randomized clinical trial. *JAMA Oncology, 7*, 709–717.

West, H., et al. (2019). Atezolizumab in combination with carboplatin plus nab-paclitaxel chemotherapy compared with chemotherapy alone as first-line treatment for metastatic non-squamous non-small-cell lung cancer (IMpower130): A multicentre, randomised, open-label, phase 3 trial. *The Lancet Oncology, 20*, 924–937.

Yang, Y., et al. (2020). Efficacy and safety of Sintilimab plus pemetrexed and platinum as first-line treatment for locally advanced or metastatic nonsquamous NSCLC: A randomized, double-blind, phase 3 study (Oncology pRogram by InnovENT anti-PD-1-11). *Journal of Thoracic Oncology, 15*, 1636–1646.

Yang, H., et al. (2022). EGFR mutation status in non-small cell lung cancer receiving PD-1/PD-L1 inhibitors and its correlation with PD-L1 expression: A meta-analysis. *Cancer Immunology, Immunotherapy, 71*, 1001–1016.

Zhao, B., Qi, H., Wu, J., & Ma, W. (2023). Cemiplimab plus chemotherapy could be a first-line option for advanced and metastatic NSCLC: Results from the phase 3 EMPOWER-lung 3 part 2 trial. *Journal of Thoracic Oncology, 18*, e72–e73.

Zhou, C., et al. (2021). Sintilimab plus platinum and gemcitabine as first-line treatment for advanced or metastatic squamous NSCLC: Results from a randomized, double-blind, phase 3 trial (ORIENT-12). *Journal of Thoracic Oncology, 16*, 1501–1511.

Zhou, C., et al. (2023). Camrelizumab plus carboplatin and pemetrexed as first-line treatment for advanced nonsquamous NSCLC: Extended follow-up of CameL phase 3 trial. *Journal of Thoracic Oncology, 18*, 628–639.

Chapter 10
Immunotherapy in Breast Cancer

Jenna Hoppenworth and Roberto A. Leon-Ferre

Abstract Breast cancer affects 12% of women worldwide. Although advances in systemic, surgical, and radiation therapy approaches will cure a large proportion of women with breast cancer, a significant subset will experience disease relapse and die as a result of their disease. Of the three main breast cancer subtypes, triple-negative breast cancer poses a special challenge to clinicians and researchers due to its aggressive features and the paucity of targetable alterations. Recent progress in immunotherapy and novel therapeutics has transformed the treatment of this breast cancer subtype. In this chapter, we introduce the reader to the biology and classification of breast cancer and review the modern multidisciplinary approaches to management, with special emphasis on the incorporation of immunotherapy in the early-stage and metastatic settings. We also review the emerging role of immunotherapy biomarkers and other modern treatments, including monoclonal antibodies and antibody-drug conjugates.

Keywords Breast cancer · Risk factors · Breast cancer subtypes · Triple-negative breast cancer · HER2-negative breast cancer · Early-stage breast cancer · Metastatic breast cancer · Immunotherapy · Chemotherapy · PD-L1 · KEYNOTE-522 · KEYNOTE-355 · Antibody-drug conjugates · Monoclonal antibodies · Tumor-infiltrating lymphocytes

Introduction

Breast cancer will affect approximately 313,510 people in the Unites States in 2024. Of those affected with breast cancer in 2024, 42,780 will die as a result of their breast cancer diagnosis (Siegel et al., 2024). Despite the prevalence, the death rate has steadily declined since the 1990s, mostly credited to early detection and more

J. Hoppenworth · R. A. Leon-Ferre (✉)
Division of Medical Oncology, Mayo Clinic, Rochester, MN, USA
e-mail: leonferre.roberto@mayo.edu

effective treatments (Siegel et al., 2024). The recent introduction of immunotherapy has transformed the way we are treating patients with breast cancer, particularly the triple-negative breast cancer (TNBC) subtype. This chapter will look at the current role of immunotherapy strategies in the treatment of localized and of metastatic breast cancer, with special emphasis on TNBC, as well as novel approaches being investigated that may be incorporated into the clinical management of breast cancer in the future.

Risk Factors

One in eight women will be diagnosed with breast cancer in their lifetime (Siegel et al., 2024). The risk of developing breast cancer may increase under certain circumstances, such as older age, history of benign breast disease, dense breast tissue, and being a carrier for inherited genetic mutations such as BRCA 1/BRCA 2, PALB2, and others (Antoniou et al., 2003; Rahman et al., 2007); having a family history of breast or ovarian cancer (Collaborative Group on Hormonal Factors in Breast Cancer, 2001); prior receipt of hormone replacement therapy; reproductive factors such as earlier onset of menses, late menopause (Collaborative Group on Hormonal Factors in Breast Cancer, 2012), older age at first full-time pregnancy, or nulliparity (Rosner et al., 1994); postmenopausal obesity (Morimoto et al., 2002); excessive alcohol use or smoking (Gram et al., 2015; Cao et al., 2015); and prior radiation to the chest at a young age (Henderson et al., 2010); among others. Risk-reducing measures include maintaining a healthy weight, abstaining from the use of alcohol/tobacco, and limiting estrogen replacement therapy, among others.

Basics of Breast Cancer

Breast cancer evolves when atypical cells develop and divide in an uncontrolled manner. Benign breast diseases such as atypical ductal or lobular hyperplasia may progress into ductal or lobular carcinoma in situ or eventually become invasive diseases (with the potential to spread to distant organs). To decrease the risk of potential spread, invasive cancers may require treatment with chemotherapy. Ductal carcinoma in situ and lobular carcinoma in situ are noninvasive cancers (without the potential to spread) and are often referred to as stage 0 cancer. Given that they typically remain localized, chemotherapy is not recommended.

Breast cancers are classified biologically by the presence or absence of several markers, most importantly estrogen, progesterone, and HER2 (human epidermal growth factor receptor 2) receptors. Other features such as their appearance under the microscope (known as histologic subtype), grade (how mature or immature cells look in a biopsy specimen), and Ki-67 (a marker of cell proliferation) help breast cancer specialists determine the most effective and appropriate treatment.

Breast Cancer Subtypes

Breast cancer can be categorized into three major subtypes, according to the presence of three major markers within tumors, as outlined in Fig. 10.1 and below:

- *Hormone receptor-positive breast cancer*: It is characterized by the expression of the estrogen and/or progesterone receptors. In this subtype, growth is stimulated by estrogen and the activation of its receptor. Antiestrogen therapy is a major component of the treatment of patients with this tumor subtype. In certain situations, chemotherapy may also be necessary.
- *HER2-positive breast cancer*: These tumors are characterized by excessive amounts of HER2, a normal protein involved in normal cell division. In this breast cancer subtype, the presence of an abnormally high number of HER2 proteins contributes to excessive growth of cancer cells. To treat these tumors, therapies targeting the HER2 signaling pathway have been developed. These drugs are typically combined with chemotherapy.
- *Triple-negative breast cancer*: These tumors are characterized by absence of the estrogen and progesterone receptor and lack HER2 overexpression. This subtype

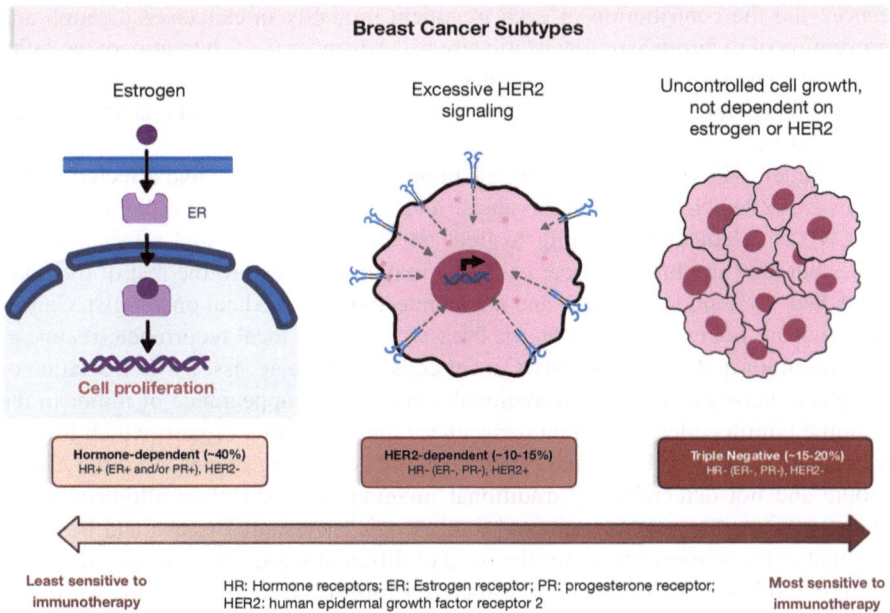

Fig. 10.1 Breast cancer subtypes. The three main breast cancer subtypes are classified according to the presence or absence of the hormone receptors (estrogen and progesterone receptors) and the presence or absence of excessive HER2 signaling. Hormone receptor-positive breast cancers are the least susceptible to the effects of the immune system, while triple-negative breast cancers (lacking all three features) are the most susceptible to the effects of the immune system

is the most aggressive type of breast cancer. For many years, chemotherapy has been the main form of treatment. However, this subtype has benefitted the most from the development of immunotherapy.

Each of these subtypes of breast cancer has a different biology and clinical behavior, requiring different treatment approaches as introduced briefly here. Importantly, immunotherapy approaches have demonstrated the greatest degree of clinical activity in the TNBC subtype. Given this, we will focus our subsequent discussions primarily on TNBC.

Early-Stage Breast Cancer: Multidisciplinary Approaches to Treatment

Early-stage breast cancer (breast cancer that is confined to the breast and regional lymph nodes and has not spread distantly) can be eradicated and treated with the goal of cure. To achieve this, specialists from different medical disciplines work together. These include surgical oncologists, radiation oncologists, medical oncologists, geneticists, physical therapists, and plastic surgeons, among others. It is important to understand the role each discipline plays in the treatment of breast cancer and the contribution of each treatment modality in cancer eradication and prevention of recurrence or metastatic disease. Advances in each treatment modality and in the integration of multidisciplinary care have led to substantial improvements in recurrence rates and breast cancer survival (Poortmans et al., 2015; Whelan et al., 2015).

Treatments specifically targeting the tumor within the breast and affected lymph nodes are called "locoregional therapies" and include surgery and radiation therapy (Fig. 10.2). Medications aiming to treat not only the breast and affected lymph nodes but also any breast cancer cells that may have spread to the rest of the body are called "systemic therapies" and are managed by the medical oncologist. Cancer cells that are not eradicated from the breast can lead to local recurrence (reappearance of tumor in the same breast). Cancer cells that have accessed the circulation or lymphatic networks can lead to regional recurrence (reappearance of tumor in the draining lymph nodes) or distant recurrence (spread to other organs, which is often incurable). Cancer cells that have spread before colonizing organs are often microscopic and not detectable by traditional imaging. As such, the multidisciplinary team evaluates the risk for potential microscopic metastatic disease and based on this makes recommendations for the need of different treatment modalities.

Immunotherapy is primarily considered a form of systemic therapy, with their main goal being to help activate the immune system's inherent ability to recognize and eliminate abnormal cells (in this case cells that have become cancerous). However, certain local immunotherapies have also been developed and are under investigation (examples of these include injections of medications or immune stimulants into the tumor or lymph nodes).

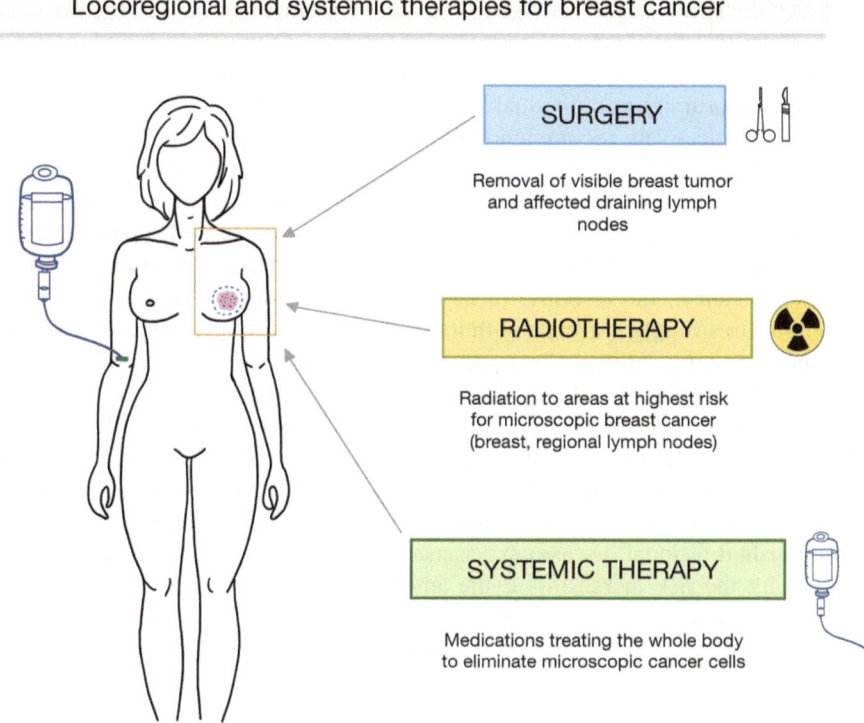

Fig. 10.2 Locoregional and systemic therapies for breast cancer. Surgery and radiotherapy are considered locoregional therapies, while medications including chemotherapy, immunotherapy, and targeted therapies are considered systemic therapies

How Are the Different Treatment Modalities Integrated?

Over the last decade, the multidisciplinary management paradigm of early-stage breast cancer, particularly for TNBC and HER2-positive breast cancer, has shifted away from doing surgery first and systemic therapy after surgery (called "adjuvant" systemic therapy) to a preference for administering systemic therapy before surgery (called "neoadjuvant" systemic therapy). This strategy of giving systemic therapy first has allowed clinicians to evaluate the sensitivity of the cancer to the treatment as it is administered and make adjustments as needed. The administration of neoadjuvant chemotherapy has several direct benefits to the patient with breast cancer, including (1) potential for less extensive breast and axillary surgery, in turn leading to decreased surgical morbidity and complications, given that tumors and lymph nodes often shrink or even disappear after neoadjuvant chemotherapy (Piltin et al., 2020; Boughey et al., 2018), allowing surgeons to remove smaller amounts of affected tissue; (2) better ability to estimate future risk of recurrence (Cortazar et al., 2014; Symmans et al., 2007; Boughey et al., 2017; Symmans et al., 2017; Yau et al., 2022), given that the degree of response of the breast tumor and lymph nodes to systemic therapy is strongly associated with the subsequent risk of cancer recurrence; (3) opportunity to individualize postoperative treatment decisions, allowing clinicians to selectively recommend additional medications to patients with more resistant tumors, and avoiding those medicines in patients with more sensitive tumors that were eradicated prior to surgery; and (4) more rapid evaluation of newer drugs, as clinical trials testing new drugs while the tumor has not been removed yet allows to quickly evaluate their efficacy (Masuda et al., 2017; Tutt et al., 2021a).

In breast cancer, the response to neoadjuvant systemic therapy has repeatedly been shown to strongly correlate with long-term outcomes, including risk of recurrence and long-term survival (Cortazar et al., 2014; Symmans et al., 2007; Boughey et al., 2017; Symmans et al., 2017; Yau et al., 2022). Patients whose tumors are completely eradicated by the end of neoadjuvant systemic therapy (called a pathologic complete response or pCR) enjoy very favorable long-term survival, with recurrence and mortality rates of <10% (Symmans et al., 2017). On the other hand, patients whose tumors or parts of their tumors survive after neoadjuvant systemic therapy (called residual disease) experience higher rates of disease recurrence and death—with the risk increasing as the amount of residual disease increases (Yau et al., 2022). This risk can be mitigated by administering additional medications after surgery for patients who have residual disease.

Breast Cancer and the Immune System

As elaborated throughout this book, immunotherapy has transformed the treatment landscape and prognosis of aggressive malignancies that previously had limited systemic therapy options. In breast cancer, patients with TNBC have derived the largest benefits from immunotherapy. This is in part due to TNBC tumors being better able to trigger immune system responses than HER2-positive or hormone receptor-positive breast cancer (Cortes et al., 2020; Loibl et al., 2019; Mittendorf et al., 2020; Nanda et al., 2020; Schmid et al., 2020). Importantly, TNBC tumors that generate more robust immune responses generally have better clinical outcomes than TNBC tumors with weaker immune responses. For example, a measure of the ability of a tumor to trigger immune responses is the observation of immune system cells such as lymphocytes invading within the tumor tissues. These immune system cells, often called "tumor-infiltrating lymphocytes" (TILs), have the ability to recognize cancer cells and—if appropriately stimulated—eradicate them. Compared with TNBC that contains low levels of TILs, patients with TNBC that contains high levels of TILs have better survival following adjuvant systemic therapy (Loi et al., 2019), higher rates of pCR following neoadjuvant systemic therapy (Denkert et al., 2018), and in select cases (such as in stage I TNBC) better survival even without systemic therapy (Leon-Ferre et al., 2018; Park et al., 2019; de Jong et al., 2022;

Leon-Ferre et al., 2024). TIL levels are also associated with prognosis and response to systemic therapy in HER2-positive breast cancer (Loi et al., 2014) but less so in hormone receptor-positive breast cancer (Criscitiello et al., 2020). As such, TILs and other features of immune activation are promising biomarkers that may allow clinicians to optimize systemic therapy for TNBC and possibly HER2-positive breast cancer in the future.

In the clinic, expression of a protein called programmed death-ligand 1 (PD-L1) in the tumor microenvironment is currently used to identify patients with metastatic TNBC who may benefit from immunotherapy. This protein can be found on the surface of tumor cells and in immune cells. When activated and through interactions with another protein (called programmed cell death protein 1 or PD-1), it sends a signal to T cells from the immune system to stop attacking the tumor cells, shielding them from eradication by the immune system. PD-1 and PD-L1 blocking medications effectively release the breaks from the immune system and restore the ability of T cells to recognize and attack breast cancer tumor cells.

Several studies have shown that in patients with metastatic TNBC, the addition of immunotherapy to chemotherapy only benefits patients whose tumors express PD-L1, whereas patients with tumors that are negative for PD-L1 do not appear to derive benefit. However, in patients with localized TNBC treated with multimodality approaches, the use of immunotherapy appears to benefit patients regardless of whether their tumors express PD-L1 or not. For this reason, testing for PD-L1 expression is only recommended in the setting of metastatic TNBC and not in early-stage TNBC. However, challenges with this biomarker remain, as there are multiple assays, methodologies and cutoff points to determine "positivity" versus "negativity" (Gonzalez-Ericsson et al., 2020).

Chemoimmunotherapy for Early-Stage Triple-Negative Breast Cancer

TNBC is more aggressive than other breast cancer subtypes and has historically been associated with higher and earlier rates of disease recurrence and death (Lin et al., 2012; Cortes et al., 2022; Bardia et al., 2021a). TNBC represents approximately 15% of all breast cancer cases and more often affects younger women and racial and ethnic minority groups including Black, Latina, and Indian women (Lin et al., 2012; Friebel-Klingner et al., 2021; DeSantis et al., 2019; Du, 2022; Kulkarni et al., 2020). As elaborated previously, modern management of early-stage TNBC generally favors administration of systemic therapy prior to surgery for several reasons, including the ability to assess the effect of the treatment on the tumor cells prior to being surgically removed. In TNBC, it has become very clear that attainment of pCR is strongly associated with lower recurrence rates and decreased mortality (Cortazar et al., 2014; Symmans et al., 2007; Boughey et al., 2017; Symmans et al., 2017; Yau et al., 2022). As such, one of the major goals of systemic therapy optimization has been to incorporate drugs that can increase pCR and subsequently improve long-term outcomes. Patients who do not achieve pCR can then be offered additional systemic therapy to further decrease risk of recurrence (Masuda et al., 2017).

Until recently, the mainstay of systemic therapy for TNBC was cytotoxic chemotherapy, often including a combination of an anthracycline (such as doxorubicin or epirubicin, among others) paired with cyclophosphamide and followed by (or preceded by) a taxane (such as paclitaxel or docetaxel). Several studies tested whether incorporating additional agents could improve the rates of pCR and long-term outcomes. The incorporation of immunotherapy agents (particularly pembrolizumab) to neoadjuvant chemotherapy has been one of the major advances of the management of early-stage TNBC, leading to improvements both on pCR rates and event-free survival (the time between treatment and the occurrence of a new "event" such as recurrence, a new primary cancer or death). The KEYNOTE-522 clinical trial evaluated the addition of pembrolizumab to a chemotherapy backbone consisting of carboplatin + paclitaxel followed by an anthracycline and cyclophosphamide (Schmid et al., 2020). In this trial, 1174 patients with newly diagnosed stage 2 or 3 TNBC were randomly assigned (in a 2:1 fashion) to receive IV pembrolizumab plus chemotherapy (paclitaxel and carboplatin followed by doxorubicin and cyclophosphamide) versus standard of care with chemotherapy plus placebo. Eligibility patients had newly diagnosed node-positive TNBC or tumors measuring ≥2 cm (regardless of nodal involvement). Patients with both PD-L1-positive and PD-L1-negative TNBC were eligible (although 84% in the treatment arm were PD-L1 positive). Following surgery, patients received nine additional cycles of adjuvant pembrolizumab or placebo every three weeks regardless of treatment response.

The incorporation of pembrolizumab to neoadjuvant chemotherapy increased the proportion of patients achieving a pCR (63%) compared to chemotherapy alone (56%), leading to an improvement in pCR rates of 7%. Furthermore, patients who received pembrolizumab displayed an improved event-free survival (85% with pembrolizumab compared to 77% with chemotherapy alone, an improvement of 8%). While patients who achieved pCR in either treatment arm had very similarly favorable outcomes (three-year EFS of 94% vs. 93% with or without immunotherapy), patients who had residual disease following treatment with immunotherapy had improved three-year event-free survival (67%) compared to those who received chemotherapy alone (57%).

As previously mentioned, PD-L1 expression does not appear to help distinguish which patients with early-stage TNBC benefit from the addition of pembrolizumab (unlike in the metastatic setting). However, in KEYNOTE-522, patients with TNBC expressing higher levels of PD-L1 demonstrated higher rates of pCR (both with and without immunotherapy).

Several outstanding questions remain in the field regarding the optimal incorporation of immunotherapy for early-stage TNBC. These are being actively research and include the following:

1. Can we identify who derives the most benefit from immunotherapy (i.e., are there other biomarkers beyond PD-L1 that can be used to select patients for treatment?)?
2. If immunotherapy is incorporated, can we use less intensive chemotherapy and maintain the same efficacy?
3. For patients who achieve pCR, do we need to continue immunotherapy after surgery?
4. For patients who do not achieve pCR, can we improve outcomes further by adding other drugs to pembrolizumab after surgery?

Regarding this last point, patients who have residual disease after neoadjuvant systemic therapy are often offered additional systemic therapy after surgery. Prior to the routine incorporation of immunotherapy in the neoadjuvant setting, the CREATE-X trial had demonstrated that administration of capecitabine (an oral chemotherapy drug) after surgery improved disease-free and overall survival in patients with TNBC and residual disease. In the CREATE-X trial, 910 patients with HER-2 negative residual invasive breast cancer, who were previously treated with an anthracycline/taxane-based regimen, were randomized to receive capecitabine versus control. Among patients with TNBC, disease-free survival in the capecitabine arm was 70% versus 56% in the control group. Overall survival was 79% in the capecitabine group and 70% in the placebo group. The question remains whether capecitabine paired with immunotherapy leads to better outcomes, but it is routinely done in clinical practice (Masuda et al., 2017). Additional options for gBRCA carriers with TNBC (or hormone receptor-positive breast cancer) include adjuvant PARP (poly adenosine diphosphate-ribose) inhibitors. Those with residual HER-2 negative disease after standard neoadjuvant chemotherapy were included in this trial of 1836 patients randomized in a 1:1 ratio to olaparib or placebo. Olaparib is associated with a 9% improvement in the three-year invasive disease-free survival (Tutt et al., 2021b).

Incorporation of immunotherapy is associated with additional toxicity that needs to be considered. Unlike other treatment settings, such as in metastatic cancers where long-term survival may be limited, or where the outcomes of patients are significantly worse without incorporation of immunotherapy, early-stage TNBC can be cured in most women. Immunotherapy toxicities, as elaborated in Chap. 15, can be long-lasting and life-altering. As such, the incremental improvement of pCR and event-free survival rates in the early-stage setting need to be carefully weighed against the potential for such toxicities. In KEYNOTE-522, the frequency of all treatment-related adverse events was similar between two treatment arms (nearly all patients experienced adverse events). However, the frequency of severe adverse events was higher with the incorporation of immunotherapy (77% with pembrolizumab, 72% without). Most of the severe adverse events happened during the preoperative systemic therapy phase.

Chemoimmunotherapy for Metastatic Triple-Negative Breast Cancer

Metastatic breast cancer (when cancer spreads beyond the breast and regional lymph nodes) remains incurable. When focusing specifically on TNBC, overall survival remains shorter than two years for most patients. For many years, the standard treatment remained limited to cytotoxic chemotherapy. Recently, progress in the understanding of TNBC has led to the identification of subgroups of patients with TNBC that may have tumors that are sensitive to specific targeted therapies, including immunotherapy. Unlike in the early-stage setting, and for reasons that are still not well understood, immunotherapy appears to offer a benefit only in patients whose tumors express higher levels of PD-L1 (recall that in the early-stage setting, a benefit was seen in all groups, whether tumors expressed or did not express PD-L1). Additionally, several studies have shown that in TNBC, immunotherapy appears to only improve outcomes when combined with traditional chemotherapy—unlike in other tumors like melanoma, where immunotherapy is effective even when used without chemotherapy—and when used as first-line therapy. Approximately 40–50% of TNBC tumors have high levels of PD-L1 and are eligible for immunotherapy. At the time of this writing, the only immunotherapy agent that is clinically used in the United States for metastatic TNBC is pembrolizumab and is used in combination with one of three chemotherapy options: paclitaxel, nab-paclitaxel, or a combination of gemcitabine and carboplatin. This is based on the KEYNOTE-355 trial (Cortes et al., 2020), which demonstrated that the addition of pembrolizumab to chemotherapy led to a significant improvement in progression-free survival and overall survival in patients with PD-L1-positive TNBC. A total of 847 participants with new diagnosis of metastatic TNBC (and who had not received prior treatment in the metastatic setting) were randomly assigned (in a 2:1 fashion) to receive pembrolizumab plus chemotherapy (physicians could choose between the three options mentioned previously) or chemotherapy alone (with placebo instead of pembrolizumab). Patients who had previously been treated for early-stage breast cancer and later developed metastatic disease were eligible if at least six months had elapsed since completion of curative intent therapy and development of metastatic disease.

KEYNOTE-355 also evaluated whether expression of PD-L1 would help identify patients who would benefit from the addition of pembrolizumab versus not but allowed enrollment of patients with tumors that were PD-L1 positive or negative. PD-L1 positivity was determined using a scoring method called the "combined positive score" (CPS). Patients whose tumors demonstrated a PD-L1 CPS ≥10 had the best overall outcomes and derived significant improvement with the addition of immunotherapy compared to chemotherapy alone. The median overall survival in this subset was 23 months with chemotherapy + pembrolizumab compared to 16 months with chemotherapy + placebo. At 18 months, the overall survival rate with chemotherapy + pembrolizumab was 58% compared to 45% with chemotherapy + placebo. Progression-free survival (time from study enrollment to cancer progression) was 9.7 months with chemotherapy + pembrolizumab compared to 5.6 months with chemotherapy + placebo. In comparison, patients whose tumors expressed lower levels of PD-L1 (CPS 1–9) or were PD-L1 negative did not appear to benefit from the addition of immunotherapy. For patients with PD-L1 CPS of 1–9, overall survival and progression-free survival were similar with or without pembrolizumab (14 vs. 16 months, respectively, for overall survival, and approximately 6 months for both groups for progression-free survival). Likewise, similar outcomes with or without pembrolizumab were seen for the PD-L-negative (CPS <1) subgroup (16 vs. 15 months, respectively, for overall survival; approximately 6 months for both groups for progression-free survival).

Atezolizumab + Chemotherapy in Metastatic TNBC

The first immunotherapy drug to be approved for metastatic PD-L1-positive TNBC was the PD-L1 inhibitor atezolizumab, in March 2019. However, in August 2021, Genentech (the manufacturer of atezolizumab) voluntarily withdrew the indication for TNBC, after conflicting results observed in two clinical trials. Initially, atezolizumab received accelerated approval by the FDA based on the phase 3 IMpassion130 trial (Schmid et al., 2018), which showed that the median progression-free survival was improved modestly (by approximately 2.5 months in both the entire population and in the PD-L1-positive group). However, while the median overall survival was numerically superior in the entire population (21 months with atezolizumab vs. 18 months without), these results were not statistically significant, precluding statistical assertions about the PD-L1 subgroup per protocol design. Nevertheless, given the numerically superior outcomes of patients treated with atezolizumab plus chemotherapy, the FDA granted accelerated approval of this regimen, with definitive approval being contingent on the results of a subsequent clinical trial: IMpassion131 (Miles et al., 2021). In this follow-up study, neither progression-free nor overall survival were improved in the PD-L1-positive subgroup or in the entire study population. After these results, Genentech decided to withdraw their indication for breast cancer in the United States. However, the drug continues to be approved by the European Medical Agency and continues to be available for metastatic PD-L1-positive TNBC in Europe. Atezolizumab is still being evaluated in clinical trials of breast cancer worldwide, including in the United States.

Monoclonal Antibodies and Antibody-Drug Conjugates

While not traditionally thought as a form of immunotherapy in the modern sense of the term, one of the first approaches leveraging tools from the immune system to treat cancer was the development of monoclonal antibodies. Antibodies are proteins made by a subset of immune cells (plasma cells, derived from the B lymphocytes) that function as the "bullets" of the immune system. These proteins attach to specific targets present in bacteria, viruses, and other entities that the immune system detects as different than "self" (including cancer cells). Using this framework, manmade modified versions of antibodies designed to target proteins present in cancer cells have been developed.

The first monoclonal antibody to find success in breast cancer was trastuzumab, which targets HER2, a protein that is overexpressed (present in excessive amounts) in 15–20% of breast cancers. Trastuzumab attaches to the portion of the HER2 protein that is outside of cancer cells and prevents the activation of its signaling pathway, halting the signals that lead to uncontrolled cell growth. Additionally, monoclonal antibodies can trigger a response from the immune system in a process called antibody-dependent cell-mediated cytotoxicity.

Building upon the success of monoclonal antibodies recognizing cell surface proteins in tumor cells, a new generation of drugs called antibody-drug conjugates (ADC) were developed. These drugs consist of "charged" monoclonal antibodies, where monoclonal antibodies targeting a specific protein are linked to a chemotherapy drug (known as the payload). This allows tumor-selective delivery of chemotherapy, concentrating the chemotherapy at tissues where the target protein is expressed in the highest quantities. The three key elements of the drug, the antibody, the linker, and the payload, define the spectrum of activity of the drug (which tumors they can target), their potency, their side effect profile, and the ability to affect neighboring cells that may not harbor the target antigen (known as bystander effect).

While HER2-targeted therapies have significantly contributed to the improvement of the outcomes of patients with HER2-positive breast cancer, the benefit of these drugs has been historically restricted to patients harboring tumors with high levels of HER2 expression (traditionally HER2-overexpressed or HER2-amplified tumors). However, next-generation ADCs with improved linkers and payloads exhibiting an ability to diffuse through cancer cell membranes have challenged this paradigm, demonstrating high antitumor efficacy even in tumors with lower levels of HER2 expression (previously categorized as HER2 "negative" or not amplified). These ADCs, such as trastuzumab deruxtecan (Cortés et al., 2022), are now approved for any HER2-expressing breast cancer (regardless of level of expression) and are changing the way we think about HER2 expression in breast cancer tumors. Furthermore, the activity of these drugs appears to be broad, with efficacy being shown in other tumor types, including gastrointestinal and pulmonary cancers. A major challenge remains the development of severe pulmonary toxicities with these agents, which have led to deaths in the initial clinical trials.

The technologies that led to the development of ADCs targeting HER2 have been leveraged to target other antigens in breast cancer and expand their benefit to other breast cancer subtypes. Sacituzumab govitecan, an ADC targeting Trop2, was the first ADC to demonstrate both a progression-free and overall survival in metastatic TNBC, demonstrating superiority over traditional cytotoxic chemotherapy (Bardia et al., 2021b). This drug has now demonstrated to also benefit patients with hormone-receptor-positive, HER2 not overexpressed breast cancer (Rugo et al., 2022). Furthermore, sacituzumab govitecan is being evaluated in patients with early-stage TNBC with residual disease after NAC, to determine whether it can improve cure rates compared to traditional therapy with pembrolizumab +/− capecitabine. Additionally, several ADCs are being studied in combination with immune checkpoint inhibitors (a few examples listed in Table 10.1).

Table 10.1 Select novel immunotherapy approaches under investigation for breast cancer

Intervention	Breast cancer population	Phase of trial	NCT
Immune checkpoint inhibitors			
Durvalumab + olaparib	Metastatic breast cancer with germline BRCA mutation	II	NCT02734004
Pembrolizumab + niraparib	Metastatic TNBC	II	NCT02657889
Durvalumab + olaparib + paclitaxel	Nonmetastatic HER2-negative	II	NCT01042379
Dostarlimab + niraparib	Nonmetastatic HER2-negative breast cancer with germline BRCA or PALB2 mutation	II	NCT04584255
Magrolimab + taxane or sacituzumab govitecan	Metastatic TNBC	II	NCT04958785
Pembrolizumab + sacituzumab govitecan	Metastatic PD-L1+ TNBC	III	NCT05382286
Bispecific antibodies			
Zanidatamab (targeting two distinct extracellular domains of HER2) + docetaxel	Metastatic HER2+ breast cancer	I	NCT04276493
Zanidatamab + endocrine therapy	Nonmetastatic, low-risk HER2+ breast cancer	II	NCT05035836
PF-07260437 (targeting B7-H4 and CD3)	Metastatic HER2-negative breast cancer	I	NCT05067972
Cellular therapies			
CAR-T targeting mesothelin	Mesothelin expressing metastatic breast cancer	I	NCT02792114
CAR-T targeting c-met	c-met expressing metastatic breast cancer	I	NCT03060356
CAR-T targeting MUC1	MUC1 expressing metastatic breast cancer	I	NCT04020575
CAR-T targeting ROR1	ROR1 expressing metastatic TNBC	I	NCT05274451
NKR-2 cells	Metastatic TNBC	I	NCT03018405
Autologous TILs (LN-145)	Metastatic TNBC	II	NCT04111510
Oncolytic viruses			
T-VEC + chemotherapy	Nonmetastatic TNBC	I/II	NCT02779855
T-VEC + atezolizumab	Metastatic TNBC	Ib	NCT03256344
Adenovirus (ADV/HSV-tk) + SBRT + pembrolizumab	Metastatic TNBC	II	NCT03004183
Modified measles virus (MV-s-NAP)	Metastatic breast cancer (all subtypes)	I	NCT04521764
LTX-315 + ipilimumab or pembrolizumab	Metastatic TNBC	I	NCT01986426
Vaccinia virus (TBio-6517) + pembrolizumab	Metastatic TNBC	I/II	NCT04301011
Vaccines			
Folate receptor alpha (multi-peptide)	Nonmetastatic TNBC	II	NCT03012100

(continued)

Table 10.1 (continued)

Intervention	Breast cancer population	Phase of trial	NCT
P10s-PADRE +/− chemotherapy	Nonmetastatic TNBC	II	NCT02938442
AE37 + pembrolizumab (peptide)	Metastatic TNBC	II	NCT04024800
PVX-410 + durvalumab (multi-peptide)	Non-metastatic TNBC	Ib	NCT02826434
PVX-410 +/− pembrolizumab (multi-peptide)	Metastatic TNBC	Ib	NCT03362060
Galinpepimut (WT1, multi-peptide)	Metastatic TNBC (and other cancers)	I/II	NCT03761914
Anti-HER2/HER3 DC	Metastatic TNBC or HER2+	II	NCT04348747

Future Directions of Immunotherapy for Breast Cancer

Beyond targeting the PD-1/PD-L1 axis, several novel approaches to immunotherapy are being actively investigated in breast cancer, particularly in the metastatic setting and for TNBC. These approaches include targeting other immune checkpoints (reviewed in more detail in Chap. 2), bispecific antibodies (reviewed in Chap. 3), cellular therapies (i.e., CAR-T cell therapy and TILs expanded ex vivo, reviewed in Chap. 4), virotherapy (reviewed in Chap. 5), and vaccine strategies. Select novel immunotherapy approaches are summarized in Table 10.1.

References

Antoniou, A., et al. (2003). Average risks of breast and ovarian cancer associated with BRCA1 or BRCA2 mutations detected in case series unselected for family history: A combined analysis of 22 studies. *The American Journal of Human Genetics, 72*(5), 1117–1130.

Bardia, A., et al. (2021a). Sacituzumab Govitecan in metastatic triple-negative breast cancer. *The New England Journal of Medicine, 384*(16), 1529–1541.

Bardia, A., et al. (2021b). Sacituzumab govitecan in metastatic triple-negative breast cancer. *New England Journal of Medicine, 384*(16), 1529–1541.

Boughey, J. C., et al. (2017). Tumor biology and response to chemotherapy impact breast cancer-specific survival in node-positive breast cancer patients treated with neoadjuvant chemotherapy: Long-term follow-up from ACOSOG Z1071 (Alliance). *Annals of Surgery, 266*(4), 667.

Boughey, J. C., et al. (2018). Surgical standards for management of the axilla in breast cancer clinical trials with pathological complete response endpoint. *npj Breast Cancer, 4*(1), 1–5.

Cao, Y., et al. (2015). Light to moderate intake of alcohol, drinking patterns, and risk of cancer: Results from two prospective US cohort studies. *BMJ, 351*, h4238.

Collaborative Group on Hormonal Factors in Breast Cancer. (2001). Familial breast cancer: Collaborative reanalysis of individual data from 52 epidemiological studies including 58 209 women with breast cancer and 101 986 women without the disease. *The Lancet, 358*(9291), 1389–1399.

Collaborative Group on Hormonal Factors in Breast Cancer. (2012). Menarche, menopause, and breast cancer risk: Individual participant meta-analysis, including 118 964 women with breast cancer from 117 epidemiological studies. *The Lancet Oncology, 13*(11), 1141–1151.

Cortazar, P., et al. (2014). Pathological complete response and long-term clinical benefit in breast cancer: The CTNeoBC pooled analysis. *The Lancet, 384*(9938), 164–172.

Cortes, J., et al. (2020). Pembrolizumab plus chemotherapy versus placebo plus chemotherapy for previously untreated locally recurrent inoperable or metastatic triple-negative breast cancer (KEYNOTE-355): A randomised, placebo-controlled, double-blind, phase 3 clinical trial. *The Lancet, 396*(10265), 1817–1828.

Cortes, J., et al. (2022). Pembrolizumab plus chemotherapy in advanced triple-negative breast cancer. *The New England Journal of Medicine, 387*(3), 217–226.

Cortés, J., et al. (2022). Trastuzumab deruxtecan versus trastuzumab emtansine for breast cancer. *New England Journal of Medicine, 386*(12), 1143–1154.

Criscitiello, C., et al. (2020). Tumor-infiltrating lymphocytes (TILs) in ER+/HER2− breast cancer. *Breast Cancer Research and Treatment, 183*(2), 347–354.

Denkert, C., et al. (2018). Tumour-infiltrating lymphocytes and prognosis in different subtypes of breast cancer: A pooled analysis of 3771 patients treated with neoadjuvant therapy. *The Lancet Oncology, 19*(1), 40–50.

DeSantis, C. E., et al. (2019). Breast cancer statistics, 2019. *CA: a Cancer Journal for Clinicians, 69*(6), 438–451.

Du, X. (2022). Racial disparities in health insurance, triple-negative breast cancer diagnosis, tumor stage, treatment and survival in a large nationwide SEER cohort in the United States. *Molecular and Clinical Oncology, 16*(4), 95.

Friebel-Klingner, T. M., et al. (2021). Risk factors for breast cancer subtypes among black women undergoing screening mammography. *Breast Cancer Research and Treatment, 189*(3), 827–835.

Gonzalez-Ericsson, P., et al. (2020). 1: CAS: 528: DC% 2BB3cXnvFKnu7w% 3D: The path to a better biomarker: Application of a risk management framework for the implementation of PD-L1 and TILs as immuno-oncology biomarkers in breast cancer clinical trials and daily practice. *The Journal of Pathology, 250*(5), 667–684.

Gram, I. T., et al. (2015). Smoking and risk of breast cancer in a racially/ethnically diverse population of mainly women who do not drink alcohol: The MEC study. *American Journal of Epidemiology, 182*(11), 917–925.

Henderson, T. O., et al. (2010). Systematic review: Surveillance for breast cancer in women treated with chest radiation for childhood, adolescent, or young adult cancer. *Annals of Internal Medicine, 152*(7), 444–455.

de Jong, V. M. T., et al. (2022). Prognostic value of stromal tumor-infiltrating lymphocytes in young, node-negative, triple-negative breast cancer patients who did not receive (neo)adjuvant systemic therapy. *Journal of Clinical Oncology, 40*(21), 2361–2374.

Kulkarni, A., et al. (2020). Meta-analysis of prevalence of triple-negative breast cancer and its clinical features at incidence in Indian patients with breast cancer. *JCO Global Oncology, 6*, 1052–1062.

Leon-Ferre, R. A., et al. (2018). Impact of histopathology, tumor-infiltrating lymphocytes, and adjuvant chemotherapy on prognosis of triple-negative breast cancer. *Breast Cancer Research and Treatment, 167*(1), 89–99.

Leon-Ferre, R., et al. (2024). Tumor-Infiltrating Lymphocytes in Triple-Negative Breast Cancer. *JAMA, 331*(13), 1135–1144. https://doi.org/10.1001/jama.2024.3056

Lin, N. U., et al. (2012). Clinicopathologic features, patterns of recurrence, and survival among women with triple-negative breast cancer in the National Comprehensive Cancer Network. *Cancer, 118*(22), 5463–5472.

Loi, S., et al. (2014). Tumor infiltrating lymphocytes are prognostic in triple negative breast cancer and predictive for trastuzumab benefit in early breast cancer: Results from the FinHER trial. *Annals of Oncology, 25*(8), 1544–1550.

Loi, S., et al. (2019). Tumor-infiltrating lymphocytes and prognosis: A pooled individual patient analysis of early-stage triple-negative breast cancers. *Journal of Clinical Oncology, 37*(7), 559–569.

Loibl, S., et al. (2019). A randomised phase II study investigating durvalumab in addition to an anthracycline taxane-based neoadjuvant therapy in early triple-negative breast cancer: Clinical results and biomarker analysis of GeparNuevo study. *Annals of Oncology, 30*(8), 1279–1288.

Masuda, N., et al. (2017). Adjuvant capecitabine for breast cancer after preoperative chemotherapy. *New England Journal of Medicine, 376*(22), 2147–2159.

Miles, D., et al. (2021). Primary results from IMpassion131, a double-blind, placebo-controlled, randomised phase III trial of first-line paclitaxel with or without atezolizumab for unresectable locally advanced/metastatic triple-negative breast cancer. *Annals of Oncology, 32*(8), 994–1004.

Mittendorf, E. A., et al. (2020). Neoadjuvant atezolizumab in combination with sequential nab-paclitaxel and anthracycline-based chemotherapy versus placebo and chemotherapy in patients with early-stage triple-negative breast cancer (IMpassion031): A randomised, double-blind, phase 3 trial. *The Lancet, 396*(10257), 1090–1100.

Morimoto, L. M., et al. (2002). Obesity, body size, and risk of postmenopausal breast cancer: The Women's Health Initiative (United States). *Cancer Causes & Control, 13*, 741–751.

Murthy, R. K., et al. (2020). Tucatinib, trastuzumab, and capecitabine for HER2-positive metastatic breast cancer. *New England Journal of Medicine, 382*(7), 597–609.

Nanda, R., et al. (2020). Effect of pembrolizumab plus neoadjuvant chemotherapy on pathologic complete response in women with early-stage breast cancer: An analysis of the ongoing phase 2 adaptively randomized I-SPY2 trial. *JAMA Oncology, 6*(5), 676–684.

Park, J. H., et al. (2019). Prognostic value of tumor-infiltrating lymphocytes in patients with early-stage triple-negative breast cancers (TNBC) who did not receive adjuvant chemotherapy. *Annals of Oncology, 30*(12), 1941–1949.

Piltin, M. A., et al. (2020). Oncologic outcomes of sentinel lymph node surgery after neoadjuvant chemotherapy for node-positive breast cancer. *Annals of Surgical Oncology, 27*(12), 4795–4801.

Poortmans, P. M., et al. (2015). Internal mammary and medial supraclavicular irradiation in breast cancer. *New England Journal of Medicine, 373*(4), 317–327.

Rahman, N., et al. (2007). PALB2, which encodes a BRCA2-interacting protein, is a breast cancer susceptibility gene. *Nature Genetics, 39*(2), 165–167.

Rosner, B., Colditz, G. A., & Willett, W. C. (1994). Reproductive risk factors in a prospective study of breast cancer: The Nurses' Health Study. *American Journal of Epidemiology, 139*(8), 819–835.

Rugo, H. S., et al. (2022). Sacituzumab govitecan in hormone receptor–positive/human epidermal growth factor receptor 2–negative metastatic breast cancer. *Journal of Clinical Oncology, 40*(29), 3365–3376.

Schmid, P., et al. (2018). Atezolizumab and nab-paclitaxel in advanced triple-negative breast cancer. *New England Journal of Medicine, 379*(22), 2108–2121.

Schmid, P., et al. (2020). Pembrolizumab for early triple-negative breast cancer. *The New England Journal of Medicine, 382*(9), 810–821.

Siegel, R. L., et al. (2024). Cancer statistics, 2023. *CA: a Cancer Journal for Clinicians, 73*(1), 17–48. https://doi.org/10.3322/caac.21820

Symmans, W. F., et al. (2007). Measurement of residual breast cancer burden to predict survival after neoadjuvant chemotherapy. *Journal of Clinical Oncology, 25*(28), 4414–4422.

Symmans, W. F., et al. (2017). Long-term prognostic risk after neoadjuvant chemotherapy associated with residual cancer burden and breast cancer subtype. *Journal of Clinical Oncology, 35*(10), 1049.

Tutt, A. N. J., et al. (2021a). Adjuvant Olaparib for patients with BRCA1- or BRCA2-mutated breast cancer. *The New England Journal of Medicine, 384*(25), 2394–2405.

Tutt, A. N., et al. (2021b). Adjuvant olaparib for patients with BRCA1-or BRCA2-mutated breast cancer. *New England Journal of Medicine, 384*(25), 2394–2405.

Whelan, T. J., et al. (2015). Regional nodal irradiation in early-stage breast cancer. *New England Journal of Medicine, 373*(4), 307–316.

Yau, C., et al. (2022). Residual cancer burden after neoadjuvant chemotherapy and long-term survival outcomes in breast cancer: A multicentre pooled analysis of 5161 patients. *The Lancet Oncology, 23*(1), 149–160.

Chapter 11
Immunotherapy in Genitourinary Malignancies

Jacob Orme

Abstract Different genitourinary cancers—that is, the cancers of the urinary tract (kidney and bladder/urothelial) and male genitalia (prostate, testicles, and penis)—respond differently to immunotherapy. Currently, immunotherapies are most important in kidney and bladder/urothelial cancers and are often the first-line therapy. There are fewer current indications for prostate and penile cancers and no current role for immunotherapy in testicular cancer.

Keywords Kidney · Urothelial · Bladder · Testicular · Prostate · Penile · Enfortumab · Adjuvant · Neoadjuvant · Unresectable · Muscle invasive

Kidney/Renal Cell Carcinomas

Introduction

Renal cell carcinoma (RCC) is a heterogeneous group of kidney cancers that exhibit distinct histological features and biological behaviors. The classification of RCC is based on histological subtypes and tumor grades, which provide valuable information about prognosis, treatment strategies, and likely outcomes.

Clear cell renal cell carcinoma (ccRCC) is the most common RCC subtype, accounting for approximately 75% of cases. Microscopically, ccRCC is characterized by a clear or pale cytoplasm due to the accumulation of lipids and glycogen within the tumor cells. ccRCC tends to be aggressive and higher grade than other histologic types, with a higher likelihood of metastasis. However, it is also known to respond well to a combination of ICI and a type of targeted therapy termed tyrosine kinase inhibitors (TKIs).

J. Orme (✉)
Department of Oncology, Mayo Clinic, Rochester, MN, USA
e-mail: orme.jacob@mayo.edu

© The Author(s), under exclusive license to Springer Nature Switzerland AG 2024   141
H. Dong, S. N. Markovic (eds.), *The Basics of Cancer Immunotherapy*,
https://doi.org/10.1007/978-3-031-59475-5_11

The remaining 25% of RCC cases are termed non-clear cell RCC (nccRCC). Papillary carcinoma accounts for about 10–15% of RCC cases. It is further classified into types 1 and 2. Type 1 papillary carcinoma has a more indolent course, while type 2 is associated with a higher risk of progression and metastasis. Papillary RCCs exhibit a papillary growth pattern and display varying degrees of nuclear atypia. They are often linked to genetic mutations in the MET proto-oncogene. They tend to be less responsive to traditional immunotherapy than ccRCC.

Chromophobe carcinoma constitutes approximately 5% of RCC cases. Histologically, chromophobe RCC comprises large cells pale and granular cytoplasm. Other rare subtypes of RCC include collecting duct carcinoma and renal medullary carcinoma. These are less common and may require specialized management approaches. In addition, there are renal-collecting duct carcinomas—a subset of which are renal medullary carcinomas that are aggressive and sometimes associated with sickle cell anemia—that tend to resemble urothelial carcinomas and are usually treated with chemotherapy.

Renal Cell Carcinoma Grade, Stage, and Risk

Selecting treatment and determining prognosis of common RCC histologies depends on grade, stage, and overall risk of disease. Tumor grading in RCC is typically assessed using the Fuhrman grading system (Fuhrman et al., 1982), which assigns a grade from 1 to 4 based on cancer cell nuclear diameter, shape, lobe count, and overall consistency. Higher grades indicate more aggressive tumor behavior and worse prognosis. Often, systemic therapy can be deferred for grade 1–2 tumors even when metastatic.

Staging is the next essential component of determining the appropriate approach to treatment in RCC (Motzer et al., 2022). Staging is most commonly performed with the TNM system comprising size and extent of the primary tumor (T), involvement of lymph nodes (N), and distant metastatic spread (M). In stage I disease, the tumor is confined to the kidney and is 7 cm or smaller in size (T1) without regional lymph node involvement (N0) or distant metastasis (M0). In stage II disease, the tumor may be larger than 7 cm (T2) but is confined to the kidney (N0M0). Stage III is reached when the tumor involves the renal vein, perinephric fat, adrenal gland, or other nearby structures including the renal vein or vena cava above the diaphragm (T3) or when any regional lymph node is involved (N1). Stage IV disease is reached when the tumor extends beyond Gerota's fascia, involves an ipsilateral adrenal gland, or has distant metastases (M1). These metastases most commonly involve distant lymph nodes, bones, lungs, liver, or other organs.

Treatment options change significantly for ccRCC and some nccRCC depending on stage (see Fig. 11.1). Broadly, stage I disease usually does not benefit from systemic therapy (including immunotherapy) after surgery. In contrast, some patients with certain risk factors with stage II/stage III disease may benefit from

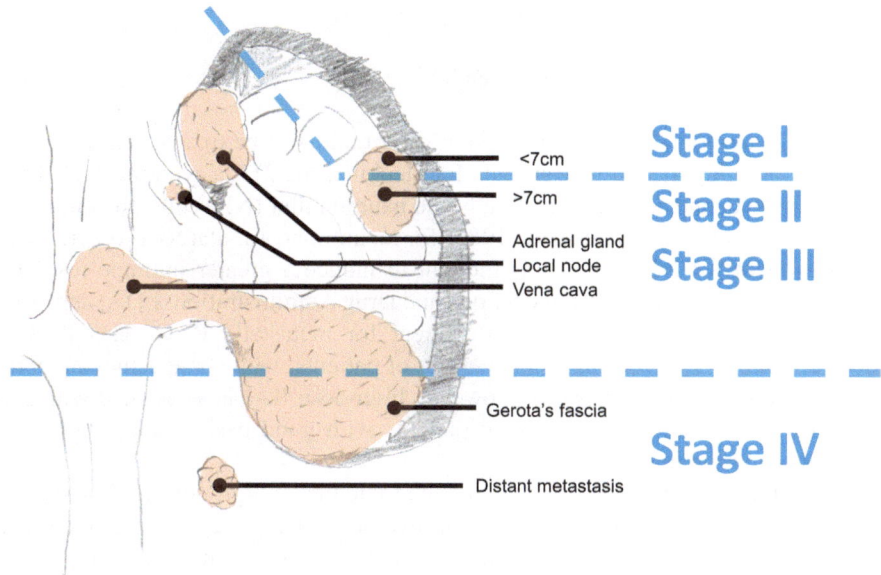

Fig. 11.1 Kidney cancers are commonly divided by stage depending on size and involvement of local and/or distant structures, which inform treatment options

immunotherapy after surgery in some circumstances (see "Adjuvant Immunotherapy in ccRCC"). Patients with unresectable and/or stage IV disease usually derive the most benefit from systemic therapy depending on tumor grading, risk factors, and comorbidities.

Risk stratification beyond grade and stage plays a crucial role in predicting prognosis, selecting appropriate treatment strategies, and guiding clinical decision-making. Two commonly used risk stratification systems for RCC are the Motzer Score (previously known as the Memorial Sloan Kettering Cancer Center or MKSCC score) (Motzer et al., 2002) and the International Metastatic Renal Cell Carcinoma Database Consortium (IMDC) Heng Risk score (Heng et al., 2009).

The Motzer Score takes into account clinical and laboratory parameters to classify patients into three risk categories: favorable, intermediate, and poor. Patients with poor Karnofsky performance status (KPS), delayed treatment, low hemoglobin (anemia), elevated corrected calcium levels, and increased LDH are expected to experience a worse prognosis. The IMDC Heng Risk score similarly includes KPS, delayed treatment, hemoglobin, and corrected calcium but also neutrophil/platelet levels (and does not include LDH). Both scores have demonstrated utility in risk stratification and predicting outcomes in advanced or metastatic RCC and can be used to guide treatment for metastatic disease.

Immunotherapy in Renal Cell Carcinoma

History of Immune Modulation in RCC

Renal cell carcinoma was one of the first solid tumors to be treated with systemic therapies targeting the immune system. Interleukin 2 (IL-2) is a cytokine that stimulates the growth and activation of T cells and natural killer (NK) cells. Recombinant IL-2 was used clinically first in the 1980s for its immunostimulatory properties and as a treatment for RCC. IL-2 was thought to induce a greater immune response against cancer cells. In 1992, the US Food and Drug Administration (FDA) approved high-dose IL-2 (aldesleukin) as a treatment for metastatic RCC. This therapy showed durable responses in a small subset of patients, with some achieving complete and long-lasting remissions. However, high-dose IL-2 is associated with significant toxicities and was limited to patients with good performance status and normal organ function.

Due to the limited efficacy and significant toxicities of high-dose IL-2, researchers explored combination therapies to improve outcomes. IL-2 was combined with other immunotherapies, such as interferon-alpha, to enhance response rates. However, toxicity remained a challenge. In the 2000s, targeted therapies revolutionized the treatment of RCC, and alternative treatments like tyrosine kinase inhibitors (TKIs) targeting vascular endothelial growth factor (VEGF) receptors and mammalian target of rapamycin (mTOR) inhibitors showed improved response rates and progression-free survival compared to IL-2. These targeted therapies became the standard of care for most patients with advanced RCC.

Immunotherapy in Metastatic ccRCC

The advent of immune checkpoint inhibitors, specifically Programmed death-1 (PD-1) and Programmed death ligand-1 (PD-L1) inhibitors, ushered in a new era of immune modulation in RCC. Pembrolizumab and nivolumab, PD-1 inhibitors, were approved for advanced RCC patients who progressed on prior targeted therapies. These inhibitors effectively reinvigorated the immune response against cancer cells. Most of the evidence for immunotherapy in RCC has been for ccRCC. Papillary and chromophobe subtypes are commonly treated with TKI alone or with an mTOR inhibitor, as nccRCC experience demonstrably poorer responses to immunotherapy (McDermott et al., 2021).

Clinical trials have gone on to evaluate the combination of immune checkpoint inhibitors with targeted therapies in ccRCC. The combination of immune checkpoint inhibitors (e.g., avelumab, nivolumab, pembrolizumab) with VEGF inhibitors (e.g., axitinib, cabozantinib, lenvatinib, also called tyrosine kinase inhibitors or TKIs) has repeatedly shown improved overall survival and progression-free survival compared to sunitinib, a standard VEGF-targeted therapy in clinical trials (Table 11.1).

Table 11.1 Current clinical trials of combination therapy in renal cell carcinoma

Regimen	ORR (%)	Risk group	Trial
Avelumab + axitinib	55%	Any	JAVELIN Renal-101 (NCT02684006) Motzer et al. (2019)
Pembrolizumab + axitinib	60%	Any	KEYNOTE-426 (NCT02853331) Powles et al. (2020a)
Nivolumab + cabozantinib	56%	Any	CheckMate-9ER (NCT03141177) Choueiri et al. (2021a)
Pembrolizumab + lenvatinib	71%	Any	CLEAR (NCT02811861) Motzer et al. (2021)
Atezolizumab and cabozantinib	58%	Not yet approved	COSMIC-021 (NCT03170960) Pal et al. (2021)
Nivolumab/ipilimumab (no TKI)	42%	Intermediate/poor	CheckMate-214 (NCT02231749)

In clinical practice, four combinations (in alphabetical order: avelumab/axitinib, nivolumab/cabozantinib, pembrolizumab/axitinib, pembrolizumab/lenvatinib) are commonly used for any risk metastatic ccRCC. None of these regimens have been compared head-to-head and are thought to be similarly efficacious.

JAVELIN Renal-101 (NCT02684006) was a phase III clinical trial that evaluated the efficacy and safety of avelumab in combination with axitinib as a first-line treatment for advanced RCC (Motzer et al., 2019). The trial compared avelumab/axitinib combination therapy to sunitinib and demonstrated improved progression-free survival (median 13.8 months, HR 0.69 [95% CI 0.56–0.84]) and response rate (55.2%) in patients receiving avelumab plus axitinib compared to sunitinib, leading to the approval of this regimen for certain patients with advanced RCC.

Similarly, KEYNOTE-426 (NCT02853331) compared pembrolizumab/axitinib in first-line treatment to sunitinib (Powles et al., 2020a). The trial demonstrated significantly improved overall survival (median not reached, HR 0.53 [95% CI 0.38–0.74]), progression-free survival (median 15.1 months, HR 0.69 [95% CI 0.57–0.84]), and objective response rate (59.3%) in patients receiving pembrolizumab plus axitinib compared to sunitinib, leading to the approval of this regimen for certain patients with advanced ccRCC.

Also similarly, CheckMate-9ER (NCT03141177) compared nivolumab/cabozantinib to sunitinib in ccRCC (Choueiri et al., 2021a). The trial demonstrated superior overall survival (median not reached, HR 0.60 [reported 98.89% CI 0.40–0.89]), progression-free survival (median 16.6 months, HR 0.51 [95% CI 0.41–0.6]), and objective response rate (55.7%) in patients receiving nivolumab plus cabozantinib compared to sunitinib, leading to the approval of this regimen for certain patients with advanced ccRCC.

Lastly, CLEAR (NCT02811861) compared pembrolizumab/lenvatinib to both lenvatinib/everolimus and sunitinib in ccRCC (Motzer et al., 2021). The trial demonstrated significantly improved overall survival (median not reached, HR 0.66

[95% CI 0.48–0.88]), progression-free survival (median 23.9 months, HR 0.47 [95% CI 0.38–0.58]), and objective response rate (71%) in patients receiving lenvatinib plus pembrolizumab compared to sunitinib, leading to the approval of this regimen for certain patients with advanced ccRCC.

The above clinical trials have not been compared head-to-head, and we generally advocate selecting treatment based on the clinician's experience, drug availability/affordability, and convenience of administration. Side effects from TKIs are generally similar and can include diarrhea, blood pressure elevation, hand/foot syndrome (a red rash on the palms and soles), voice changes, and increased risk of bleeding. The doses of each of these TKIs can be adjusted to minimize side effects.

An additional trial, CheckMate-214, has also shown ICI efficacy without a TKI in intermediate- and poor-risk ccRCC (NCT02231749) (Motzer et al., 2018). In this phase III clinical trial, nivolumab was combined with ipilimumab, a cytotoxic T-lymphocyte-associated protein 4 (CTLA-4) inhibitor, as a first-line treatment for advanced RCC. Notably, patients with good risk (by Heng/IMDC) disease were excluded from this trial. The trial demonstrated improved overall survival and objective response rates in patients receiving nivolumab plus ipilimumab compared to sunitinib, leading to the approval of this combination. In clinical practice, some clinicians advocate the use of this combination in young patients with good risk disease not requiring a dramatic response.

A particularly important question in the field of ccRCC is whether immunotherapy should be used in the second-line after the failure of a first-line immunotherapy. For instance, after failure of combination pembrolizumab/axitinib, should a patient start atezolizumab/cabozantinib or simply use single-agent cabozantinib? This question was at least partially addressed in the phase III CONTACT-03 trial (NCT04338269) in which an interim overall survival analysis showed no significant benefit of combined atezolizumab/cabozantinib versus cabozantinib alone in the second-line after prior immunotherapy (ORR 40.5% versus 40.9%, PFS 10.6 versus 10.8 months, $p = 0.784$ and OS 25.7 months versus NE, $p = 0.690$) (Albiges et al., 2023). Many clinicians advise against reexposure to immunotherapy given these data, although other ICI combinations have not been tested in this setting.

Adjuvant Immunotherapy in ccRCC

The most common treatment for stage I through stage III kidney cancer is nephrectomy—surgical resection of all or part of the involved kidney. Surgical resection has been extremely important. Most kidney cancers do not respond well to chemotherapy. For patients with certain characteristics, however, there is a very high risk of disease recurrence. Thus, adjuvant (i.e., postsurgical) treatments to prevent recurrence may be useful in some circumstances. Pembrolizumab was tested in the adjuvant setting for patients with ccRCC in KEYNOTE 564 (NCT03142334) (Choueiri et al., 2021b). Patients with high-risk features including stage II disease with high-grade (i.e., grade 4 of 4) or sarcomatoid features, any stage III disease, or M1 disease rendered NED (no evidence of disease) by surgery and were included in the study. They were randomized to receive up to 1 year (or 17 cycles) pembrolizumab or placebo. Patients in the pembrolizumab group experienced an improved two-year disease-free survival (77.3%) than those in the placebo group (68.1%) in the study (DFS HR 0.68, [95% CI 0.53–0.87], $p = 0.002$). In addition, there was a small overall survival benefit (HR 0.54, 95% CI 0.3–0.96).

While KEYNOTE 564 was a positive study reaching its prespecified endpoint, the disease-free survival at 3 years was nearly identical. Nineteen percent of patients receiving pembrolizumab experienced grade 3 AEs. In clinical practice, each patient is different and each has different preferences. Commonly, we see young patients who wish to be as aggressive as possible take the added risk of immunotherapy while older patients with competing comorbidities often defer systemic therapy in hopes of never requiring it.

Bladder/Urothelial Cancers

Introduction

Bladder cancer is the most common urinary system cancer with over 80,000 cases and nearly 17,000 deaths each year (Siegel et al., 2023). Most bladder cancers are urothelial (also known as transitional cell) carcinomas. Most of the available data on immunotherapy in bladder cancers is based on urothelial cancers that arise directly from the bladder. However, some bladder cancers comprise other histologies (e.g., squamous cell carcinoma, small cell carcinoma, adenocarcinoma, and mixed), and some urothelial cancers also arise from outside the bladder, including from the ureters and renal pelvis (together termed upper tract urothelial cancers or UTUC).

Associated risk factors for bladder cancer include tobacco use, occupational exposures to aniline dyes, and inflammatory conditions of the bladder such as schistosomiasis. Any chronic bladder inflammation can lead to bladder cancer, including chronic urinary tract infections, consumption of aristolochic acid, and exposure to arylamines, benzene, plastics, and petrochemicals. Some medical treatments, including cyclophosphamide, thorium dioxide, and radiation therapy, can also elevate the risk of developing bladder and urothelial cancers. Similarly, genetic syndromes like Balkan nephropathy have been associated with increased bladder cancer risk.

Staging

Bladder cancer staging—that is, determination of the extent of the cancer—is critical for selecting appropriate treatment (Flaig et al., 2022). Staging is most commonly performed with the TNM system comprising size and extent of the primary tumor (T), involvement of lymph nodes (N), and distant metastatic spread (M). A numerical stage from I to IV is assigned based on TNM results. Two critical thresholds are reached when urothelial carcinoma becomes muscle-invasive (T2a), termed muscle-invasive bladder cancer (MIBC) as distinct from non-muscle-invasive bladder cancer (NMIBC), and when urothelial carcinoma either invades adjacent organs like the prostate, vagina, uterus, or bowel (T4b) or becomes distantly metastatic (M1), which is termed unresectable (Abu-Rustum et al., 2023). Notably, not all lymph node or metastatic involvement is truly unresectable and will depend on surgical consultation. For treatment decisions, it is useful to think of bladder cancers as either NMIBC, MIBC, or unresectable (Fig. 11.2). However, there are nuances that a qualified medical oncologist will consider for any given treatment.

Broadly speaking, NMIBC and MIBC may be curable with a combination of systemic and localized (i.e., surgical or radiotherapeutic) modalities. However, patients with unresectable disease are rarely rendered "no evidence of disease" (NED) and thus have much poorer outcomes. For this reason, most clinicians aggressively treat NMIBC and MIBC with a goal of definitive surgical resection. In most cases, immunotherapy is used alongside other treatment types—commonly platinum-containing chemotherapy regimens—in order to provide the greatest opportunity to achieve NED. This is particularly important in bladder cancer, because unresectable disease is associated with poor overall survival.

Urothelial carcinoma can exhibit variant histologies, which are characterized by distinct morphological patterns and behavior. These variants include squamous cell

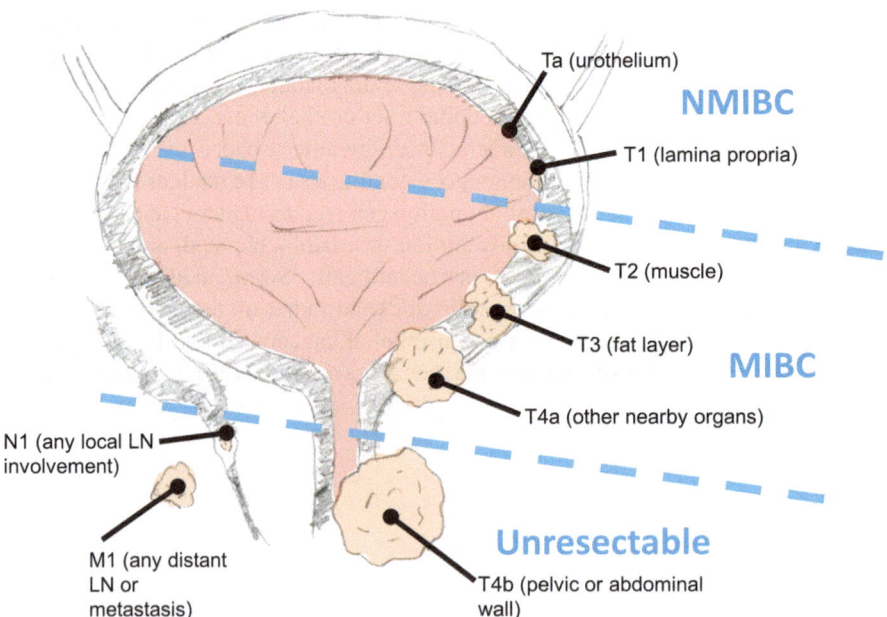

Fig. 11.2 Bladder and urothelial cancers are divided into non-muscle invasive, muscle-invasive, and unresectable for treatment selection

carcinoma, adenocarcinoma, small cell carcinoma, micropapillary carcinoma, and plasmacytoid carcinoma. The location along the urinary tract (e.g., in the bladder itself versus UTUC arising from the upper tracts or from the urethra) is also important to consider, as biologically different tumors may arise from a different embryonic source in each location. These variants have unique clinical characteristics and treatment approaches compared to typical urothelial carcinoma arising from the bladder.

Immunotherapy in Bladder Cancer

Immunotherapy in Non-muscle-Invasive Bladder Cancer (NMIBC)

Bacillus Calmette-Guérin (BCG) is a weakened strain of mycobacterium that is commonly instilled in the bladder for patients with localized NMIBC. This intravesicular BCG treatment incites an immune response in the bladder environment that helps clear remaining tumor cells. Most commonly, BCG is given in weekly instillations in an induction phase of approximately 6 weeks followed by 3-week maintenance courses thereafter. Risks include local reactions like bladder irritability, dysuria, and hematuria as well as systemic flu-like symptoms, fever, and malaise. In very rare instances, systemic infection with BCG has been observed. BCG is not recommended in cases of traumatic catheterization, bacteriuria, persistent gross hematuria, persistent severe local symptoms, or systemic symptoms. Alternatively, some localized bladder cancers are treated with instilled chemotherapy rather than BCG.

Approximately 30% of localized NMIBC do not respond to BCG immunotherapy, while others experience disease recurrence or progression despite initial response. In cases where cancers are unresponsive or recur without muscle invasion, immunotherapy with immune checkpoint inhibitor (ICI) pembrolizumab has been studied in the KEYNOTE-057 trial (NCT02625961) (Balar et al., 2021). In this study, patients with carcinoma in situ with Eastern Cooperative Oncology Group (ECOG) performance status 0–2 received 200 mg intravenous pembrolizumab every 3 weeks for up to 2 years or until disease persistence, recurrence, or progression or until discontinuation for any reason. The primary endpoint was complete response rate (defined as no persistence or progression of disease) assessed by cystoscopy after 3 months. Of 96 patients with BCG-unresponsive bladder cancer who received pembrolizumab on the study, 39 (41%) had a complete response at 3 months. Of those, approximately 50% of patients enjoyed disease-free survival for at least 1 year and 98% were alive after 1 year. Thirteen percent of patients experienced grade 3 or 4 treatment-related adverse events. The median duration of treatment on study was 4.2 months. Notably, there are other non-immunotherapy options available in this setting that should also be considered.

Immunotherapy in Localized Muscle-Invasive Bladder Cancer (MIBC)

Muscle invasion significantly elevates the risk of death from bladder cancer and, consequently, increases the importance of curative-intent therapy where possible. The most common treatment approach for MIBC is neoadjuvant (i.e., before surgery) chemotherapy including cisplatin where possible with the goals of (A) simplifying and improving surgical efficacy as measured by improved disease-free survival, (B) determining the risk of recurrence based on post-chemotherapy pathology characteristics, and (C) ensuring that the disease is truly resectable before undergoing an intensive surgery.

It is known that residual disease—particularly postchemotherapy T2-T4 or node-positive (N1)—in the surgical specimen after chemotherapy portends a higher risk of recurrence. For patients with these characteristics, the CheckMate-274 study sought to determine whether adjuvant (i.e., post-surgery) nivolumab could improve a 6-month disease-free survival (DFS) (NCT02632409) (Bajorin et al., 2021). In brief, this study enrolled 709 patients who either (A) had received neoadjuvant platinum-containing chemotherapy and had residual T2–T4 or node-positive (N1) disease or (B) had not received neoadjuvant chemotherapy and had T3, T4, or N1 disease. Patients were randomized to receive nivolumab or placebo. The median disease-free survival in patients treated with nivolumab was 20.8 months (95% CI 16.5–27.6 months) versus 10.8 months (95% CI 8.3–13.9 months) with placebo (p < 0.001). Interestingly, this was not significantly different for patients with PD-L1-positive (defined as PD-L1 expression of 1% or more) versus those with PD-L1-negative disease. Overall survival results are not yet mature for this study.

It is uncertain how broadly these observations apply to other circumstances. For instance, relatively few patients with upper tract urothelial cancers (UTUC, that is, urothelial cancers above the bladder in the ureters or close to the kidneys) were included in CheckMate-274 (21% of patients). It is thought that these tumors may be *less* responsive to immunotherapy than regular bladder cancers, and clinical trials addressing appropriate immunotherapies in UTUC are ongoing. Many patients with UTUC have Lynch syndrome with alterations in DNA mismatch repair genes such as MLH1 and MSH2, which may increase the likelihood of response. Genetic testing in advanced bladder cancer is advised to help direct targeted therapies, including immunotherapy.

Notably, some immunotherapies have also been ineffective in this adjuvant setting. In the IMvigor010 trial, which enrolled patients very similar to the CheckMate-274 trial, patients with bladder cancers were randomized to receive atezolizumab versus observation (Bellmunt et al., 2021). Median disease-free survival was not significantly improved (19.4 versus 16.6 months, HR 0.89 [95% CI 0.74–1.08]). Atezolizumab is not approved for adjuvant use in bladder cancer.

Immunotherapy in Unresectable Bladder Cancer

Bladder cancer that is unresectable—whether due to wide metastatic spread or contraindications to localized therapies—presents a significant and dangerous disease. Until recently, cisplatin-based chemotherapy remains the most commonly used first-line therapy (Flaig et al., 2022). However, immunotherapy-based approaches are gaining traction in three broad groups: (A) as co-therapies with targeted chemotherapy, (B) as maintenance therapies after response to chemotherapy, and (C) as later-line monotherapies for patients with contraindications to chemotherapy (e.g., in patients with kidney disease that makes cisplatin and/or carboplatin chemotherapy untenable).

The combination of pembrolizumab with enfortumab vedotin in EV103/KEYNOTE-869 (NCT03288545) has recently led to approval from the FDA as a first-line therapy in unresectable bladder cancer (Hoimes et al., 2023). Enfortumab vedotin is a chemotherapy-conjugated anti-Nectin-4 therapeutic antibody (also termed an antibody-drug conjugate or ADC). In this early-phase trial, 45 patients who were not eligible for or refused platinum-based chemotherapy received enfortumab vedotin (1.25 mg/kg) on days 1 and 8 and pembrolizumab (200 mg) intravenously once every 3 weeks. The confirmed objective response rate after a median of nine cycles was 73.3%, with a complete response rate of 15.6%. The median duration of response and overall survival were 25.6 months and 26.1 months, respectively. As a result, many oncologists use combination enfortumab vedotin and pembrolizumab as a first- or second-line treatment in cisplatin-ineligible or refractory settings, respectively. However, in clinical practice, the rates of peripheral neuropathy, rash, and fatigue can limit the added value of enfortumab vedotin.

Similar emerging data may suggest a further role for combining chemotherapy and immunotherapy in unresectable bladder cancer. CheckMate-901 (NCT03036098) tested multiple immunotherapy combinations to standard of care cisplatin/gemcitabine. In previously reported results, nivolumab/ipilimumab failed to improve overall or progression-free survival. However, although the official results have not been reported formally, it has been confirmed that nivolumab/cisplatin/gemcitabine met its combined overall and progression-free survival endpoint and is superior to cisplatin/gemcitabine alone. Additional data are pending and the combination has not yet been evaluated for approval by the FDA.

Maintenance therapies are treatments with favorable toxicity that are used to maintain therapeutic gains after harsher treatments such as cisplatin-based chemotherapy. Avelumab is an approved immunotherapy for patients with partial response (PR), complete response (CR), or stable disease (SD) after platinum-based chemotherapy as studied in the JAVELIN BLADDER 100 trial (NCT02603432) (Powles et al., 2020b). In this clinical trial, 700 patients were randomized to receive avelumab maintenance therapy versus observation after 4–6 cycles of gemcitabine/cisplatin or gemcitabine/carboplatin. Only patients who experienced SD or better were included in the study. A striking improvement in a 1-year overall survival (71.3% in the avelumab group and 58.4% in the control group) was observed. Median overall survival was 21.4 months versus 14.3 months (HR 0.69 [95% CI 0.56–0.86], $p = 0.001$). While these gains are meaningful and we recommend maintenance immunotherapy in patients who fit these criteria, most patients in both arms experienced eventual disease progression.

Many patients cannot receive platinum-containing chemotherapies, and these chemotherapies eventually fail for most patients with advanced bladder cancers. In the absence or failure of prior chemotherapy regimens, ICI therapies offer important additional approaches. Pembrolizumab, studied in the KEYNOTE-045 trial (NCT02256436), showed promising results in patients with advanced urothelial carcinoma who experienced progression after cisplatin-based chemotherapy (Bellmunt et al., 2017). It was further studied in the KEYNOTE-052 in patients who were not eligible to receive cisplatin-based chemotherapy (Vuky et al., 2020). Both studies demonstrated a favorable objective response rate, indicating that pembrolizumab has the potential to induce tumor shrinkage and improve disease control in these patient populations. Atezolizumab, evaluated in the IMvigor 210 trial, demonstrated efficacy in patients with metastatic bladder cancer who expressed high levels of PD-L1 (greater than 5%) who were not eligible for cisplatin (NCT02108652) (Balar et al., 2017). Nivolumab, studied in the CheckMate-275 trial (NCT02387996) (Sharma et al., 2017), showed modest but clinically meaningful responses in patients with metastatic bladder cancer who had progressed after platinum-based chemotherapy. These findings offer ICI as an important alternative treatment option for patients whose tumors do not respond, who cannot tolerate, or who are ineligible for cisplatin-based chemotherapy. It is yet unknown whether rechallenge with a second ICI after prior failure of ICI has utility in bladder cancer.

Prostate, Testicular, and Penile Cancers

Immunotherapy in Prostate Cancer

Prostate cancer is the most common cancer in men, affecting one in eight, and poses a significant health concern worldwide. Over the years, significant advancements have been made in the understanding, diagnosis, and treatment of this disease, leading to improved outcomes and enhanced quality of life for patients. Surgical or radiotherapeutic interventions are most important in localized prostate cancer, whereas treatments targeting the androgen receptor (AR) are essential components of treatment in metastatic disease. Prostate cancers are often subdivided into castration-sensitive (meaning they respond to androgen deprivation therapy or ADT, which has been a mainstay of systemic treatment for over 80 years) and castration-resistant (meaning they no longer respond to ADT) and are designated CSPC and CRPC, respectively.

Large clinical trials of ICI immunotherapy in both CSPC and CRPC have been generally disappointing. KEYNOTE-199 (NCT02787005) (Antonarakis et al., 2020) and CheckMate-650 (NCT02985957) (Sharma et al., 2020) are the largest of these trials evaluating pembrolizumab and combined nivolumab/ipilimumab, respectively. Prostate cancers are uniquely refractory to immunotherapy and exhibit relatively low tumor mutation burden (TMB). One proposed reason why immunotherapy may not work effectively in prostate cancer is the activity of AR that significantly curtails innate immune signaling. Unfortunately, newer medications that target the AR pathway (AR pathway inhibitors or ARPI) have not enhanced prostate cancer response to immunotherapy. Similarly, chemotherapy, radiotherapy, PARP inhibitors, and cellular immune therapies have also failed to significantly improve the response to ICI in prostate cancer (Yu et al., 2023; Dorff et al., 2021; McNeel et al., 2022; Stein et al., 2022). However, it has been reported that a combination of atezolizumab and a tyrosine kinase inhibitor, cabozantinib, has met its primary endpoint of PFS in the CONTACT-02 study (NCT044446117). At this time, ICI are approved only for use in prostate cancers with high TMB on genetic testing. PD-L1 immunohistochemistry has no role in clinical decision-making in prostate cancer.

Beyond ICI therapy, the immune system does play a role in prostate cancer outcomes. The OPeRATIC trial (NCT02816983) showed that patients with metastatic CRPC who experienced increases in $CD8^+CD11a^{high}$ T cells enjoyed favorable long-term outcomes (Zhang et al., 2021). Notably, one non-ICI immunotherapy is approved in refractory prostate cancer in some settings. Sipuleucel-T is an autologous cellular immunotherapy in which a patient's white blood cells are collected and exposed to PA2024, which is a fusion of prostatic acid phosphatase (PAP) and immune-stimulating molecule granulocyte-macrophage colony-stimulating factor (GM-CSF). This exposure helps activate the patient's immune system against prostate cancer cells. The activated immune cells are then reinfused back into the patient. In the IMPACT trial (NCT00065442), 127 patients with metastatic CRPC with Gleason 7 or less, no visceral metastases, and an expected survival of at least 6 months were treated with either sipuleucel-T or placebo (Kantoff et al., 2010). Although the treatment did not show a substantial effect on slowing disease progression, it did extend survival by a mean 4.1 months (25.8 versus 21.7 months). This finding was particularly noteworthy considering the limited treatment options available at that time for mCRPC. This led to the approval of Sipuleucel-T in CRPC with bone metastases. Clinical use is limited due to the stringent criteria in this study and its approval (for instance, the exclusion of visceral metastases) and the availability of newer therapies.

Additional immunotherapies attempted in prostate cancer include a PSA-targeting viral vector vaccine in the PROSTVAC trial (NCT01322490) and other combination therapies. Unfortunately, the no trial has demonstrated a significant improvement in overall survival compared to placebo. ICI treatment in prostate cancer aside from TMB-selected patients should only be pursued in a clinical trial.

Immunotherapy in Testicular Cancer

Testicular cancers, also termed germ cell tumors (GCT), may present as a painless lump or swelling in the testicles, often accompanied by a feeling of heaviness. Other symptoms may include testicular pain, back pain, abdominal pain, or enlargement of the breasts due to hormonal changes. The prognosis for testicular or germ cell tumors is generally favorable, with a high cure rate, especially when detected at an early stage. Even when the cancer has spread beyond the testicles, it can often be effectively treated with a combination of surgery, chemotherapy, and radiation therapy.

Clinical trials investigating immunotherapy in testicular cancer are relatively limited compared to other cancer types. This likely relates to their exquisite sensitivity to—and high cure rates from—chemotherapy even in late-stage disease. Although chemotherapies carry significant toxicities, it is considered unethical to compare alternative potentially non-curative therapies such as immunotherapy in this setting. Small trials of immunotherapy have been performed in the relapsed or refractory setting. Avelumab (Mego et al., 2019), durvalumab (Necchi et al., 2018), nivolumab (Zschäbitz et al., 2017), and pembrolizumab (Zschäbitz et al., 2017; Adra et al., 2018) monotherapies have each failed to achieve any meaningful clinical benefit. Immunotherapy with ICI for testicular cancers is not advisable outside of a clinical trial.

Immunotherapy in Penile Cancer

Penile cancer is extremely rare. As such, clinical trials specifically investigating immunotherapy in penile cancer are limited. Urothelial cancer trials KEYNOTE-045 (NCT02256436) and JAVELIN Bladder 100 (NCT02603432) both included small subsets of patients with penile cancer.

Given the scarcity of data in this area, further research and clinical trials are needed to explore the potential benefits and efficacy of immunotherapy in penile cancer treatment. Immunotherapy with ICI for penile cancers is not advisable outside of a clinical trial.

References

Abu-Rustum, N., et al. (2023). Uterine neoplasms, version 1.2023, NCCN clinical practice guidelines in oncology. *Journal of the National Comprehensive Cancer Network, 21*(2), 181–209.

Adra, N., et al. (2018). Phase II trial of pembrolizumab in patients with platinum refractory germ-cell tumors: A Hoosier cancer research network study GU14-206. *Annals of Oncology, 29*(1), 209–214.

Albiges, L., et al. (2023). Efficacy and safety of atezolizumab plus cabozantinib vs cabozantinib alone after progression with prior immune checkpoint inhibitor (ICI) treatment in metastatic renal cell carcinoma (RCC): Primary PFS analysis from the phase 3, randomized, open-label CONTACT-03 study. *Journal of Clinical Oncology, 41*(17_suppl), LBA4500.

Antonarakis, E. S., et al. (2020). Pembrolizumab for treatment-refractory metastatic castration-resistant prostate cancer: Multicohort, open-label phase II KEYNOTE-199 study. *Journal of Clinical Oncology, 38*(5), 395–405.

Bajorin, D. F., et al. (2021). Adjuvant nivolumab versus placebo in muscle-invasive urothelial carcinoma. *New England Journal of Medicine, 384*(22), 2102–2114.

Balar, A. V., et al. (2017). Atezolizumab as first-line treatment in cisplatin-ineligible patients with locally advanced and metastatic urothelial carcinoma: A single-arm, multicentre, phase 2 trial. *The Lancet, 389*(10064), 67–76.

Balar, A. V., et al. (2021). Pembrolizumab monotherapy for the treatment of high-risk non-muscle-invasive bladder cancer unresponsive to BCG (KEYNOTE-057): An open-label, single-arm, multicentre, phase 2 study. *The Lancet Oncology, 22*(7), 919–930.

Bellmunt, J., et al. (2017). Pembrolizumab as second-line therapy for advanced urothelial carcinoma. *New England Journal of Medicine, 376*(11), 1015–1026.

Bellmunt, J., et al. (2021). Adjuvant atezolizumab versus observation in muscle-invasive urothelial carcinoma (IMvigor010): A multicentre, open-label, randomised, phase 3 trial. *The Lancet Oncology, 22*(4), 525–537.

Choueiri, T. K., et al. (2021a). Nivolumab plus Cabozantinib versus sunitinib for advanced renal-cell carcinoma. *New England Journal of Medicine, 384*(9), 829–841.

Choueiri, T. K., et al. (2021b). Adjuvant pembrolizumab after nephrectomy in renal-cell carcinoma. *New England Journal of Medicine, 385*(8), 683–694.

Dorff, T., et al. (2021). Phase Ib study of patients with metastatic castrate-resistant prostate cancer treated with different sequencing regimens of atezolizumab and sipuleucel-T. *Journal for Immunotherapy of Cancer, 9*(8), e002931.

Flaig, T. W., et al. (2022). NCCN guidelines® insights: Bladder cancer, version 2.2022. *Journal of the National Comprehensive Cancer Network, 20*(8), 866–878.

Fuhrman, S. A., Lasky, L. C., & Limas, C. (1982). Prognostic significance of morphologic parameters in renal cell carcinoma. *The American Journal of Surgical Pathology, 6*(7), 655–663.

Heng, D. Y., et al. (2009). Prognostic factors for overall survival in patients with metastatic renal cell carcinoma treated with vascular endothelial growth factor-targeted agents: Results from a large, multicenter study. *Journal of Clinical Oncology, 27*(34), 5794–5799.

Hoimes, C. J., et al. (2023). Enfortumab Vedotin plus pembrolizumab in previously untreated advanced urothelial cancer. *Journal of Clinical Oncology, 41*(1), 22–31.

Kantoff, P. W., et al. (2010). Sipuleucel-T immunotherapy for castration-resistant prostate cancer. *New England Journal of Medicine, 363*(5), 411–422.

McDermott, D. F., et al. (2021). Open-label, single-arm, phase II study of pembrolizumab monotherapy as first-line therapy in patients with advanced non-clear cell renal cell carcinoma. *Journal of Clinical Oncology, 39*(9), 1029–1039.

McNeel, D. G., et al. (2022). Phase 2 trial of T-cell activation using MVI-816 and pembrolizumab in patients with metastatic, castration-resistant prostate cancer (mCRPC). *Journal for Immunotherapy of Cancer, 10*(3), e004198.

Mego, M., et al. (2019). Phase II study of avelumab in multiple relapsed/refractory germ cell cancer. *Investigational New Drugs, 37*(4), 748–754.

Motzer, R. J., et al. (2002). Interferon-alfa as a comparative treatment for clinical trials of new therapies against advanced renal cell carcinoma. *Journal of Clinical Oncology, 20*(1), 289–296.

Motzer, R. J., et al. (2018). Nivolumab plus ipilimumab versus sunitinib in advanced renal-cell carcinoma. *New England Journal of Medicine, 378*(14), 1277–1290.

Motzer, R. J., et al. (2019). Avelumab plus Axitinib versus sunitinib for advanced renal-cell carcinoma. *New England Journal of Medicine, 380*(12), 1103–1115.

Motzer, R., et al. (2021). Lenvatinib plus pembrolizumab or everolimus for advanced renal cell carcinoma. *New England Journal of Medicine, 384*(14), 1289–1300.

Motzer, R. J., et al. (2022). Kidney cancer, version 3.2022, NCCN clinical practice guidelines in oncology. *Journal of the National Comprehensive Cancer Network, 20*(1), 71–90.

Necchi, A., et al. (2018). Abstract CT102: APACHE: An open label, randomized, phase II study of durvalumab (Durva), alone or in combination with Tremelimumab (Treme), in patients (pts) with advanced germ cell tumors (GCT): Results at the end of first stage. *Cancer Research, 78*(13_Supplement), CT102.

Pal, S. K., et al. (2021). Cabozantinib in combination with atezolizumab for advanced renal cell carcinoma: Results from the COSMIC-021 study. *Journal of Clinical Oncology, 39*(33), 3725–3736.

Powles, T., et al. (2020a). Pembrolizumab plus axitinib versus sunitinib monotherapy as first-line treatment of advanced renal cell carcinoma (KEYNOTE-426): Extended follow-up from a randomised, open-label, phase 3 trial. *The Lancet Oncology, 21*(12), 1563–1573.

Powles, T., et al. (2020b). Avelumab maintenance therapy for advanced or metastatic urothelial carcinoma. *New England Journal of Medicine, 383*(13), 1218–1230.

Sharma, P., et al. (2017). Nivolumab in metastatic urothelial carcinoma after platinum therapy (CheckMate-275): A multicentre, single-arm, phase 2 trial. *The Lancet Oncology, 18*(3), 312–322.

Sharma, P., et al. (2020). Nivolumab plus ipilimumab for metastatic castration-resistant prostate cancer: Preliminary analysis of patients in the CheckMate-650 trial. *Cancer Cell, 38*(4), 489–499.e3.

Siegel, R. L., et al. (2023). Cancer statistics, 2023. *CA: a Cancer Journal for Clinicians, 73*(1), 17–48.

Stein, M. N., et al. (2022). ADXS31142 immunotherapy ± pembrolizumab treatment for metastatic castration-resistant prostate cancer: Open-label phase I/II KEYNOTE-046 study. *The Oncologist, 27*(6), 453–461.

Vuky, J., et al. (2020). Long-term outcomes in KEYNOTE-052: Phase II study investigating first-line pembrolizumab in cisplatin-ineligible patients with locally advanced or metastatic urothelial cancer. *Journal of Clinical Oncology, 38*(23), 2658–2666.

Yu, E. Y., et al. (2023). Pembrolizumab plus Olaparib in patients with metastatic castration-resistant prostate cancer: Long-term results from the phase 1b/2 KEYNOTE-365 cohort a study. *European Urology, 83*(1), 15–26.

Zhang, H., et al. (2021). Phase II evaluation of stereotactic ablative radiotherapy (SABR) and immunity in 11C-choline-PET/CT–identified oligometastatic castration-resistant prostate cancer. *Clinical Cancer Research, 27*(23), 6376–6383.

Zschäbitz, S., et al. (2017). Response to anti-programmed cell death protein-1 antibodies in men treated for platinum refractory germ cell cancer relapsed after high-dose chemotherapy and stem cell transplantation. *European Journal of Cancer, 76*, 1–7.

Chapter 12
Immunotherapy for Gastrointestinal Malignancies

Mojun Zhu

Abstract Gastrointestinal (GI) malignancies comprise esophageal, stomach, liver, biliary tract, pancreatic, small bowel, appendiceal, colorectal, and anal cancer. All of them originate from the GI tract; however, their disease course and management vary significantly. To date, only a small number of GI cancers respond well to immunotherapy that has been approved by the US Food and Drug Administration. Their different sensitivity to immunotherapy may be due to the type of cancer cells involved (e.g., adenocarcinoma versus squamous cell carcinoma), primary location of the cancer (e.g., pancreatic versus anal cancer), potential causes of cancer (e.g., acid reflux for esophageal cancer versus bacterial infection for stomach cancer), and so on. Altogether, these factors shape the interactions among cancer cells, immune cells, and adjacent normal cells, which ultimately determine the treatment response to immunotherapy. In this chapter, we will discuss the current state of immunotherapy in the field of GI cancers by reviewing the most pertinent concept and landmark clinical trials that guide the use of immunotherapy to treat GI cancers.

Keywords Immunotherapy · Aanti-PD-1 · Checkpoint · GI cancer · Colorectal cancer · Anal cancer · Esophageal cancer · Stomach cancer · Liver cancer · Biliary tract cancer · Pancreatic cancer · Clinical trial

Colorectal, Appendiceal, and Small Bowel Cancer

Colorectal cancer (CRC) is the most common type of GI cancer worldwide. In the USA, it is the third most commonly diagnosed cancer and the third leading cause of cancer-related death. Localized, stage I–III CRC is primarily treated by surgical resection. Advanced, stage IV CRC that is not amenable to surgical resection or has metastasized to a different organ or distant lymph nodes is treated with systemic

M. Zhu (✉)
Department of Oncology, Mayo Clinic, Rochester, MN, USA
e-mail: zhu.mojun@mayo.edu

therapy. Chemotherapy remains the preferred, first-line systemic therapy for most patients with advanced CRC as immunotherapy has been found efficacious only in patients with CRC that have defective DNA mismatch repair (MMR) mechanism (Cercek et al., 2022; Lenz et al., 2022; Diaz Jr. et al., 2022). At the time of diagnosis, standardized tests will be performed to assess whether the tumor is MMR-deficient (dMMR), which is commonly found in patients who carry an inherited genetic condition such as Lynch syndrome predisposing its carriers to cancer development (Moreira et al., 2012). dMMR can also occur sporadically to patients without any known genetic conditions. Only ~15% of CRC are dMMR; sporadic acquirement of this feature is more common than having an hereditary disorder (Kim et al., 1994; Leclerc et al., 2021). Following evaluation of dMMR status, patients will be assessed to make sure that they do not have any medical conditions particularly autoimmune disorders that can be worsened by immunotherapy.

Treatment with immune checkpoint inhibitors (ICI) that targets the PD-1/PD-L1 axis (i.e., anti-PD-1 and anti-PD-L1) as discussed in previous chapters is recommended as the first-line therapy for patients with dMMR CRC. This recommendation is based on data from phase 3 clinical trials, which demonstrated that patients who received anti-PD-1 for dMMR CRC lived longer (i.e., longer survival) and had higher chances of tumor shrinkage (i.e., higher response rates) compared with those who received chemotherapy (Diaz Jr. et al., 2022; André et al., 2020). In general, all types of dMMR cancers can be treated with ICI (Le et al., 2015). These cancers are enriched by immune cells known as tumor-infiltrating lymphocytes (TIL), which are reinvigorated by ICI to kill cancer cells (Smyrk et al., 2001). ICI alone as a first-line therapy is only recommended for the treatment of dMMR CRC, certain types of lung cancer, and melanoma because longer survival and higher response rates were demonstrated by phase 3 clinical trials comparing ICI with chemotherapy in these cancers.

In addition to dMMR, other biomarkers such as tumor mutational burden (TMB) and PD-L1 expression scores can help to predict treatment response to anti-PD-1; however, utility and reliability of these biomarkers are more limited than dMMR. For instance, CRC with a high TMB (i.e., TMB $\geq$ 10 mutations per megabase) did not appear to respond well to anti-PD-1 despite FDA approval of using pembrolizumab, an anti-PD-1 therapy, to treat solid tumors with TMB $\geq$ 10 that have progressed on prior therapy (Rousseau et al., 2021). Biomarkers that are associated with favorable treatment response to immunotherapy indicate that one's immune system can be potentiated by this therapy to kill cancer cells; however, none of the exiting biomarkers are perfect due to the presence of false-positive and false-negative errors. As a result, the search for novel biomarkers and testing algorithms that better predict efficacy of anticancer therapy including immunotherapy is an area of active research in the era of personalized medicine.

Cancers that arise from the appendix and small bowel are rare; therefore, there are much less experimental data and clinical trials that have investigated immunotherapy in these cancers. Their management is largely based on our clinical experience with CRC. Similarly, ICI should be considered for dMMR cancers. Anti-PD-1 was shown to be effective in dMMR small bowel cancer that was previously treated with first-line chemotherapy (Pedersen et al., 2021). The best approach to incorporating immunotherapy to the treatment of appendiceal and small bowel cancer remains to be determined.

Anal Cancer

In contrast to colorectal, appendiceal, and small bowel cancer that is predominantly adenocarcinoma, most anal cancers are squamous cell carcinoma (SCC). Human papillomavirus (HPV) infection is detected in ~90% of anal SCC (Daling et al., 2004). These two features probably make anal cancer more sensitive to immunotherapy.

As background, localized anal cancer is primarily treated with concurrent chemotherapy and radiotherapy (i.e., chemoradiation). Surgical resection that makes permanent colostomy construction inevitable is only considered when the cancer if refractory to chemoradiation.

Advanced anal cancer is treated with systemic therapy. Although dMMR is rare in anal cancer, anal SCC seems more susceptible to ICI than CRC. HPV positivity and increased TIL are associated with improved survival and treatment response to chemoradiation in anal cancer, suggesting that HPV infection may trigger immune response and enhance the efficacy of immunotherapy (Balermpas et al., 2017). These trends were also observed in clinical trials with anti-PD-1 in SCC of the head and neck (Ferris et al., 2016). Retifanlimab, an anti-PD-1 therapy, in combination with chemotherapy is being actively evaluated as a first-line therapy for advanced anal SCC (Rao et al., 2022). Currently, two other anti-PD-1 agents (i.e., nivolumab and pembrolizumab) have been endorsed by the National Comprehensive Cancer Network as second-line therapy for anal SCC after disease progression on first-line chemotherapy (Morris et al., 2017; Marabelle et al., 2020a). Yet, none have received FDA approval.

Esophageal and Stomach Cancer

Esophageal cancer can be either SCC or adenocarcinoma while stomach cancer and cancer arising from the gastroesophageal junction (GEJ, that is, the part of GI tract where the esophagus connects to the stomach) are predominantly adenocarcinoma. These upper GI cancers are more resistant to chemotherapy than CRC and are associated with a poor prognosis. Less than 10% of patients are alive five years after they have been diagnosed with an advanced upper GI cancer based on data provided by the Surveillance, Epidemiology, and End Results Program.

The advent of immunotherapy has enriched our treatment options for upper GI cancers but has only improved clinical outcomes modestly. In general, upper GI cancers appear more sensitive to immunotherapy than CRC; esophageal SCC

(ESCC) appears more sensitive to immunotherapy than esophageal, GEJ, and stomach adenocarcinoma. In advanced ESCC, anti-PD-1 in combination with chemotherapy is more efficacious than chemotherapy alone as a first-line therapy regardless of prerequisite biomarker expression (Sun et al., 2021; Doki et al., 2022).

In esophageal, GEJ, and stomach adenocarcinoma, combined positive score (CPS) that measures the amount of PD-L1 expression by tumor and immune cells is a critical biomarker that predicts treatment response to anti-PD-1. The higher the CPS score, the higher the likelihood that the cancer is going to respond to anti-PD-1. In these cancers, first-line nivolumab or pembrolizumab in combination with chemotherapy was found more efficacious than chemotherapy alone in patients with CPS ≥ 5 and 10, respectively (Sun et al., 2021; Janjigian et al., 2021). In addition, first-line pembrolizumab in combination with chemotherapy and trastuzumab, which is a monoclonal antibody targeting HER2 expression in tumor cells, was found more efficacious than chemotherapy and trastuzumab in HER2-overexpressing GEJ and stomach adenocarcinoma with CPS ≥ 1(Janjigian et al., 2023).

Similar to CRC, dMMR also predicts favorable response to immunotherapy in upper GI cancers. It is found in ~2% and ~ 15% of esophageal and stomach cancers, respectively (Bonneville et al., 2017). ICI alone or in combination with chemotherapy should be considered as a first-line therapy for these tumors (Kim et al., 2018). Overall, these data indicate that patients with advanced upper GI cancers that harbor dMMR or high CPS scores benefit from first-line therapy that contains anti-PD-1.

Furthermore, ICI is found to enhance the therapy for localized upper GI cancers, which are generally treated with multimodality therapy consisting of chemotherapy, radiotherapy, and surgery. In the adjuvant setting (i.e., postoperative), nivolumab was shown to improve disease-free survival of patients with esophageal and GEJ cancer with residual disease after receiving chemoradiation and surgery and its use has already been approved by FDA (Kelly et al., 2021). In the neoadjuvant setting (i.e., preoperative), several studies have demonstrated the safety and potential efficacy of combining anti-PD-1 with chemoradiation and surgery (van den Ende et al., 2021; Zhu et al., 2022). Larger, phase 3 studies are currently underway to confirm the efficacy of perioperative use of ICI (Eads et al., 2020; Janjigian et al., 2022; Shitara et al., 2023).

Liver Cancer

Incidence and mortality rates of liver cancer, also known as hepatocellular carcinoma (HCC), have been rising (Ryerson et al., 2016). Viral hepatitis, alcoholic cirrhosis, and nonalcoholic fatty liver disease are known risk factors for HCC, highlighting the importance of disease prevention and screening (Akinyemiju et al., 2017). For patients with limited amount of tumor burden, partial hepatectomy and locoregional therapies are promising (Llovet et al., 2021). Liver transplantation as a curative therapy is reserved for only a small group of patients with early-stage HCC (Mazzaferro et al., 1996).

Historically, first-line therapy with tyrosine kinase inhibitors (TKI) such as sorafenib has limited efficacy in HCC, prolonging patients' overall survival by ~3 months compared with placebo (Llovet et al., 2008). Given the understanding that chronic inflammation can drive development of HCC (Ringelhan et al., 2018), immunotherapy has become an area of active research. In patients with advanced HCC, atezolizumab (anti-PD-L1) in combination with bevacizumab (monoclonal antibody targeting vascular endothelial growth factor [VEGF]) (Finn et al., 2020a) and durvalumab (anti-PD-1) in combination with tremelimumab (ICI targeting CTLA-4) (Abou-Alfa et al., 2022), respectively, improved response rates and overall survival compared with first-line sorafenib. Based on these studies, both combinations have been approved by FDA as first-line therapy for HCC. In addition, anti-PD-1 therapy also demonstrated efficacy in HCC that was previously treated with sorafenib (El-Khoueiry et al., 2017; Finn et al., 2020b). Currently, there is no conclusive data to guide the sequence of systemic therapy (i.e., ICI to be followed by TKI versus vice versa) for HCC.

Biliary Tract Cancer

Biliary tract cancer (BTC) encompasses gallbladder cancer and cholangiocarcinoma, which can be further divided into intrahepatic and extrahepatic cholangiocarcinoma. BTC is often diagnosed at an advanced stage and is associated with a poor prognosis (Hundal & Shaffer, 2014). Durvalumab (anti-PD-1) in combination with chemotherapy improved overall survival compared with chemotherapy alone, and this combination was hence approved by FDA as a first-line therapy for advanced BTC (Oh et al., 2022).

Although dMMR is found in less than 3% of BTC (Bonneville et al., 2017; Abrha et al., 2020), anti-PD-1 was shown to have significant antitumor activity in these tumors (Marabelle et al., 2020b). As a result, it is important to perform MMR testing at diagnosis. In addition, emerging data from genetic testing have revealed other genetic alterations that can be targeted by novel therapy, underscoring the need for comprehensive molecular testing to guide treatment recommendations for BTC (Valle et al., 2017).

Pancreatic Cancer

Pancreatic ductal adenocarcinoma (PDAC) accounts for 90% of pancreatic cancer and has a poor prognosis (Siegel et al., 2023). Chemotherapy currently remains first-line therapy for advanced PDAC as immunotherapy and targeted therapy have not demonstrated reasonable efficacy.

PDAC appears much more resistant to immunotherapy compared with other GI cancers. The rates of dMMR and high TMB are low in PDAC (Bonneville et al., 2017; Abrha et al., 2020). Treatment with anti-PD-1 led to tumor shrinkage in only 18.2% of patients with previously treated dMMR PDAC (versus 45.8% of patients with previously treated dMMR gastric cancer) (Marabelle et al., 2020b). ICI combinations also demonstrated poor antitumor activity (O'Reilly et al., 2019). The resistance of PDAC to ICI has been attributed to a tumor microenvironment that is devoid of TIL (O'Donnell et al., 2019; Osipov et al., 2019). In addition, targeted therapy against common somatic mutations in PDAC including KRAS, TP53, SMAD4, and CDKN2A showed limited efficacy (Waddell et al., 2015; Ho et al., 2020), which may be mediated by desmoplasia consisting of dense fibrosis produced by pancreatic stellate cells, impairing drug penetration (Whatcott et al., 2015). Overall, future studies should perhaps focus on strategies that reprogram PDAC tumor microenvironment to enable the actions of ICI and small molecule inhibitors.

Neuroendocrine Tumor and Carcinoma

Neuroendocrine tumors (NET) of GI origin comprise a diverse group of malignancies. They are divided into high, intermediate, and low grade based on the rate of cancer cell proliferation: high-grade NET grow the fastest and therefore are the most aggressive (Nagtegaal et al., 2020). Neuroendocrine carcinomas (NEC) are distinct from NET as NEC are poorly differentiated and much more aggressive (Nagtegaal et al., 2020). Although dMMR is rare in this disease (0% of pancreatic NET (Salem et al., 2018), 3.6% of NET of all origins (Vanderwalde et al., 2018), and 12.4% of all NEC (Sahnane et al., 2015)), anti-PD-1 may be considered selectively in high-grade NET and NEC based on data from phase 2 clinical trials (Patel et al., 2020, 2021; Yao et al., 2021).

Summary

The FDA approval of anti-PD-1 as a therapy for dMMR cancers marks a paradigm shift in medical oncology. In comparison to chemotherapy, immunotherapy such as ICI appears less toxic and more efficacious in the long term. GI cancers have demonstrated varied sensitivity to immunotherapy (Table 12.1), and this is mediated by interactions among cancer cells, immune cells, and adjacent normal cells, which constitute a distinct tumor immune microenvironment. Active research is underway to crack the code of tumor immune microenvironment, which holds the key to successful development of immunotherapy in the near future.

Table. 12.1 FDA-approved immunotherapy for treatment of GI cancers

Type of GI cancer	Prerequisite biomarker	Treatment
Colorectal adenocarcinoma	MMR deficient	Anti-PD-1 monotherapy or in combination with anti-CTLA-4
Esophageal squamous cell carcinoma	None	Anti-PD-1 in combination with chemotherapy
Esophageal, gastroesophageal, and gastric adenocarcinoma	PD-L1 expression	Anti-PD-1 in combination with chemotherapy
Hepatocellular carcinoma	None	Anti-PD-1 in combination with anti-VEGF or anti-CTLA-4
Cholangiocarcinoma	None	Anti-PD-1 in combination with chemotherapy

References

Abou-Alfa, G. K., Lau, G., Kudo, M., et al. (2022). Tremelimumab plus Durvalumab in Unresectable Hepatocellular Carcinoma. *NEJM Evidence, 1*, EVIDoa2100070.

Abrha, A., Shukla, N. D., Hodan, R., et al. (2020). Universal screening of gastrointestinal malignancies for mismatch repair deficiency at Stanford. *JNCI Cancer Spectrum, 4*(5), pkaao54.

Akinyemiju, T., Abera, S., Ahmed, M., et al. (2017). The burden of primary liver cancer and underlying etiologies from 1990 to 2015 at the global, regional, and National level: Results from the global burden of disease study 2015. *JAMA Oncology, 3*, 1683–1691.

André, T., Shiu, K.-K., Kim, T. W., et al. (2020). Pembrolizumab in microsatellite-instability–high advanced colorectal cancer. *New England Journal of Medicine, 383*, 2207–2218.

Balermpas, P., Martin, D., Wieland, U., et al. (2017). Human papilloma virus load and PD-1/PD-L1, CD8(+) and FOXP3 in anal cancer patients treated with chemoradiotherapy: Rationale for immunotherapy. *Oncoimmunology, 6*, e1288331.

Bonneville, R., Krook, M. A., Kautto, E. A., et al. (2017). Landscape of microsatellite instability across 39 cancer types. *JCO Precision Oncology, 2017*, 1–15.

Cercek, A., Lumish, M., Sinopoli, J., et al. (2022). PD-1 blockade in mismatch repair–Deficient, locally advanced rectal cancer. *New England Journal of Medicine, 386*, 2363–2376.

Daling, J. R., Madeleine, M. M., Johnson, L. G., et al. (2004). Human papillomavirus, smoking, and sexual practices in the etiology of anal cancer. *Cancer, 101*, 270–280.

Diaz, L. A., Jr., Shiu, K.-K., Kim, T.-W., et al. (2022). Pembrolizumab versus chemotherapy for microsatellite instability-high or mismatch repair-deficient metastatic colorectal cancer (KEYNOTE-177): Final analysis of a randomised, open-label, phase 3 study. *The Lancet Oncology, 23*, 659–670.

Doki, Y., Ajani, J. A., Kato, K., et al. (2022). Nivolumab combination therapy in advanced esophageal squamous-cell carcinoma. *New England Journal of Medicine, 386*, 449–462.

Eads, J. R., Weitz, M., Gibson, M. K., et al. (2020). A phase II/III study of perioperative nivolumab and ipilimumab in patients (pts) with locoregional esophageal (E) and gastroesophageal junction (GEJ) adenocarcinoma: A trial of the ECOG-ACRIN cancer research group (EA2174). *Journal of Clinical Oncology, 38*, TPS4651.

El-Khoueiry, A. B., Sangro, B., Yau, T., et al. (2017). Nivolumab in patients with advanced hepatocellular carcinoma (CheckMate 040): An open-label, non-comparative, phase 1/2 dose escalation and expansion trial. *Lancet, 389*, 2492–2502.

van den Ende, T., de Clercq, N. C., van Berge Henegouwen, M. I., et al. (2021). Neoadjuvant chemoradiotherapy combined with atezolizumab for resectable esophageal adenocarcinoma: A single-arm phase II feasibility trial (PERFECT). *Clinical Cancer Research, 27*(12), 3351–3359.

Ferris, R. L., Blumenschein, G., Jr., Fayette, J., et al. (2016). Nivolumab for recurrent squamous-cell carcinoma of the head and neck. *The New England Journal of Medicine, 375*, 1856–1867.

Finn, R. S., Qin, S., Ikeda, M., et al. (2020a). Atezolizumab plus Bevacizumab in Unresectable Hepatocellular Carcinoma. *New England Journal of Medicine, 382*, 1894–1905.

Finn, R. S., Ryoo, B. Y., Merle, P., et al. (2020b). Pembrolizumab as second-line therapy in patients with advanced hepatocellular carcinoma in KEYNOTE-240: A randomized, double-blind, phase III trial. *Journal of Clinical Oncology, 38*, 193–202.

Ho, W. J., Jaffee, E. M., & Zheng, L. (2020). The tumour microenvironment in pancreatic cancer – clinical challenges and opportunities. *Nature Reviews. Clinical Oncology, 17*, 527–540.

Hundal, R., & Shaffer, E. A. (2014). Gallbladder cancer: Epidemiology and outcome. *Clinical Epidemiology, 6*, 99–109.

Janjigian, Y. Y., Shitara, K., Moehler, M., et al. (2021). First-line nivolumab plus chemotherapy versus chemotherapy alone for advanced gastric, gastro-oesophageal junction, and oesophageal adenocarcinoma (CheckMate 649): A randomised, open-label, phase 3 trial. The Lancet, 398, 27–40

Janjigian, Y. Y., Custem, E. V., Muro, K., et al. (2022). MATTERHORN: phase III study of durvalumab plus FLOT chemotherapy in resectable gastric/gastroesophageal junction cancer. *Future Oncology, 18*(20), 2465–2473.

Janjigian, Y. Y., Kawazoe, A., Bai, Y., et al. (2023). Pembrolizumab plus trastuzumab and chemotherapy for HER2-positive gastric or gastro-oesophageal junction adenocarcinoma: interim analyses from the phase 3 KEYNOTE-811 randomised placebo-controlled trial. *The Lancet, 402*(10418), 2197–2208.

Kelly, R. J., Ajani, J. A., Kuzdzal, J., et al. (2021). Adjuvant nivolumab in resected Esophageal or gastroesophageal junction cancer. *New England Journal of Medicine, 384*, 1191–1203.

Kim, H., Jen, J., Vogelstein, B., et al. (1994). Clinical and pathological characteristics of sporadic colorectal carcinomas with DNA replication errors in microsatellite sequences. *The American Journal of Pathology, 145*, 148–156.

Kim, S. T., Cristescu, R., Bass, A. J., et al. (2018). Comprehensive molecular characterization of clinical responses to PD-1 inhibition in metastatic gastric cancer. *Nature Medicine, 24*, 1449–1458.

Le, D. T., Uram, J. N., Wang, H., et al. (2015). PD-1 blockade in tumors with mismatch-repair deficiency. *New England Journal of Medicine, 372*, 2509–2520.

Leclerc, J., Vermaut, C., & Buisine, M. P. (2021). Diagnosis of lynch syndrome and strategies to distinguish lynch-related tumors from sporadic MSI/dMMR Tumors. *Cancers (Basel), 13*(3), 467.

Lenz, H. J., Van Cutsem, E., Luisa Limon, M., et al. (2022). First-line nivolumab plus low-dose ipilimumab for microsatellite instability-high/mismatch repair-deficient metastatic colorectal cancer: The phase II CheckMate 142 study. *Journal of Clinical Oncology, 40*, 161–170.

Llovet, J. M., Ricci, S., Mazzaferro, V., et al. (2008). Sorafenib in advanced hepatocellular carcinoma. *New England Journal of Medicine, 359*, 378–390.

Llovet, J. M., De Baere, T., Kulik, L., et al. (2021). Locoregional therapies in the era of molecular and immune treatments for hepatocellular carcinoma. *Nature Reviews Gastroenterology & Hepatology, 18*, 293–313.

Marabelle, A., Cassier, P. A., Fakih, M., et al. (2020a). Pembrolizumab for advanced anal squamous cell carcinoma (ASCC): Results from the multicohort, phase II KEYNOTE-158 study. *Journal of Clinical Oncology, 38*, 1–1.

Marabelle, A., Le, D. T., Ascierto, P. A., et al. (2020b). Efficacy of pembrolizumab in patients with noncolorectal high microsatellite instability/mismatch repair-deficient cancer: Results from the phase II KEYNOTE-158 study. *Journal of Clinical Oncology, 38*, 1–10.

Mazzaferro, V., Regalia, E., Doci, R., et al. (1996). Liver transplantation for the treatment of small hepatocellular carcinomas in patients with cirrhosis. *The New England Journal of Medicine, 334*, 693–699.

Moreira, L., Balaguer, F., Lindor, N., et al. (2012). Identification of lynch syndrome among patients with colorectal cancer. *JAMA, 308*, 1555–1565.

Morris, V. K., Salem, M. E., Nimeiri, H., et al. (2017). Nivolumab for previously treated unresectable metastatic anal cancer (NCI9673): A multicentre, single-arm, phase 2 study. *The Lancet Oncology, 18*, 446–453.

Nagtegaal, I. D., Odze, R. D., Klimstra, D., et al. (2020). The 2019 WHO classification of tumours of the digestive system. *Histopathology, 76*, 182–188.

O'Donnell, J. S., Teng, M. W. L., & Smyth, M. J. (2019). Cancer immunoediting and resistance to T cell-based immunotherapy. *Nature Reviews. Clinical Oncology, 16*, 151–167.

Oh, D.-Y., He, A. R., Qin, S., et al. (2022). Durvalumab plus gemcitabine and cisplatin in advanced biliary tract cancer. *NEJM Evidence, 1*, EVIDoa2200015.

O'Reilly, E. M., Oh, D. Y., Dhani, N., et al. (2019). Durvalumab with or without tremelimumab for patients with metastatic pancreatic ductal adenocarcinoma: A phase 2 randomized clinical trial. *JAMA Oncology, 5*, 1431–1438.

Osipov, A., Zaidi, N., & Laheru, D. A. (2019). Dual checkpoint inhibition in pancreatic cancer: Revealing the limitations of synergy and the potential of novel combinations. *JAMA Oncology, 5*, 1438–1439.

Patel, S. P., Othus, M., Chae, Y. K., et al. (2020). A phase II basket trial of dual anti–CTLA-4 and anti–PD-1 blockade in rare tumors (DART SWOG 1609) in patients with nonpancreatic neuroendocrine tumors. *Clinical Cancer Research, 26*, 2290–2296.

Patel, S. P., Mayerson, E., Chae, Y. K., et al. (2021). A phase II basket trial of dual anti-CTLA-4 and anti-PD-1 blockade in rare tumors (DART) SWOG S1609: High-grade neuroendocrine neoplasm cohort. *Cancer, 127*, 3194–3201.

Pedersen, K. S., Foster, N. R., Overman, M. J., et al. (2021). ZEBRA: A multicenter phase II study of pembrolizumab in patients with advanced small-bowel adenocarcinoma. *Clinical Cancer Research, 27*, 3641–3648.

Rao, S., Jones, M., Bowman, J., et al. (2022). POD1UM-303/InterAACT 2: A phase III, global, randomized, double-blind study of retifanlimab or placebo plus carboplatin-paclitaxel in patients with locally advanced or metastatic squamous cell anal carcinoma. *Frontiers in Oncology, 12*, 935383.

Ringelhan, M., Pfister, D., O'Connor, T., et al. (2018). The immunology of hepatocellular carcinoma. *Nature Immunology, 19*, 222–232.

Rousseau, B., Foote, M. B., Maron, S. B., et al. (2021). The spectrum of benefit from checkpoint blockade in hypermutated Tumors. *New England Journal of Medicine, 384*, 1168–1170.

Ryerson, A. B., Eheman, C. R., Altekruse, S. F., et al. (2016). Annual report to the nation on the status of cancer, 1975-2012, featuring the increasing incidence of liver cancer. *Cancer, 122*, 1312–1337.

Sahnane, N., Furlan, D., Monti, M., et al. (2015). Microsatellite unstable gastrointestinal neuroendocrine carcinomas: A new clinicopathologic entity. *Endocrine-Related Cancer, 22*, 35–45.

Salem, M. E., Puccini, A., Grothey, A., et al. (2018). Landscape of tumor mutation load, mismatch repair deficiency, and PD-L1 expression in a large patient cohort of gastrointestinal cancers. *Molecular Cancer Research, 16*, 805–812.

Shitara, K., Rha, S. Y., Wyrwicz, L. S., et al. (2023). Neoadjuvant and adjuvant pembrolizumab plus chemotherapy in locally advanced gastric or gastro-oesophageal cancer (KEYNOTE-585): an interim analysis of the multicentre, double-blind, randomised phase 3 study, *The Lancet Oncology, 25*(2), 212–224.

Siegel, R. L., Miller, K. D., Wagle, N. S., et al. (2023). Cancer statistics, 2023. *CA: a Cancer Journal for Clinicians, 73*, 17–48.

Smyrk, T. C., Watson, P., Kaul, K., et al. (2001). Tumor-infiltrating lymphocytes are a marker for microsatellite instability in colorectal carcinoma. *Cancer, 91*, 2417–2422.

Sun, J.-M., Shen, L., Shah, M. A., et al. (2021). Pembrolizumab plus chemotherapy versus chemotherapy alone for first-line treatment of advanced oesophageal cancer (KEYNOTE-590): A randomised, placebo-controlled, phase 3 study. *The Lancet, 398*, 759–771.

Valle, J. W., Lamarca, A., Goyal, L., et al. (2017). New horizons for precision medicine in biliary tract cancers. *Cancer Discovery, 7*, 943–962.

Vanderwalde, A., Spetzler, D., Xiao, N., et al. (2018). Microsatellite instability status determined by next-generation sequencing and compared with PD-L1 and tumor mutational burden in 11,348 patients. *Cancer Medicine, 7*, 746–756.

Waddell, N., Pajic, M., Patch, A.-M., et al. (2015). Whole genomes redefine the mutational landscape of pancreatic cancer. *Nature, 518*, 495–501.

Whatcott, C. J., Diep, C. H., Jiang, P., et al. (2015). Desmoplasia in primary tumors and metastatic lesions of pancreatic cancer. *Clinical Cancer Research, 21*, 3561–3568.

Yao, J. C., Strosberg, J., Fazio, N., et al. (2021). Spartalizumab in metastatic, well/poorly differentiated neuroendocrine neoplasms. *Endocrine-Related Cancer, 28*, 161–172.

Zhu, M., Chen, C., Foster, N. R., et al. (2022). Pembrolizumab in combination with neoadjuvant chemoradiotherapy for patients with resectable adenocarcinoma of the gastroesophageal junction. *Clinical Cancer Research, 28*, 3021–3031.

Chapter 13
Immunotherapy in the Solid Organ Transplant Recipient

Alex Liu, Elena Barbir, Aleksandra Kukla, and Kymberly D. Watt

Abstract Checkpoint inhibitor immunotherapy has limited data in the immuno-suppressed solid organ transplant recipient population as early use in this popula-tion was associated with notable organ rejection risk. Over time experience with these anticancer agents has been associated with lower rejection risk by altering the immunosuppression management strategy with these immunotherapy agents. This chapter reviews the experience with immunotherapy in this population to date. Prospective data with adequate immunosuppression will move this practice forward.

Keywords Solid organ transplant · Transplantation · Immunosuppression · Organ rejection · Immunotherapy · Checkpoint inhibitor · PD-1 · PD-L1

Introduction

Immune checkpoint inhibitors (ICIs) have revolutionized cancer treatment, offering hope where there were previously few therapeutic options. As their use becomes increasingly generalized, a growing subset of ICI therapy recipients will be solid organ transplant recipients. There are two primary concerns associated with the use of ICI in solid organ transplant recipients, namely, the risk of allograft rejection associated with disruption of co-inhibitory T cell mechanisms which contribute to allograft tolerance and the risk of blunting the antitumor activity of checkpoint

A. Liu
Department of Internal Medicine, Mayo Clinic, Rochester, MN, USA

E. Barbir · A. Kukla
Department of Medicine, Division of Nephrology and Hypertension, Mayo Clinic, Rochester, MN, USA

K. D. Watt (✉)
Department of Medicine, Division of Gastroenterology/Hepatology, Mayo Clinic, Rochester, MN, USA
e-mail: watt.kymberly@mayo.edu

inhibitors through the concomitant use of maintenance immunosuppression (Murakami et al., 2021). This chapter will review indications and outcomes for ICI use in solid organ transplant, with a focus on kidney and liver transplantation.

Solid organ transplant recipients have a higher mortality compared to the general population (Acuna et al., 2016). Part of the reason for this is the higher rate of malignancy compared to those in the general population (Collett et al., 2010; Yeh et al., 2020), due to the immunosuppression regimen required posttransplant. Calcineurin inhibitors (tacrolimus and cyclosporine) are the backbone of transplant immunosuppression and have been shown to be correlated with increased malignancy risk posttransplant, with several studies in both kidney and liver transplant showing this dose-dependent relationship (Lichtenberg et al., 2017; Rodríguez-Perálvarez et al., 2022; Carenco et al., 2015). Suspected mechanisms behind this immunosuppression-related phenomenon include creating a biologically favorable environment for tumor proliferation. The attenuation of T cell responses to viral antigens and mutation-associated antigens results in decreased immune surveillance, allowing for tumor immune evasion, and an increased risk of oncogenic viral infections. Worse cancer-related outcomes after transplantation also relate, in part, to less aggressive cancer care due to comorbidities and the possibility of organ rejection (specifically pertaining to ICI) (Miao et al., 2009).

The chronic immunosuppression medications, particularly the calcineurin inhibitors required in organ transplantation, decrease T cell activity to allow for graft survival (Sehgal, 2003; Kelly et al., 1995; Allison, 2005). This mechanism of action of these immunosuppressants acts in opposition to ICI therapy, which increases T cell activity. Thus, ICI therapy via activation of T cells may precipitate allograft rejection (Fig. 13.1). Due to the perceived high risk of organ failure, patients with solid organ transplants are rarely offered ICI therapy in clinical practice and have been excluded from the clinical trials utilizing ICIs (Portuguese et al., 2022). The majority of data currently available regarding ICI use in solid organ transplant recipients have originated only from case reports and case series, and there are a paucity of data regarding their use as first- or second-line versus salvage therapy (in most cases) (Murakami et al., 2021; Zhuang et al., 2020; Rossi et al., 2022; Manohar et al., 2020).

The kidney is the most frequently transplanted organ in the United States, with 25,487 kidney transplants performed in 2021 alone (Lentine et al., 2023); thus kidney transplant recipients make up most of the organ transplant population that has been studied to date. Liver transplants are increasing over time as well, with 9234 recipients in 2021. Moreover, as the immunological risk of these transplant recipients has decreased, and immunosuppressive regiments have become more nuanced, both liver and kidney transplant recipients have benefited from longer allograft survival which translates to longer exposure to maintenance immunosuppression (Hariharan et al., 2022). However, cancer-related mortality is highly prevalent in this population, accounting for almost one-third of deaths after the first year posttransplant (Hariharan et al., 2022; Watt et al., 2010).

Transplant recipients have not experienced any improvement in cancer-related outcomes over the decades despite substantial improvement in cancer-related

A: Host T cell and donor cell interaction without ICI therapy

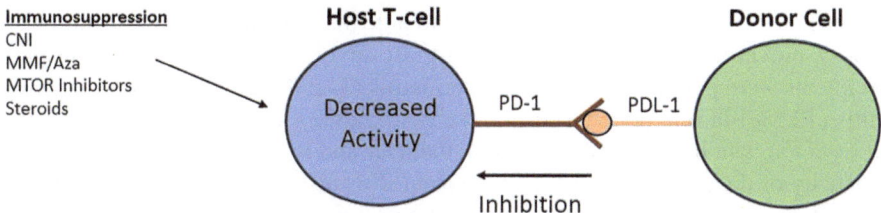

B: Host T cell and donor cell interaction with ICI therapy

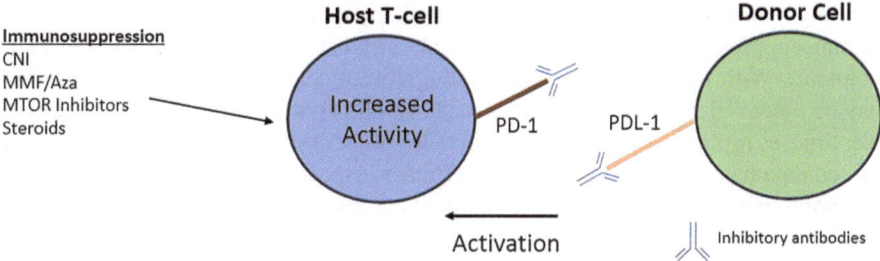

Fig. 13.1 Mechanism for ICI medication allograft rejection. Abbreviations: CNI calcineurin inhibitor, MMF mycophenolate mofetil, Aza azathioprine, MTOR mammalian target of rapamycin, PD-1 programmed cell death protein 1, PDL-1 programmed death ligand 1

prognosis in non-transplant population (Blosser et al., 2021). To ensure transplant recipients experience similar gains in prognosis and life years gained through improved anti-cancer regimens, it is important to ensure that transplant recipients have access to the best available treatments for their malignant complications, which includes ICI therapy. Notably, there are first-line indications for the use of ICI therapy in advanced forms of the most common cancers seen in kidney transplant patients—squamous cell carcinoma and melanoma (Murakami et al., 2021; Portuguese et al., 2022; Garrett et al., 2017; Ho, 2023; Lamba et al., 2022).

Outcomes and Complications of ICI Use in Solid Organ Transplant Recipients

General ICI Adverse Event Overview

ICI-associated toxicity is a well-described phenomenon and can present in a variety of ways such as pneumonitis, colitis, and hepatitis, which are detailed in other chapters. However, the most common and concerning adverse event in the transplant recipient has been allograft rejection. A systematic review found that rejection has occurred in 42.2% of the transplant recipients with a median time to rejection of approximately three weeks, with almost all cases occurring within the first seven weeks (81.8%) (Fig. 13.2). It is important to note that not all cases of rejection were biopsy proven. The most common non-graft adverse events in these transplant recipients were pneumonitis (37.5%), dermatitis (31.3%), colitis (25.0%), and hepatitis (12.5%) in this review (Portuguese et al., 2022). It is important to note that most of the data in this analysis were in the liver and kidney transplant and there is a paucity of data in heart and lung transplant. It is also important to recognize that all systematic reviews of case reports and case series lack a definite denominator and percentages may be misleading. In general, when a transplant recipient is diagnosed with cancer, their transplant provider will reduce immunosuppression to the lowest feasible dose. There has been a learning curve related to immunosuppression handling with concurrent ICI therapy, recognizing that these patients need increased immunosuppression (relative to the normal circumstance of cancer in a transplant recipient). With this in mind, assessing the more recent years of data (case series) may be more reflective of the rejection risk, and this will likely continue to improve over time, as immunosuppression optimization work continues (Fig. 13.3). However, limited data has also demonstrated less efficacy, especially if more than two immunosuppressive agents are used (Murakami et al., 2021).

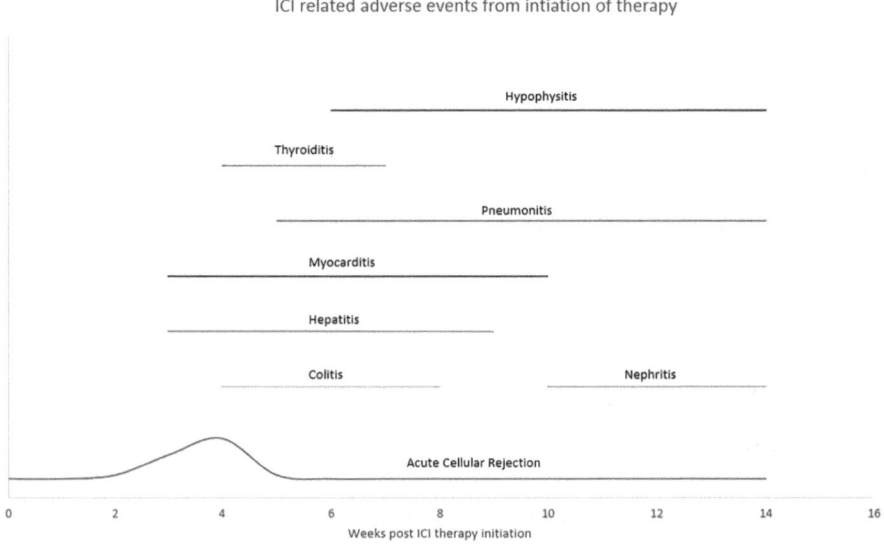

Fig. 13.2 ICI-related adverse events from initiation of therapy. Figure depicts median time of onset from initiation of therapy. Acute cellular rejection occurs most often around weeks 3–4 but can occur anytime after therapy is initiated

A: Percent of Cases Reporting Rejection in Kidney Transplant Recipients

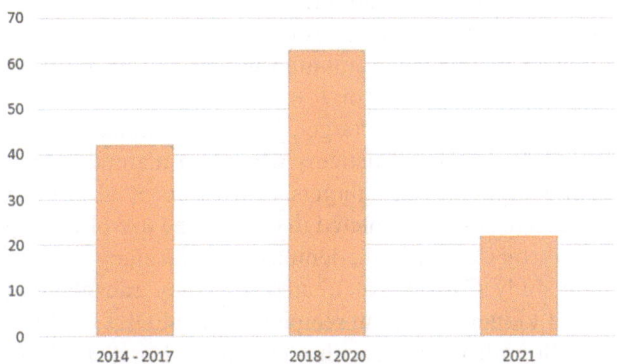

B: Percent of Cases Reporting Rejection in Liver Transplant Recipients

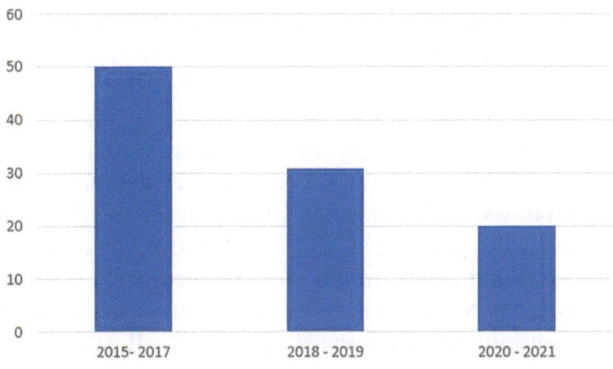

Fig. 13.3 Cases reporting rejection after ICI initiation over time

Outcomes and Adverse Effects by Organ

Kidney

The risk of kidney allograft rejection with initiation of ICI therapy is reported in the range of 40–50% with subsequent allograft failure occurring in 50–65% of those who experienced an initial episode of rejection (Murakami et al., 2021; Portuguese et al., 2022; Manohar et al., 2020; Alzahrani et al., 2023). However, the retrospective data we have available to date is heterogeneous—the rejection rate is influenced by the type of ICI therapy (anti-PD1, PDL1, or CTLA4 monotherapy vs. combination therapy), the number and type of immunosuppressive agents the patient is continued on at the time of ICI therapy, and whether the patient has a prior history of rejection (Murakami et al., 2021; Portuguese et al., 2022; Delyon et al., 2021). The comparatively low rate of rejection observed in Owoyemi et al.'s single-center analysis at the Mayo Clinic further emphasizes the existing hetero-geneity of the data. They observed acute allograft rejection in one of seven kidney transplant patients included in their case series (14%). While all of their patients experienced a reduction in maintenance immunosuppression at the time of ICI initiation, only one of seven patients was on low-dose prednisone alone, one was on Sirolimus alone with a higher trough target, and the remainder were on two agents (4/7) and three agents (1/7). All patients who were maintained on mTOR inhibitors were targeting higher trough targets (Owoyemi et al., 2020). More recently, the only prospective study completed to date on the use of ICI therapy in kidney transplant patients, by Carroll et al., demonstrated a kidney allograft rejec-tion rate of 12%. In their study, Carroll et al. treated 16 kidney transplant recipients with PD1 inhibitors and 1 kidney transplant recipient with a PDL1 inhibitor. These patients all had stable allograft function with a creatinine less than 2 mg/dl and were defined as low or intermediate immunologic risk based on the concentration of pre-formed donor-specific antibodies at the time of ICI therapy initiation (Carroll et al., 2022). None of these patients underwent pre-emptive reduction in their maintenance immunosuppression prior to initiation of ICI therapy, and nota-bly, the response to therapy was comparable to that seen in the general population of patients with cancer (Carroll et al., 2022). Carroll et al. described 24% complete responses and 29% partial responses with a 27.7 month median duration of response (Carroll et al., 2022). Comparably, in their recent systematic review of ICI use in all solid organ transplant recipients, Portuguese et al. reported an objec-tive response rate (ORR) of 68.2% in cutaneous SCC patients and 35.7% in cuta-neous melanoma patients (Portuguese et al., 2022). Objective response rate is the sum of complete responses and partial responses. These reported response rates are better than that reported in Murakami et al.'s earlier retrospective study look-ing at ICI use for the management of advanced squamous cell carcinoma (SCC) and cutaneous melanoma in 66 kidney transplant recipients (ORR 28.9%), many of whom did undergo a reduction in maintenance immunosuppression (Murakami et al., 2021).The lower rejection rates described by both Owoyemi et al. and Carroll et al. are likely attributable to the higher baseline maintenance immuno-suppression through ICI therapy. The systematic review by Portuguese et al. con-firmed that the rejection rate decreased as the number of maintenance immunosuppressive agents increased (Portuguese et al., 2022). Moreover, multi-ple studies have associated a switch to a mammalian target of rapamycin (mTOR) inhibitors at the time of ICI therapy initiation with a decreased risk of allograft rejection while maintaining the antitumor response of the ICI (Murakami et al., 2021; Portuguese et al., 2022; Esfahani et al., 2019; Barnett et al., 2017). Lastly, the use of steroid minipulses prior to initiation of ICI therapy, termed dynamic immunosuppression, has also shown potential benefit in patients with a decreased incidence of allograft rejection (25%), while maintaining antitumor effect. However, sample size was small (n = 8, with 4 patients on dynamic immunosup-pression and 4 on maintenance dose prednisone), and immunosuppression regi-men at the initiation of ICI therapy was not standardized between the patients (Danesh et al., 2020).

It is difficult to compare ORR across studies as they involve heterogeneous populations—it is likely that timing from transplantation, lifetime cumulative degree of immunosuppression, the type of maintenance immunosuppression agents used, and the cancer types all affect the ORR. Perhaps most importantly, the timing of ICI therapy initiation in relation to progression of the malignancy certainly influences response rates. Most patients, particularly in the earlier experience, received ICI only after multiple failed attempts to treat the cancer. As the use of ICI therapy in transplant populations is slowly increasing over time, the delay to ICI initiation may be less in the more recent cohort, perhaps contributing to the improved ORR described by Carroll et al. and Portuguese et al. when comparing to prior studies. Most importantly, we now have evidence that continuation of maintenance immune suppression does not severely mitigate the antitumor effect of ICI therapy.

The type of rejection typically triggered by ICI therapy is acute cellular rejection, with or without concomitant antibody-mediated rejection, often with arteritis (Murakami et al., 2021; Carroll et al., 2022). There is no clear guidance on the approach to treating ICI-mediated rejections, though most approaches will involve ICI therapy cessation and high doses of steroids. Carroll et al. advocate for the use of plasma exchange to eliminate the circulating ICI monoclonal antibodies that could perpetuate enhanced T cell cytotoxicity (Carroll et al., 2022).

Of the different immune checkpoint inhibitor targets, PD1 inhibitors, and combination therapy (PD1/CTLA4) have been associated with higher rejection rates (Portuguese et al., 2022). The PD1/PDL1 pathway is thought to play a central role in the development of allograft tolerance, with upregulation of PDL1 expression by human renal tubular epithelial cells leading to suppressed alloreactivity of class II human leukocyte antigens expressed on the same tubular epithelial cells (Manohar et al., 2020; Riella et al., 2012). Allograft PD-L1 staining may be a useful method to risk stratify transplant recipients prior to ICI initiation in the future.

Allograft rejection is not the only potential renal limited adverse effect of ICI therapy initiation. ICI-associated acute kidney injury (AKI) is a well-known complication of ICI use in native kidneys. Its incidence is much lower, occurring in less than 5% of patients, and with a comparatively delayed timing of onset—occurring at a median of 14–16 weeks post ICI therapy initiation. The most common histologic lesion seen with ICI-associated AKI is acute interstitial nephritis (AIN) (Cortazar et al., 2020). AIN is challenging to distinguish from Banff grade 1 acute cellular rejection. Both lesions involve a lymphocyte predominant tubulointerstitial infiltrate. Given the limited ability to distinguish these two lesions using histology alone, Adam et al. have attempted to utilize gene expression profiling to differentiate the two (Adam et al., 2021). They observed significant molecular overlap between immune checkpoint inhibitor-associated acute interstitial nephritis, ICI-associated T cell-mediated rejection, and drug-induced AIN—suggesting a potential central role of hypersensitivity mechanisms in these entities. Despite the overlap between the three entities, they were able to identify and validate an IFN-a-induced transcript, IFI27, as a novel biomarker for differentiating immune checkpoint inhibitor-associated T cell-mediated rejection from immune checkpoint inhibitor-associated acute interstitial nephritis (Hope et al., 2015).

Liver

Within the realm of liver transplantation, the use of ICI posttransplant has been limited to case reports and case series of limited single institutional experiences which have been summarized in review articles. To this date, there are no clinical trials or prospective studies published in the literature. The most common cancers studied were hepatocellular carcinoma and melanoma. ICIs were, on average, used as third-line therapies and nivolumab was the most used drug (Kayali et al., 2023). Patients who responded to ICI had improved survival outcomes compared to those without. Responders tended to be further out from transplant, and not surprisingly, the nonresponders experienced more graft rejection. Notably, overall mortality was most commonly due to malignancy progression as opposed to graft loss from rejection (Kayali et al., 2023; Zhang et al., 2022). As the data is derived entirely from case reports and case series, it makes it difficult to estimate the true prevalence of these events. What this data does suggest is that ICIs may be introduced too late in the disease to optimally affect outcomes. More studies are sorely needed in this field with a broader range of malignancies.

Acute rejection continues to be a significant concern. Rejection rates are quoted in systematic reviews inclusive of the early experience close to 40% but are lower than originally described and approximate 20%, when early experience has been removed (Portuguese et al., 2022; Kayali et al., 2023). Systematic reviews have found that rejection-free survival was improved in patients receiving at least immunosuppressant other than steroids (d'Izarny-Gargas et al., 2020). Patients with positive PD-L1 expression on liver biopsy (8 out of 12 patients in the literature) experienced more rejection compared to those with negative PD-L1 staining (Zhang et al., 2022). However, these stains were not performed in all patients, again making it difficult to estimate the true significance or role for PDL-1 staining as a predictor for rejection. Immune-related adverse effects in this population have not been well studied as well. Hepatitis and cholestatic liver injury have been reported in some series but not in others (Owoyemi et al., 2020; Anugwom et al., 2022).

Unfortunately, the liver transplant literature is limited given its derivation from case reports and case series. This makes it difficult to estimate the true prevalence of acute cellular rejection as well as immune-related adverse events as these are less likely to be reported. Likewise, it is unclear what the true success rate of ICI in the liver transplant population as they are used only as salvage therapy and patients tend to die from their malignancy. More studies are sorely needed within this population.

Heart and Lung

Even less data exist in the heart (ten cases) and lung transplant (three cases) literature (Kawashima et al., 2022). Heart and lung transplant recipients have higher immune suppression requirements as rejection is more common in these individuals. Cancer is a dominant cause of posttransplant mortality in this population as well. Preliminary results for ICI in this population suggest that the outcomes are poor, related to rejection or immune-mediated disease of the allografts (Kawashima et al., 2022). There is a registry being developed which encapsulates thoracic organ transplant (Daud et al., 2020).

Summary

Transplant recipients have not experienced any improvement in cancer-related outcomes over the decades despite substantial improvement in cancer-related prognosis in nontransplant population (Blosser et al., 2021). Within current clinical practice, initiation of ICI in solid organ transplant recipients is currently done as salvage therapy. It is worth discussing with patients that their risk of disease progression is high and that in the absence of alternative cancer-directed therapies, their therapeutic alternatives are limited. Reduction of immunosuppression alone, outside of posttransplant lymphoproliferative disease, has not been shown to improve cancer-free survival (Hope et al., 2015). Accordingly, multiple studies in transplant recipients undergoing ICI therapy have demonstrated that cancer progression is the most frequent cause of premature death, rather than allograft failure post rejection (Delyon et al., 2021; Owoyemi et al., 2020; Carroll et al., 2022). This may be a feature more unique to kidney transplant patients due to the availability of organ replacement therapy with dialysis. On the other hand, rejection risk in a transplant recipient is real, and whether it is 12%, 20%, or 40%, it is high and efforts to mitigate this risk are needed.

Given the paucity of prospective data, and the heterogeneity of the retrospective data available, counselling kidney or liver transplant recipients with advanced or metastatic cancer on the best path forward is challenging. An individualized discussion is paramount in these cases, stressing the risks and benefits of initiating ICI therapy. Research on patient's preferences post-kidney transplant have demonstrated that patients are both concerned about cancer as well as graft health (failure and rejection) (Howell et al., 2016; Sautenet et al., 2017). A qualitative analysis of post-kidney transplant patients' expectations revealed that patients worry about the longevity of the allograft, with some not wanting to resume dialysis if their allograft fails (Tucker et al., 2019).

Patients would benefit from a multidisciplinary care team, with their oncologists and transplant physicians working closely together to determine the potential benefits of pursuing ICI therapy in terms of the likelihood of response to therapy, and the risks to their allograft, utilizing the most current data and not historic data. Knowledge on this domain is continuing to evolve and should improve with active intervention. Ultimately, the final decision will hinge on the patient's willingness to accept the potential risk of allograft failure in exchange for further cancer-directed therapy.

References

Acuna, S. A., Fernandes, K. A., Daly, C., et al. (2016). Cancer mortality among recipients of solid-organ transplantation in Ontario, Canada. *JAMA Oncology, 2*(4), 463–469. https://doi.org/10.1001/jamaoncol.2015.5137

Adam, B. A., Murakami, N., Reid, G., et al. (2021). Gene expression profiling in kidney transplants with immune checkpoint inhibitor-associated adverse events. *Clinical Journal of the American Society of Nephrology, 16*(9), 1376–1386. https://doi.org/10.2215/cjn.00920121

Allison, A. C. (2005). Mechanisms of action of mycophenolate mofetil. *Lupus, 14*(Suppl 1), s2–s8. https://doi.org/10.1191/0961203305lu2109oa

Alzahrani, N., Al Jurdi, A., & Riella, L. V. (2023). Immune checkpoint inhibitors in kidney transplantation. *Current Opinion in Organ Transplantation, 28*(1), 46–54. https://doi.org/10.1097/mot.0000000000001036

Anugwom, C. M., Leventhal, T. M., & Debes, J. D. (2022). Understanding immune perspectives and options for the use of checkpoint immunotherapy in HCC post liver transplant. *Hepatoma Research, 8*, 7. https://doi.org/10.20517/2394-5079.2021.123

Barnett, R., Barta, V. S., & Jhaveri, K. D. (2017). Preserved renal-allograft function and the PD-1 pathway inhibitor nivolumab. *The New England Journal of Medicine, 376*(2), 191–192. https://doi.org/10.1056/NEJMc1614298

Blosser, C. D., Haber, G., & Engels, E. A. (2021). Changes in cancer incidence and outcomes among kidney transplant recipients in the United States over a thirty-year period. *Kidney International, 99*(6), 1430–1438. https://doi.org/10.1016/j.kint.2020.10.018

Carenco, C., Assenat, E., Faure, S., et al. (2015). Tacrolimus and the risk of solid cancers after liver transplant: A dose effect relationship. *American Journal of Transplantation, 15*(3), 678–686. https://doi.org/10.1111/ajt.13018

Carroll, R. P., Boyer, M., Gebski, V., et al. (2022). Immune checkpoint inhibitors in kidney transplant recipients: A multicentre, single-arm, phase 1 study. *The Lancet Oncology, 23*(8), 1078–1086. https://doi.org/10.1016/S1470-2045(22)00368-0

Collett, D., Mumford, L., Banner, N. R., Neuberger, J., & Watson, C. (2010). Comparison of the incidence of malignancy in recipients of different types of organ: A UK registry audit. *American Journal of Transplantation, 10*(8), 1889–1896. https://doi.org/10.1111/j.1600-6143.2010.03181.x

Cortazar, F. B., Kibbelaar, Z. A., Glezerman, I. G., et al. (2020). Clinical features and outcomes of immune checkpoint inhibitor-associated AKI: A multicenter study. *Journal of the American Society of Nephrology, 31*(2), 435–446. https://doi.org/10.1681/asn.2019070676

d'Izarny-Gargas, T., Durrbach, A., & Zaidan, M. (2020). Efficacy and tolerance of immune checkpoint inhibitors in transplant patients with cancer: A systematic review. *American Journal of Transplantation, 20*(9), 2457–2465. https://doi.org/10.1111/ajt.15811

Danesh, M. J., Mulvaney, P. M., Murakami, N., et al. (2020). Impact of corticosteroids on allograft protection in renal transplant patients receiving anti-PD-1 immunotherapy. *Cancer Immunology, Immunotherapy, 69*(9), 1937–1941. https://doi.org/10.1007/s00262-020-02644-2

Daud, A., Mehra, M. R., Siu, A., et al. (2020). Immune checkpoint inhibitors in thoracic transplant recipients: A registry initiative. *The Journal of Heart and Lung Transplantation., 39*(4, Supplement), S210. https://doi.org/10.1016/j.healun.2020.01.832

Delyon, J., Zuber, J., Dorent, R., et al. (2021). Immune checkpoint inhibitors in transplantation-a case series and comprehensive review of current knowledge. *Transplantation, 105*(1), 67–78. https://doi.org/10.1097/tp.0000000000003292

Esfahani, K., Al-Aubodah, T. A., Thebault, P., et al. (2019). Targeting the mTOR pathway uncouples the efficacy and toxicity of PD-1 blockade in renal transplantation. *Nature Communications, 10*(1), 4712. https://doi.org/10.1038/s41467-019-12628-1

Garrett, G. L., Blanc, P. D., Boscardin, J., et al. (2017). Incidence of and risk factors for skin cancer in organ transplant recipients in the United States. *JAMA Dermatology, 153*(3), 296–303. https://doi.org/10.1001/jamadermatol.2016.4920

Hariharan, S., Israni, A. K., & Danovitch, G. (2022). Long-term survival after kidney transplantation. Reply. *The New England Journal of Medicine, 386*(5), 499–500. https://doi.org/10.1056/NEJMc2115207

Ho, A. L. (2023). Immunotherapy, chemotherapy, or both: Options for first-line therapy for patients with recurrent or metastatic head and neck squamous cell carcinoma. *Journal of Clinical Oncology, 41*(4), 736–741. https://doi.org/10.1200/jco.22.01408

Hope, C. M., Krige, A. J., Barratt, A., & Carroll, R. P. (2015). Reductions in immunosuppression after haematological or solid organ cancer diagnosis in kidney transplant recipients. *Transplant International, 28*(11), 1332–1335. https://doi.org/10.1111/tri.12638

Howell, M., Wong, G., Rose, J., Tong, A., Craig, J. C., & Howard, K. (2016). Eliciting patient preferences, priorities and trade-offs for outcomes following kidney transplantation: A pilot best–worst scaling survey. *BMJ Open, 6*(1), e008163. https://doi.org/10.1136/bmjopen-2015-008163

Kawashima, S., Joachim, K., Abdelrahim, M., Abudayyeh, A., Jhaveri, K. D., & Murakami, N. (2022). Immune checkpoint inhibitors for solid organ transplant recipients: clinical updates. *Korean Journal of Transplantation, 36*(2), 82–98. https://doi.org/10.4285/kjt.22.0013

Kayali, S., Pasta, A., Plaz Torres, M. C., et al. (2023). Immune checkpoint inhibitors in malignancies after liver transplantation: A systematic review and pooled analysis. *Liver International, 43*(1), 8–17. https://doi.org/10.1111/liv.15419

Kelly, P. A., Burckart, G. J., & Venkataramanan, R. (1995). Tacrolimus: a new immunosuppressive agent. *American Journal of Health-System Pharmacy, 52*(14), 1521–1535. https://doi.org/10.1093/ajhp/52.14.1521

Lamba, N., Ott, P. A., & Iorgulescu, J. B. (2022). Use of first-line immune checkpoint inhibitors and association with overall survival among patients with metastatic melanoma in the anti-PD-1 era. *JAMA Network Open, 5*(8), e2225459. https://doi.org/10.1001/jamanetworkopen.2022.25459

Lentine, K. L., Smith, J. M., Miller, J. M., et al. (2023). OPTN/SRTR 2021 annual data report: Kidney. *American Journal of Transplantation, 23*(2 Suppl 1), S21–s120. https://doi.org/10.1016/j.ajt.2023.02.004

Lichtenberg, S., Rahamimov, R., Green, H., et al. (2017). The incidence of post-transplant cancer among kidney transplant recipients is associated with the level of tacrolimus exposure during the first year after transplantation. *European Journal of Clinical Pharmacology, 73*(7), 819–826. https://doi.org/10.1007/s00228-017-2234-2

Manohar, S., Thongprayoon, C., Cheungpasitporn, W., Markovic, S. N., & Herrmann, S. M. (2020). Systematic review of the safety of immune checkpoint inhibitors among kidney transplant patients. *Kidney International Reports, 5*(2), 149–158. https://doi.org/10.1016/j.ekir.2019.11.015

Miao, Y., Everly, J. J., Gross, T. G., et al. (2009). De novo cancers arising in organ transplant recipients are associated with adverse outcomes compared with the general population. *Transplantation, 87*(9), 1347–1359. https://doi.org/10.1097/TP.0b013e3181a238f6

Murakami, N., Mulvaney, P., Danesh, M., et al. (2021). A multi-center study on safety and efficacy of immune checkpoint inhibitors in cancer patients with kidney transplant. *Kidney International, 100*(1), 196–205. https://doi.org/10.1016/j.kint.2020.12.015

Owoyemi, I., Vaughan, L. E., Costello, C. M., et al. (2020). Clinical outcomes of solid organ transplant recipients with metastatic cancers who are treated with immune checkpoint inhibitors: A single-center analysis. *Cancer, 126*(21), 4780–4787. https://doi.org/10.1002/cncr.33134

Portuguese, A. J., Tykodi, S. S., Blosser, C. D., Gooley, T. A., Thompson, J. A., & Hall, E. T. (2022). Immune checkpoint inhibitor use in solid organ transplant recipients: A systematic review. *Journal of the National Comprehensive Cancer Network, 20*(4), 406–416.e11. https://doi.org/10.6004/jnccn.2022.7009

Riella, L. V., Paterson, A. M., Sharpe, A. H., & Chandraker, A. (2012). Role of the PD-1 pathway in the immune response. *American Journal of Transplantation, 12*(10), 2575–2587. https://doi.org/10.1111/j.1600-6143.2012.04224.x

Rodríguez-Perálvarez, M., Colmenero, J., González, A., et al. (2022). Cumulative exposure to tacrolimus and incidence of cancer after liver transplantation. *American Journal of Transplantation, 22*(6), 1671–1682. https://doi.org/10.1111/ajt.17021

Rossi, E., Schinzari, G., Maiorano, B. A., et al. (2022). Immune-checkpoint inhibitors in renal transplanted patients affected by melanoma: A systematic review. *Immunotherapy, 14*(1), 65–75. https://doi.org/10.2217/imt-2021-0195

Sautenet, B., Tong, A., Manera, K. E., et al. (2017). Developing consensus-based priority outcome domains for trials in kidney transplantation: A multinational Delphi survey with patients, caregivers, and health professionals. *Transplantation, 101*(8), 1875–1886. https://doi.org/10.1097/tp.0000000000001776

Sehgal, S. N. (2003). Sirolimus: Its discovery, biological properties, and mechanism of action. *Transplantation Proceedings, 35*(3 Suppl), 7s–14s. https://doi.org/10.1016/s0041-1345(03)00211-2

Tucker, E. L., Smith, A. R., Daskin, M. S., et al. (2019). Life and expectations post-kidney transplant: a qualitative analysis of patient responses. *BMC Nephrology, 20*(1), 175. https://doi.org/10.1186/s12882-019-1368-0

Watt, K. D., Pedersen, R. A., Kremers, W. K., Heimbach, J. K., & Charlton, M. R. (2010). Evolution of causes and risk factors for mortality post-liver transplant: Results of the NIDDK long-term follow-up study. *American Journal of Transplantation, 10*(6), 1420–1427. https://doi.org/10.1111/j.1600-6143.2010.03126.x

Yeh, C. C., Khan, A., Muo, C. H., et al. (2020). De novo malignancy after heart, kidney, and liver transplant: A Nationwide study in Taiwan. *Experimental and Clinical Transplantation, 18*(2), 224–233. https://doi.org/10.6002/ect.2019.0210

Zhang, P., Zhu, G., Li, L., et al. (2022). Immune checkpoint inhibitor therapy for malignant tumors in liver transplantation recipients: A systematic review of the literature. *Transplantation Reviews, 36*(4), 100712. https://doi.org/10.1016/j.trre.2022.100712

Zhuang, L., Mou, H. B., Yu, L. F., et al. (2020). Immune checkpoint inhibitor for hepatocellular carcinoma recurrence after liver transplantation. *Hepatobiliary & Pancreatic Diseases International, 19*(1), 91–93. https://doi.org/10.1016/j.hbpd.2019.09.011

Chapter 14
Diagnosis and Management of Immune-Related Adverse Events of Immune Checkpoint Inhibitor Therapy

Casey Fazer-Posorske, Lisa Kottschade, and Anna Schwecke

Abstract The landscape of cancer therapy has undergone a profound transformation in the last decade, shifting from traditional cytotoxic chemotherapy to the rapid rise of immune checkpoint inhibitor (ICI) therapy and combination treatments, fundamentally altering the approach to cancer treatment. However, these advancements introduce challenges in the form of unique toxicities and heightened morbidity. Unlike the side effects associated with conventional chemotherapy, ICI therapy-induced toxicity stems from the over-activation of the immune system, exhibiting delayed onset and persisting for months after treatment cessation. Prompt recognition and intervention are crucial to mitigate associated morbidity and mortality. The FDA has approved ICI drugs targeting four immune checkpoints, including CTLA-4, PD-1, PD-L1, and LAG-3, with dual therapy commonly involving anti-CTLA-4 concurrently with PD-1 or PD-L1 inhibitors. Despite variations in immune system targets, immunotherapy agents share similar and overlapping side effect profiles, necessitating a universal approach to treating immune-related adverse events (irAEs). These events, classified by organ system and severity, commonly impact dermatologic, gastrointestinal, and endocrine systems. While less frequent, toxicities affecting pulmonary, neurologic, and cardiac systems are often more severe, requiring a delicate balance in managing irAEs to attenuate immune response while preserving antitumor efficacy.

Keywords Immunotherapy · Immune-related adverse events · Immune checkpoint inhibitor · Cytotoxic T lymphocyte-associated protein 4 (CTLA-4) · Programmed death receptor 1 (PD-1) · Programmed death ligand 1 (PD-L1) · Lymphocyte activation gene 3 (LAG-3)

C. Fazer-Posorske (✉) · L. Kottschade · A. Schwecke
Division of Medical Oncology, Mayo Clinic, Rochester, MN, USA
e-mail: Fazer.casey@mayo.edu

© The Author(s), under exclusive license to Springer Nature Switzerland AG 2024   179
H. Dong, S. N. Markovic (eds.), *The Basics of Cancer Immunotherapy*,
https://doi.org/10.1007/978-3-031-59475-5_14

Introduction

The landscape of cancer therapy has undergone significant change over the past decade, transitioning from traditional cytotoxic chemotherapy and small-molecule inhibitors to the rapid emergence of immune checkpoint inhibitor (ICI) therapy and combination therapies, thus revolutionizing the paradigm of cancer treatment. Yet these advancements come with the added burden of novel toxicity and increased morbidity. The side effect profile associated with ICI therapy is distinctly different from that of chemotherapy and small-molecule therapy, as ICI toxicity is directly related to over-activation of the immune system. Unlike side effects typically observed with chemotherapy and small-molecule therapy which tend to resolve after discontinuation of treatment, toxicity from ICI therapy can exhibit delayed onset and persist for several months post-drug withdrawal. Therefore, prompt recognition and intervention are essential to mitigate morbidity and mortality.

The Food and Drug Administration (FDA) has approved ICI drugs targeting four distinct immune checkpoints: cytotoxic T lymphocyte-associated protein 4 (CTLA-4), programmed death receptor 1 (PD-1), programmed death ligand 1 (PD-L1), and lymphocyte activation gene 3 (LAG-3). Anti-CTLA-4 therapy is often administered concurrent with a PD-1 or PD-L1 inhibitor and termed dual therapy. Though the various immunotherapy agents exert their effect on different immune system targets, their side effect profiles are similar and overlapping. Thus, treatment for immune-related adverse events (irAEs) is somewhat universal across drug classes. IrAEs are typically classified by organ system and graded according to severity. Treatment of irAEs is a balancing act of attenuating the immune response to mitigate toxicity while maintaining effectiveness against the tumor. The most common irAEs affect dermatologic, gastrointestinal (GI), and endocrine systems. Although less frequent, toxicities affecting pulmonary, neurologic, and cardiac systems are often more severe.

Grading of Immunotherapy Toxicity

Immunotherapy toxicities are graded using a systematic method to evaluate severity and guide treatment and management of irAEs. Side effects are graded according to National Cancer Institute's Common Terminology Criteria for Adverse Events (CTCAE) using a 1–5 scale. Grade 1 is mild toxicity and ICI treatment can generally continue with close observation. Grade 2 indicates moderate toxicity that generally requires interruption of ICI therapy until symptoms improve and may require treatment with corticosteroids. Grade 3 denotes severe toxicity and grade 4 is a life-threatening toxicity, often necessitating further investigation and initial management within a hospital setting, and requires treatment with corticosteroids. It is common for ICI therapy to be permanently discontinued following most grade 3 or 4 adverse events. Grade 5 is a toxicity that results in death (Ramos-Casals et al., 2020).

The primary treatment for ICI toxicity is corticosteroids, such as prednisone, dexamethasone, or intravenous methylprednisolone (Brahmer et al., 2021). Steroids are indicated for most grade 2 or higher toxicity. The initial corticosteroid dosage is determined based on the severity of toxicity, with higher grades requiring higher doses. Once there is improvement in toxicity and clinical status, the steroid dose is gradually tapered facilitating safe discontinuation. A wide range of other immune suppressive and steroid-sparing agents are also used for severe, steroid-refractory, and steroid-dependent toxicity (Brahmer et al., 2021; Schneider et al., 2021; Haanen et al., 2022).

Dermatologic Toxicity

Dermatologic (cutaneous) toxicity is the most common irAE, occurring in up to 70% of patients receiving ICI therapy (Brahmer et al., 2021; Schneider et al., 2021; Haanen et al., 2022). Nonspecific maculopapular rash is the most common skin eruption (Ramos-Casals et al., 2020; Haanen et al., 2022). Less common are vitiligo, lichenoid dermatitis, psoriasis, bullous pemphigoid, granulomatous disease, drug rash with eosinophilia and systemic symptoms (DRESS), Stevens-Johnson syndrome (SJS) and toxic epidermal necrolysis (TEN), and Sweet syndrome (Ramos-Casals et al., 2020; Brahmer et al., 2021; Schneider et al., 2021; Haanen et al., 2022). Rash is often accompanied by significant pruritus (Hodi et al., 2003). Approximately 50% of patients with cutaneous toxicity will present with pruritus as the sole dermatologic manifestation with no visible skin lesions (Brahmer et al., 2021; Haanen et al., 2022). The differential diagnosis for cutaneous eruption includes drug rash from a different medication, viral illness, and infection (Haanen et al., 2022). Work-up includes physical examination, including full skin exam, and may include biopsy (Ramos-Casals et al., 2020). Clinical photographs are helpful to document cutaneous eruption, especially for grade 3 and 4 toxicity (Haanen et al., 2022).

Grading of dermatologic irAEs is based on amount of body surface area (BSA) involved and guides management (see Fig. 14.1). Patients with grade 1 toxicity, defined as less than 10% BSA involvement, can usually be managed conservatively with topical emollients, oral antihistamines, and topical corticosteroids. ICI therapy can continue cautiously, if there is no worsening of symptoms or increase in involved BSA. Patients experiencing grade 2 rash, defined as symptomatic involvement of 10% to 30% BSA or asymptomatic involvement of greater than 30% BSA, will generally require oral steroids at a dose of approximately 0.5–1 milligram per kilogram of body weight (mg/kg) of prednisone in addition to measures used in management of grade 1 cutaneous toxicity. ICI treatment should be withheld until improvement to at least grade 1, and steroid dosing has been tapered to 10 mg of prednisone. While rash may clear rapidly with introduction of oral steroids, clinicians should be cautioned that a rapid steroid taper can cause acute rebound of rash (Brahmer et al., 2021; Schneider et al., 2021; Haanen et al., 2022).

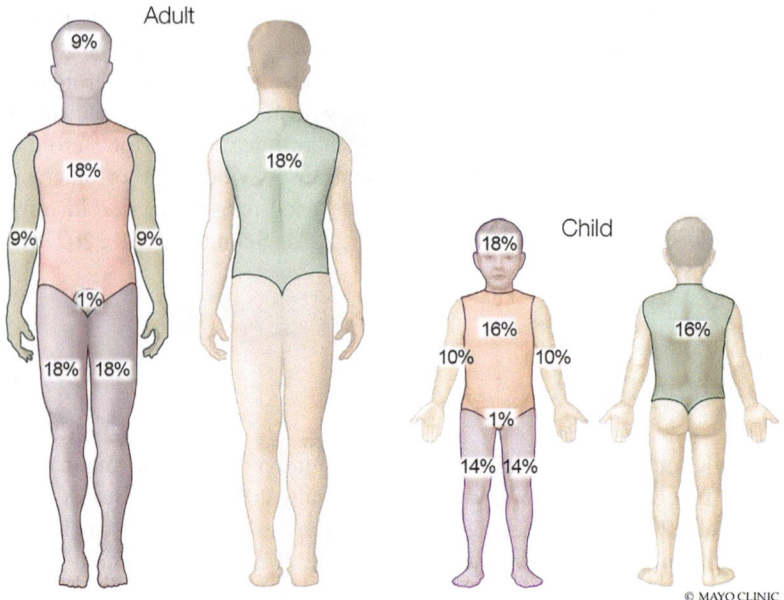

Fig. 14.1 Body surface area

Greater than 30% BSA involvement with moderate-to-severe symptoms and limitations of activities of daily living (ADLs) defines grade 3 toxicity. Grade 4 dermatologic irAE is defined as life threatening. Grades 3 and 4 require higher doses of steroids in addition to conservative measures used in the treatment of grade 1 toxicity. Dermatology referral is strongly encouraged in the setting of grade 3 and 4 toxicity and steroid-refractory irAE. ICI therapy is often permanently discontinued when patients develop grade 3 or 4 toxicity (Schneider et al., 2021; Haanen et al., 2022). Patients with blister-like lesions, fever, or lesions in the oral mucosa or genital region should be evaluated urgently to rule out more serious conditions such as SJS and TEN.

Gastrointestinal (GI) Toxicity

IrAEs of the GI system usually present as diarrhea, a manifestation of underlying immune colitis (Kottschade et al., 2016; Kim et al., 2013; Huffman et al., 2018; Hodi et al., 2014; Eigentler et al., 2016; Bertrand et al., 2015; Beck et al., 2006). Diarrhea is a symptom and is characterized by the passage of loose-to-watery stools, more frequent than a person's usual bowel habits. Where as colitis is the cause of diarrhea and a distinct condition marked by inflammation and swelling of the colon lining (Nemeth & Pfleghaar, 2023; Azer & Sun, 2023). In patients treated with dual ICI therapy, approximately 44% have reported diarrhea, while 36% of those treated with CTLA-4 monotherapy and 11% with PD-1 or PD-L1 inhibitor monotherapy encountered this symptom (Brahmer et al., 2021). Colitis, on the other hand, affects 16% of patients treated with dual ICI therapy, 8% of those treated with CTLA-4 inhibitors, and 1% of those treated with PD-1 or PD-L1 inhibitors (Brahmer et al., 2021; Wang et al., 2019; Wang et al., 2017).

Symptoms may present as a mild increase in the number of stools to severe diarrhea resulting in dehydration and electrolyte abnormalities requiring hospitalization. Although rare, fatal bowel perforations have been reported, underscoring the importance of early recognition and treatment of intestinal toxicity (Larkin et al., 2015; Eggermont et al., 2015). Assessing baseline bowel habits prior to initiation of therapy is crucial for prompt detection and intervention, considering both stool frequency and consistency. Red flag symptoms include hematochezia (bloody stool); the presence of mucus in bowel movements; fever; abdominal discomfort; dehydration, including low blood pressure and weakness (Kottschade et al., 2016). Antidiarrheal antimotility agents, such as loperamide, should be avoided as they may mask worsening symptoms without treating the underlying cause (Schneider et al., 2021).

When evaluating patients with diarrhea, consideration of the differential diagnosis is important. This should include a work-up for infections, inflammatory bowel disease (IBD), and ischemic colitis (Li et al., 2021). Additionally, medication-induced colitis, irritable bowel syndrome (IBS), GI malignancies, food allergies and intolerances, and radiation colitis should be considered in the differential diagnosis (Li et al., 2021).

The work-up and testing for diarrhea require a comprehensive approach for timely and accurate diagnosis and management. Stool testing should be performed to evaluate for infectious etiologies, including bacterial, viral, and parasitic pathogens. Laboratory testing such as complete blood count (CBC), electrolyte panel, liver function tests (LFTs), and C-reactive protein (CRP) levels provide valuable information. Flexible sigmoidoscopy or colonoscopy with biopsy is often performed to assess the severity and extent of colonic inflammation and can differentiate ICI-induced colitis from other inflammatory conditions (Brahmer et al., 2021; Schneider et al., 2021; Haanen et al., 2022). Imaging modalities such as computed tomography (CT) or magnetic resonance imaging (MRI) may be used to evaluate the extent of colonic inflammation and detect complications such as bowel perforation (Brahmer et al., 2021; Schneider et al., 2021; Haanen et al., 2022).

ICI therapy can usually be continued cautiously in patients with grade 1 diarrhea (Brahmer et al., 2021; Schneider et al., 2021; Haanen et al., 2022). Grade 1 diarrhea is defined as fewer than four stools above baseline per 24 hours, and most patients can be managed conservatively with a bland diet, increased oral fluid intake, and close monitoring for stool frequency (Kottschade et al., 2016). Patients with greater than grade 2 diarrhea will need intervention, usually with steroids to prevent further worsening of symptoms (Brahmer et al., 2021; Schneider et al., 2021; Haanen et al., 2022). ICI therapy should be held when grade 2 diarrhea occurs, defined as having 4–6 bowel movements exceeding the baseline count in a 24-hour period, until symptoms improve to grade 1 and the prednisone dosage remains 10 mg or lower. Patients experiencing grade 3 diarrhea, characterized by more than six bowel movements above baseline, will likely need to discontinue ICI treatment, with the following exception: as anti-CTLA-4 agents generally have higher rates of diarrhea, patients who have recovered to at least grade 2 and have discontinued steroids can be rechallenged with single-agent anti-PD-1 therapy, including those who developed diarrhea on dual therapy (Brahmer et al., 2021; Schneider et al., 2021; Haanen et al., 2022).

Patients with grade 3 or 4 diarrhea or those that are steroid refractory at any grade should be evaluated by a gastroenterologist and undergo flexible sigmoidoscopy or colonoscopy with random biopsies to assess the extent of colitis and assess need for biologic modifiers, such as infliximab or vedolizumab, to manage diarrhea (Brahmer et al., 2021; Kottschade et al., 2016).

Hepatic Toxicity

Hepatotoxicity is a direct result of the inflammation of hepatocytes in the liver from T-cell infiltration (Weber et al., 2013). Left untreated, autoimmune hepatitis can lead to liver failure and eventual death. Hepatitis occurs in 5% to 10% of patients receiving ICI monotherapy and in 25% to 30% receiving dual therapy (Haanen et al., 2022).

Prior to each infusion of ICI therapy, the following laboratory values should be assessed: aspartate transferase (AST), alanine aminotransferase (ALT), alkaline phosphatase, and total and direct bilirubin (Brahmer et al., 2021; Schneider et al., 2021; Haanen et al., 2022). The majority of patients who experience ICI-induced hepatotoxicity typically exhibit liver enzyme test results indicative of a hepatocellular injury pattern. This is demonstrated by the presence of asymptomatic increases in serum ALT and AST levels during routine laboratory assessments. While most patients are asymptomatic, some may occasionally present with fever, fatigue, or jaundice (Weber et al., 2013). The differential diagnosis of ICI hepatotoxicity is broad and includes infectious etiologies, such as viral hepatitis, and noninfectious etiologies such as hepatic metastases, biliary obstruction, alcohol use, non-ICI drug-induced liver injury, and others (Remash et al., 2021).

During work-up, it is essential to exclude progressive hepatic metastases and infectious hepatitis. Evaluation of infectious hepatitis includes acute hepatitis profile (hepatitis A, hepatitis B, hepatitis C), herpes simplex virus (HSV), Epstein-Barr virus (EBV), and cytomegalovirus (CMV) (Schneider et al., 2021). Specialist consultation should be sought and efforts made to limit or discontinue any hepatotoxic medications. Additionally, assessing acetaminophen usage, dietary supplement intake, and alcohol consumption can provide valuable insight into potential contributors to hepatotoxicity.

Grading of hepatotoxicity is based on degree of elevation of laboratory studies. Grade 1 is defined as less than three times upper limits of normal (ULN), warranting careful monitoring of liver enzymes on a weekly basis between ICI doses (Brahmer et al., 2021; Schneider et al., 2021; Haanen et al., 2022). Grade 2 hepatoxicity is defined as 3–5 times ULN and ICI therapy should be temporarily discontinued and steroids initiated (Brahmer et al., 2021; Schneider et al., 2021; Haanen et al., 2022). Liver enzymes should be closely monitored twice weekly until hepatotoxicity improves to grade 1. Once liver enzymes have stabilized or started to decrease, a gradual tapering of steroids can be initiated while continuing frequent monitoring of liver enzymes. It is important to exercise caution when considering rechallenging ICI therapy, as hepatotoxicity can reemerge. Therefore, careful monitoring of liver enzymes is recommended in such cases. Grade 3 is defined as five to twenty times ULN and grade 4 is greater than twenty times ULN. Patients with grade 3, 4 or with steroid-refractory hepatotoxicity should be promptly referred to a hepatologist for further management (Huffman et al., 2018). In the case of steroid-refractory hepatitis, infliximab is not recommended because of the risk of hepatotoxicity; however, mycophenolate mofetil (MMF) and tacrolimus have been used (Grover et al., 2018).

Endocrine Toxicity

The majority of endocrine irAEs fall within two categories: those involving the thyroid gland and those involving the pituitary-gonadal-adrenal (PGA) axis (Bertrand et al., 2015; Larkin et al., 2015; Gonzalez-Rodriguez et al., 2016). Type I diabetes mellitus secondary to ICI therapy is rare (Ramos-Casals et al., 2020). ICI-induced endocrinopathies can be difficult to diagnose, as many patients present with generalized constitutional symptoms, including fatigue, nausea, and headache, easily attributed to other causes, often resulting in misdiagnosis. Additionally, patients may be on steroids for other irAEs masking concurrent endocrine-related irAEs that subsequently become obvious during steroid taper (Beck et al., 2006; Ryder et al., 2014).

Thyroid Toxicity

Thyroid dysfunction is one of the most common side effects of ICI therapy, occurring in up to 6% of patients receiving ipilimumab and up to 40% of patients receiving single-agent PD-1 or PD-L1 inhibitor monotherapy (Elia et al., 2020). Thyroid toxicity occurs in two forms: hyperthyroidism and hypothyroidism. Symptoms of hyperthyroidism include weight loss, increased appetite, irritability, anxiety, diaphoresis, palpitations, and tachycardia. Conversely, symptoms of hypothyroidism include fatigue, cold sensitivity, constipation, and weight gain (Ramos-Casals et al., 2020). Hyperthyroidism is often diagnosed by routine lab monitoring demonstrating suppression of thyroid-stimulating hormone (TSH) and high free T4 in an asymptomatic patient. Some patients will have transient tachycardia associated with hyperthyroidism and will benefit from a temporary low-dose beta-blocker (Kottschade et al., 2016; Ryder et al., 2014; Elia et al., 2020).

Commonly, patients develop asymptomatic hyperthyroidism followed by rebound hypothyroidism, defined as TSH greater than 10 (Ramos-Casals et al., 2020). Patients who progress to overt hypothyroidism or present with symptomatic hypothyroidism should start thyroid replacement therapy, commonly levothyroxine (Kottschade et al., 2016; Ryder et al., 2014). Starting dose for levothyroxine is approximately 1.6 micrograms per kilogram of body weight (Ross, 2023). Lower starting dose may be considered for asymptomatic patients or those who have pre-existing cardiac comorbidities. TSH should be monitored 4–6 weeks after initiating thyroid replacement therapy and after dose adjustments with the goal of keeping TSH within normal limits (Kottschade et al., 2016; Ryder et al., 2014; Ross, 2023). Patients with isolated autoimmune thyroiditis can continue to receive ICI therapy with minimal, if any, interruption.

Pituitary-Gonad-Adrenal (PGA) Axis Toxicity

Hypophysitis, an inflammation of the pituitary gland, is the most common PGA axis dysfunction, with clinical symptoms due to secondary adrenal insufficiency (AI) (Brahmer et al., 2021; Schneider et al., 2021; Haanen et al., 2022; Elia et al., 2020). Dual ICI therapy is associated with the highest incidence of hypophysitis, ranging from 9% to 11% (Elia et al., 2020). Hypophysitis commonly presents with acute, severe headache, nausea with possible vomiting, and profound fatigue. As these symptoms mimic intracranial metastatic disease, this should be considered in the differential diagnosis. The diagnosis of hypophysitis is made based on low-to-undetectable morning cortisol and low adrenocorticotropic hormone (ACTH) levels (Corsello et al., 2013). MRI of the head is recommended to rule out intracranial metastases and other neurologic irAEs, such as encephalitis, and can assist in the diagnosis of pituitary dysfunction. Specific MRI views of the pituitary gland should be requested since these are not routinely part of a standard MRI brain exam. It is important to recognize that normal MRI cannot exclude the diagnosis of hypophysitis. During the acute phase of hypophysitis, approximately 75% of patients will have enhancement or enlargement of the pituitary gland on MRI imaging (Brahmer et al., 2021; Schneider et al., 2021; Haanen et al., 2022; Elia et al., 2020; Corsello et al., 2013).

Treatment of hypophysitis aims to decrease inflammation in the pituitary gland, thereby relieving associated symptoms. Most patients will require at least 1 mg/kg of prednisone for relief of symptoms, though patients with severe symptoms may require up to 2 mg/kg and hospitalization (Kottschade et al., 2016). Unlike other irAEs, high-dose steroids can relieve the acute symptoms of hypophysitis within 1–2 weeks. Thereafter, steroids can be rapidly tapered to physiologic replacement levels, provided other irAEs are not present (Kottschade et al., 2016). Unfortunately, the majority of patients diagnosed with hypophysitis will have permanent secondary AI and require lifetime glucocorticoid replacement. ICI therapy should be held during the acute phase of hypophysitis. Once patients are asymptomatic and have tapered to lower or physiologic doses of corticosteroids without recurrence of symptoms, ICI therapy can be safely resumed (Brahmer et al., 2021; Schneider et al., 2021; Haanen et al., 2022).

Primary AI due to ICI therapy is rare, with estimated frequency of 0.6% to 2.6% (Ramos-Casals et al., 2020; Corsello et al., 2013; Hodi et al., 2010; Hamid et al., 2013; Brahmer et al., 2012). Adrenal crisis is a life-threatening emergency that needs to be recognized and treated immediately to prevent morbidity and mortality. Symptoms of adrenal crisis include hypotension; electrolyte imbalances, notably hyponatremia and hyperkalemia; and dehydration (Ramos-Casals et al., 2020). ICI therapy is withheld until symptoms resolve, electrolytes are normal, and steroids have been tapered. Of note, it can be difficult to distinguish primary AI versus secondary AI from prolonged steroid use. Consider endocrinology consultation to assist with management of prolonged steroid tapers requiring interrogation of PGA axis prior to discontinuation of exogenous steroid (Beck et al., 2006; Ryder et al., 2014).

Diabetes Mellitus, Type 1

While rare, diabetes mellitus is a known side effect of ICI therapy and occurs more frequently in patients treated with PD-1 or PD-L1 inhibitors versus anti-CTLA4 therapy (Brahmer et al., 2021; Elia et al., 2020). The incidence of type I diabetes mellitus is 1% to 2% for patients receiving single agent PD-1 or PD-L1 inhibitor monotherapy (Brahmer et al., 2021). Type I diabetes mellitus resulting from ICI is almost always permanent and is treated according to standard guidelines. The clinician should have a low threshold to commence work-up for diabetes mellitus in a patient experiencing polydipsia, polyuria, weight loss, and nausea and vomiting, as diabetic ketoacidosis is the most common presentation (Brahmer et al., 2021). Laboratory studies, including C-peptide and antibodies (anti-glutamic acid decarboxylase, anti-insulin, anti-islet cell), are helpful to distinguish type I from type II diabetes mellitus (Elia et al., 2020).

Pulmonary Toxicity

Pulmonary toxicity, called pneumonitis, occurs less frequently than GI and dermatologic toxicity with an incidence of up to 10% of patients treated with dual ICI therapy (Brahmer et al., 2021; Schneider et al., 2021; Haanen et al., 2022). Pneumonitis rate is estimated at 1% to 5% with single-agent PD-1 or PD-L1 inhibitor monotherapy with highest incidence occurring in patients with non-small cell lung cancer and those who have received thoracic radiation (Ramos-Casals et al., 2020; Brahmer et al., 2021; Schneider et al., 2021; Haanen et al., 2022; Martins et al., 2019). Early symptoms of pneumonitis may be subtle, such as mild, persistent cough and shortness of breath with exertion, though they can progress rapidly to hypoxemia, significant respiratory compromise, and death (Brahmer et al., 2021; Schneider et al., 2021; Haanen et al., 2022; Larkin et al., 2015; Wolchok et al., 2013; Postow et al., 2015). Pneumonitis is commonly misdiagnosed and under-treated, as presenting symptoms are mistaken for bacterial pneumonia. Plain chest radiography (chest x-ray) may reveal minor changes or small consolidations inter-preted as "pneumonia." Subsequently, antibiotics are prescribed, and ICI therapy continued.

New or worsening dyspnea necessitates work-up, and the differential diagnosis includes infectious pneumonia, chronic obstructive pulmonary disease (COPD) exacerbation, progression of malignancy including pleural effusions and lymphan-gitic carcinomatosis, pulmonary embolism, and cardiac etiologies including heart failure, arrythmia, acute cardiac syndrome, myocarditis, and pericardial effusion (Haanen et al., 2022). Work-up of suspected pneumonitis includes the following: comprehensive history to assess pre-existing pulmonary and cardiac conditions that may complicate the diagnostic picture, pulse oximetry at rest and with ambulation, cross-sectional radiographic imaging of the chest (CT chest), pulmonary function tests (PFTs), and consideration of bronchoscopy with lavage to rule out infectious etiologies (Brahmer et al., 2021; Schneider et al., 2021; Haanen et al., 2022; Kottschade et al., 2016). Steroids should be started promptly once radiographic infiltrates or interstitial inflammation is identified, even before completion of infec-tious work-up, due to potential for rapid respiratory decline if pneumonitis is left untreated (Kottschade et al., 2016).

Grade 1 pneumonitis is defined as radiographic findings only in an asymptomatic patient. ICI therapy can be continued with careful monitoring, including pulse oximetry at rest and with ambulation, and consideration of more frequent cross-sectional imaging. ICI therapy should be withheld and corticosteroids started in the setting of grade 2 toxicity, which is symptomatic pneumonitis. Generally, ICI ther-apy is discontinued in the setting of grade 3 pneumonitis defined as severe symp-toms, hypoxemia, or new supplemental oxygen requirement. Grade 4 is life threatening and requires urgent medical intervention, including intubation (Schneider et al., 2021; Haanen et al., 2022). Patients with abnormal oxygen satura-tion should be hospitalized and receive high-dose IV steroids until respiratory status improves (Kottschade et al., 2016). Patients who are steroid refractory or do not improve quickly with steroids should undergo bronchoscopy with bronchoalveolar lavage for further diagnostic inquiry and to exclude infection (Brahmer et al., 2021; Schneider et al., 2021; Haanen et al., 2022; Kottschade et al., 2016).

Patients with grade 2 toxicity can be rechallenged with ICI therapy once steroids have been tapered to 10 mg of prednisone daily. Those with grade 3 or 4 toxicity should not receive further ICI therapy, due to the risk of further respiratory compro-mise (Brahmer et al., 2021; Schneider et al., 2021; Haanen et al., 2022).

Renal Toxicity

Renal toxicity from ICI therapy often manifests as acute interstitial nephritis (AIN). Incidence rates for renal toxicity are low, ranging from 2% to 7%, and are most prevalent in patients who receive dual ICI therapy (Brahmer et al., 2021; Schneider et al., 2021; Haanen et al., 2022). Routine monitoring of renal function includes measuring serum creatinine at baseline and prior to each dose of ICI therapy (Brahmer et al., 2021; Schneider et al., 2021; Haanen et al., 2022). An increase in creatinine can be an early indicator of potential renal toxicity. Other signs of acute renal failure may include azotemia, inability to maintain acid-base balance, electrolyte derangements, and changes in urine output.

Medications that can cause AIN include nonsteroidal anti-inflammatory drugs (NSAIDs), proton pump inhibitors (PPIs), various antibiotics, and diuretics (Brahmer et al., 2021). It is necessary to evaluate infectious causes such as urinary tract infections and acute pyelonephritis. Other factors to consider include drug allergies or hypersensitivity reactions, exposure to radiology contrast, exposure to toxins or heavy metals, and systemic diseases affecting the kidneys (Schneider et al., 2021).

Work-up includes monitoring kidney function with regular serum creatinine and estimated glomerular filtration rate (eGFR) measurements (Brahmer et al., 2021; Schneider et al., 2021; Haanen et al., 2022). Serum electrolytes are evaluated for electrolyte imbalances, such as hyperkalemia and hyponatremia, and acid-base disturbances. Obtain urinalysis to evaluate for proteinuria and hematuria. Patients with ICI-induced acute kidney injury (AKI) have higher levels of serum C-reactive protein (CRP) and urine retinol-binding protein to urine creatinine ratio compared to non-ICI-induced AKI (Seethapathy et al., 2021). In cases of severe or persistent renal dysfunction, a kidney biopsy may be considered to determine the underlying cause and differentiate between irAE and other renal disorders (Brahmer et al., 2021).

Patients with grade 1 creatinine elevation, defined as 1.5–2 times above baseline, can usually continue ICI therapy with close monitoring (Brahmer et al., 2021; Schneider et al., 2021; Haanen et al., 2022). For patients with grade 2 creatinine elevation, defined as 2–3 times above baseline, or higher, treatment should be withheld and nephrology consulted for further evaluation, which may include renal biopsy (Brahmer et al., 2021; Schneider et al., 2021; Haanen et al., 2022). To prevent further renal damage, steroids should be started. The recommended dosage is 0.5 mg/kg of prednisone for grade 2 toxicity and 1–2 mg/kg of prednisone for grade 3, defined as 4–6 times above baseline, or grade 4, defined as greater than six times above baseline (Schneider et al., 2021). Patients with interstitial nephritis that do not respond to steroids may receive infliximab or MMF (Brahmer et al., 2021).

Patients with grade 1 or 2 toxicity can potentially be rechallenged with ICI therapy with close monitoring. Treatment should be permanently discontinued for grade 3 and 4 nephritis (Schneider et al., 2021). Continued monitoring of renal function and vigilant management are essential to ensure early detection and prompt intervention in cases of renal toxicity.

Neurological Toxicity

Neurological toxicity encompasses a broad range of conditions, such as peripheral neuropathy (PN), aseptic meningitis, neuritis, encephalitis, Guillain-Barre syndrome (GBS) which is also called acute inflammatory-demyelinating polyneuropathy (AIDP), and myasthenia gravis (MG) (Wilgenhof & Neyns, 2011; Sznol et al., 2017; Johnson et al., 2013; Hunter et al., 2009; Bot et al., 2013; Bompaire et al., 2012). The overall incidence of neurologic irAEs is extremely rare: 3.8% with CTLA-4 inhibitors, 6% with PD-1 inhibitors, and 12% for dual therapy (Brahmer et al., 2021; Schneider et al., 2021; Haanen et al., 2022). Neurologic toxicities present with diverse clinical features, including headaches, confusion, dizziness, motor deficits, seizures, and cranial nerve palsies. The differential diagnosis involves ruling out other potential causes of neurological symptoms, such as infections, metabolic disturbances, autoimmune conditions, and central nervous system (CNS) metastatic disease (Brahmer et al., 2021; Schneider et al., 2021; Haanen et al., 2022). Prompt recognition and initiation of treatment is critical for reducing long-term morbidity and mortality of neurologic toxicities. Treatment is dependent on the toxicity type and severity and should be undertaken in collaboration with a neurologist.

Guillain-Barré Syndrome (GBS)

The hallmark symptoms of GBS include progressive ascending muscle weakness, often starting in the legs and spreading to the arms and upper body, and can lead to paralysis in severe cases. Other common symptoms include tingling sensations, loss of reflexes, and in some cases pain (Brahmer et al., 2021). GBS can progress rapidly and, in severe cases, can lead to respiratory failure and require intensive medical intervention. Work-up includes spinal MRI, electromyography (EMG), lumbar puncture (LP), serum antibody testing for GBS variants, and PFTs (Schneider et al., 2021). Immunotherapy should be permanently discontinued for all cases of GBS (Brahmer et al., 2021; Schneider et al., 2021). Pulse-dose steroids (methylprednisolone 1gram IV daily for five days) may be considered for grade 3 or 4 along with intravenous immunoglobulin (IVIG) given at 0.4G/kg/d for five days for a total dose of 2G/kg or plasmapheresis (Brahmer et al., 2021; Schneider et al., 2021). Slow steroid taper is recommended once symptoms resolve. Immunotherapy rechallenge is not recommended (Brahmer et al., 2021; Schneider et al., 2021).

Myasthenia Gravis (MG)

MG is an autoimmune neuromuscular disorder characterized by muscle weakness and fatigue, which occurs due to the body's immune system attacking the communication between nerves and muscles (Brahmer et al., 2021). Symptoms can manifest as drooping eyelids (ptosis), double vision (diplopia), difficulty swallowing (dysphagia), and weakness in limb muscles (Brahmer et al., 2021). If MG is suspected, work-up includes PFTs, EMG, and consideration of brain MRI to rule out intracranial metastatic disease (Schneider et al., 2021). Laboratory testing should include acetylcholine receptor and muscle-specific tyrosine kinase antibodies, erythrocyte sedimentation rate (ESR), CRP, creatinine phosphokinase (CPK), and aldolase for possible concomitant myositis (Schneider et al., 2021). In cases where the patient exhibits respiratory insufficiency or elevated CPK levels, a cardiac evaluation is warranted. This assessment should encompass tests such as troponin measurement and an echocardiogram to assess for potential concurrent myocarditis (Schneider et al., 2021). The standard of care for MG includes IVIG and plasmapheresis, as well as high-dose pulse corticosteroids (Brahmer et al., 2021).

Ocular Toxicity

Uveitis, episcleritis, iritis, conjunctivitis, and orbital inflammation (see Fig. 14.2) secondary to ICI therapy are reported in the literature (Brahmer et al., 2012; Wolchok et al., 2010; Robinson et al., 2004; Abdel-Rahman et al., 2017). Ocular

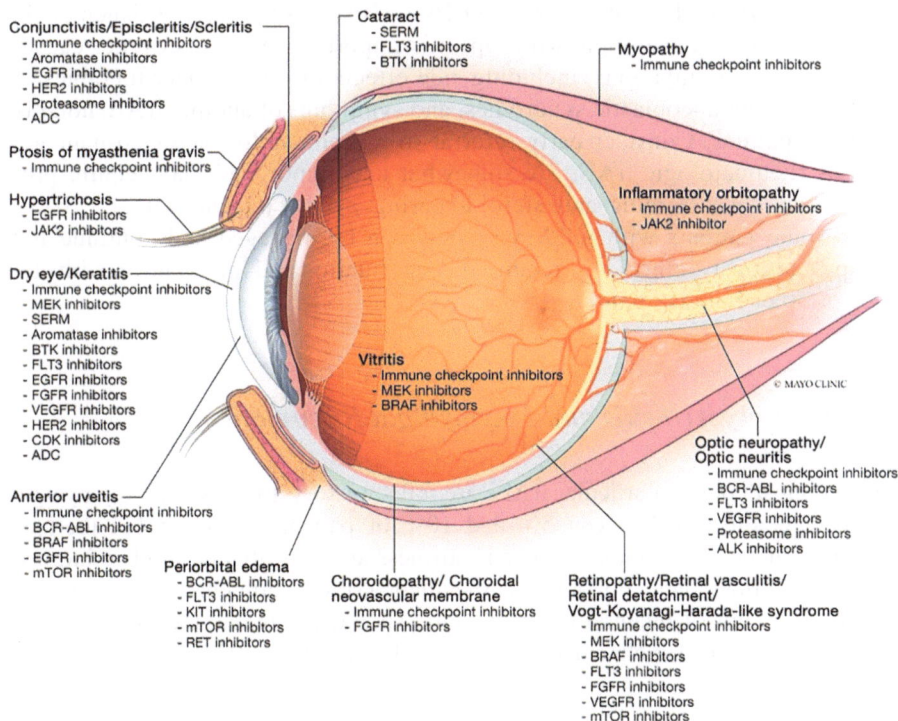

Fig. 14.2 Mechanisms of action in adverse events in the eye

toxicity occurs less frequently than other irAEs, with an incidence of approximately 1% to 4% across various immunotherapy agents (Brahmer et al., 2021; Schneider et al., 2021; Haanen et al., 2022). Patients may present with symptoms such as blurred vision, dry eyes, conjunctivitis, uveitis, or other ocular inflammatory manifestations (Brahmer et al., 2021). Distinguishing ocular toxicity from other eye disorders, such as infection or pre-existing ophthalmic conditions, is crucial. Work-up should include ophthalmologic examination, including slit lamp biomicroscopy, to identify ocular inflammation and guide management (Schneider et al., 2021). Management often involves lubricating eye drops or topical corticosteroids for mild cases and systemic corticosteroids or immunosuppressive agents for more severe presentations (Haanen et al., 2022).

Rheumatologic Toxicity

There are case reports of rheumatological-type syndromes secondary to ICI therapy, including arthralgias, inflammatory arthritis, and polymyalgia rheumatica; myalgias and myositis; Sicca syndrome, defined as dry mouth and dry eyes; granulomatous disorders; and vasculitis (Ramos-Casals et al., 2020; Sznol et al., 2017; Fadel et al., 2009). Arthralgias and myalgias occur most frequently, occurring in 1% to 43% of patients and 2% to 20%, respectively (Haanen et al., 2022). During rheumatologic work-up, it is important to consider other causes of arthralgias and myalgias, including side effects of other cancer therapies or medications, paraneoplastic syndromes, and symptoms of another irAE, notably endocrinopathies. Consider early referral to a rheumatologist for co-management as rheumatologic irAEs are somewhat uncommon and may require prolonged low-dose steroids and steroid-sparing agents (Haanen et al., 2022). While some patients with mild symptoms can be managed and continue ICI therapy cautiously, others will require discontinuation and intervention with steroids or other immune modulators.

Inflammatory Arthritis and Polymyalgia Rheumatica

The two most common articular irAEs are inflammatory arthritis and polymyalgia rheumatica, affecting between 5% and 10% of patients receiving ICI therapy. Arthritis is defined as joint swelling and stiffness and may affect a single joint, few joints, or multiple joints. Polymyalgia rheumatica (PMR) often has acute onset and classic symptoms of bilateral hip or bilateral shoulder pain and morning stiffness (Brahmer et al., 2021; Schneider et al., 2021; Haanen et al., 2022).

Work-up of inflammatory arthritis includes physical examination; count of involved joints, laboratory studies, ESR, CRP, rheumatoid factor (RF), antinuclear antibodies (ANA), anti-cyclic citrullinated peptide (CCP), plain radiographs (x-rays) of affected joints, and consideration of joint aspiration for analysis of synovial fluid. Mild arthritis can be managed with NSAIDs if there are no contraindications to this class of medication. Corticosteroid joint injections may be beneficial if arthritis is limited to one or two joints. Grade 2 and higher arthritis often require systemic corticosteroids. However, unlike other irAEs, a low dose of prednisone at 10–20 mg daily is often sufficient for mild arthritis and prednisone 40–60 mg daily sufficient for moderate symptoms. Many patients may require prolonged, low-dose prednisone to continue ICI therapy (Brahmer et al., 2021; Schneider et al., 2021; Haanen et al., 2022).

Work-up of PMR includes physical examination, laboratory studies, ESR, CRP, RF, creatine kinase (CK), anti-CCP, plain radiographs of affected joints, and consideration of ultrasound of affected joints. It is important to note that CRP may be normal and that CK is evaluated to exclude myositis as these two entities have overlapping symptoms. Grade 2 and higher PMR generally requires systemic corticosteroids, starting at a moderate dose of prednisone 10–20 mg daily. Grade 2 is defined as moderate pain, stiffness, and weakness, and symptoms limit activities of daily living (ADLs). Grade 3 is severe symptoms limiting self-care ADLs; and grade 4 is life-threatening toxicity. Grades 3 and 4 may require additional immunosuppression (Haanen et al., 2022).

Myalgias and Myositis

Myalgia refers to pain or discomfort originating from a muscle group while myositis is the inflammation of skeletal muscles and often manifests as weakness, especially in proximal muscles (NCCN, 2023). Reported incidence of myalgias varies significantly in the literature, ranging from 1% to 20%, while myositis is rare and occurs in approximately 1% of patients receiving ICI (Brahmer et al., 2021; Schneider et al., 2021; Haanen et al., 2022). Myositis can be life threatening if it involves bulbar musculature, impacts the diaphragm and respiratory muscles, or results in myocardial inflammation (Brahmer et al., 2021; Haanen et al., 2022). Work-up of myositis includes physical exam and laboratory studies, including complete metabolic panel (CMP), CK, and aldolase. Consider EMG in cases of grade 2, 3, or 4 myositis. Muscle biopsy may be indicated in severe cases. Rheumatology and neurology should be promptly consulted for co-management (Brahmer et al., 2021; Schneider et al., 2021; Haanen et al., 2022) (NCCN, 2023). IVIG and/or plasmapheresis in addition to corticosteroids are necessary in the treatment of up to 40% of patients diagnosed with immunotherapy-induced myositis (Haanen et al., 2022).

Cardiac Toxicity

Cardiac toxicity includes myocarditis, pericarditis, arrhythmias, impaired ventricular function with heart failure, vasculitis, and venous thromboembolism (Schneider et al., 2021; Haanen et al., 2022). Toxicities affecting the heart are uncommon, reported as 1%, but important due to the high mortality rate, up to 50% (Brahmer et al., 2021).

The clinical presentation of cardiac toxicities ranges from mild fatigue and muscle weakness to heart failure and fatal arrhythmia (Brahmer et al., 2021; Schneider et al., 2021; Haanen et al., 2022). It is important to rule out other causes of cardiac symptoms, such as myocardial infarction or heart failure (Brahmer et al., 2021; Schneider et al., 2021; Haanen et al., 2022).

Immediate cardiology consultation and inpatient care with telemetry monitoring is recommended. Assessment should include electrocardiogram (ECG), echocardiogram, and cardiac MRI (Brahmer et al., 2021; Schneider et al., 2021; Haanen et al., 2022). Laboratory testing should include cardiac biomarkers (CK and troponin T/I) and inflammatory biomarkers (ESR, CRP, and WBC count) (Brahmer et al., 2021; Schneider et al., 2021; Haanen et al., 2022). Biopsy should be considered for patients who are unstable or failed to respond to initial therapy (Brahmer et al., 2021; Schneider et al., 2021; Haanen et al., 2022).

All grades of cardiac toxicity warrant work-up and intervention. Grade 1 is defined as abnormal cardiac markers, without symptoms and no ECG changes (Schneider et al., 2021). In grade 2, abnormal cardiac markers are present with mild symptoms or new ECG changes (Schneider et al., 2021). In the setting of severe, grade 3, cardiac irAE, arrhythmia may be accompanied by significant echocardiogram findings without hypotension and cardiac biomarkers above the ULN (Schneider et al., 2021). Life-threatening, grade 4, cardiac irAEs are denoted by arrhythmia, hemodynamic instability, and cardiac biomarkers more than three times the ULN (Schneider et al., 2021). Permanently discontinue immunotherapy for any grade 3 or 4 cardiovascular irAEs (Schneider et al., 2021).

Treatment with IV steroids should be initiated at pulse dosing (1 gram methylprednisolone daily for 3–5 days). If there is no improvement following corticosteroid treatment within a 24-hour period, it is advisable to contemplate supplementary therapies. Options such as antithymocyte globulin (ATG), MMF, abatacept, or alemtuzumab can be considered for additional intervention (Brahmer et al., 2021; Schneider et al., 2021).

Notably, the combination of myositis, myocarditis, and MG often occurs simultaneously and is called "triple M syndrome" or "overlap syndrome." This warrants special consideration owing to its high mortality rate. Myositis and MG exhibit several overlapping symptoms and are frequently associated with myocarditis. Given the elevated fatality rates of 20% for MG and 17% for myocarditis, any suspicion of one or more of these irAEs should prompt an evaluation for all three conditions (Mahmood et al., 2018; Johnson et al., 2019).

Hematologic Toxicity

Hematologic toxicities are rare and estimated to occur in less than 5% of patients receiving ICI therapy (Brahmer et al., 2021; Haanen et al., 2022). There are a wide variety of hematologic side effects including cytopenias, acquired coagulopathies, and macrophage activation-related conditions. Of these, thrombocytopenia and hemolytic anemia occur most frequently (Brahmer et al., 2021). Differential diagnosis includes other causes of hematologic abnormalities, such as disease progression and bone marrow infiltration by malignancy, side effect of other medications, secondary myelodysplastic syndrome, and infectious sequelae (Haanen et al., 2022). Consider early hematology consultation to assist with diagnosis, which may require bone marrow aspiration and biopsy, and management (Haanen et al., 2022). Severe toxicity requires interruption of ICI therapy and high-dose IV corticosteroids and may also require blood transfusion and growth factor support. Resuming ICI therapy is done with caution as approximately 20% of patients may have persistently abnormal CBC (Haanen et al., 2022).

Principles of Corticosteroid Management

Corticosteroids are the mainstay of treatment for irAEs, with the exception of endocrinopathies. Prednisone is the most commonly used corticosteroid, and the dose is based on grade of irAE and clinical severity. Prednisone for irAEs is generally dosed in milligrams per kilogram of body weight (mg/kg). Grade 3 and 4 irAEs may require pulse-dose intravenous corticosteroid treatment initially, usually with methylprednisolone (Ramos-Casals et al., 2020). Steroids should be used at the smallest dose for the shortest period of time due to side effects of long-term use including weight gain, hyperglycemia, gastritis, osteoporosis, and opportunistic infections. GI prophylaxis with either histamine-2 receptor blockers (H2 blocker) or PPI should be started at the time steroids are prescribed. Patients are instructed to take the entire steroid dose first thing in the morning with food. Prophylaxis against pneumocystis jirovecii pneumonia (PJP) is indicated for steroid doses equal to or greater than prednisone 20 daily. Trimethoprim/sulfamethoxazole (Bactrim) is the most commonly used drug for PJP prophylaxis. For patients allergic to trimethoprim/sulfamethoxazole or for whom this drug is contraindicated, other PJP prophylaxis options include atovaquone, dapsone, and nebulized pentamidine. For prevention of osteoporosis, consideration should be given to calcium and vitamin D supplementation, especially in the setting of prolonged taper. Weight-bearing exercise is also recommended and patients may benefit from referral to physical therapy (Ramos-Casals et al., 2020; NCCN, 2023).

Once a patient demonstrates clinical improvement, steroid tapering can commence, generally over 4–6 weeks (Ramos-Casals et al., 2020). Steroid tapering is an art that requires awareness of guideline recommendations adjusted to the individual patient and toxicity (Schneider et al., 2021). Clinicians must be aware of rebound toxicity during taper and patients instructed to promptly report worsening of symptoms for reevaluation of taper pace. Clinicians must also assess for unmasking of other concurrent irAEs during the taper. If a prolonged taper is anticipated, consideration should be given to early addition of steroid-sparing strategies (Ramos-Casals et al., 2020). Steroid-refractory and steroid-dependent irAEs will require additional immunosuppression (Luo et al., 2021).

With the exception of endocrinopathies, most grade 4 toxicity often results in permanent discontinuation of ICI therapy. Grade 3 myocarditis, nephritis, pneumonitis, hepatitis, and neurologic toxicities generally result in permanent discontinuation of therapy as well. Consideration can be given to rechallenging ICI therapy with milder toxicity, using shared decision-making with each patient and evaluation of individualized risks and benefits (Ramos-Casals et al., 2020). Ideally, prednisone should be tapered to 10 mg daily or less at the time of rechallenge (Brahmer et al., 2021; NCCN, 2023). It is estimated that between 33% and 50% of patients experiencing grade greater than or equal 2 toxicity with PD-1 or PD-L1 inhibitor monotherapy developed irAE with rechallenge of the agent (Ramos-Casals et al., 2020). Colitis, hepatitis, and pneumonitis seem to be associated with higher recurrence rates than other irAEs (Schneider et al., 2021).

Conclusion

The advent of immune checkpoint inhibitors has brought a ray of hope to cancer patients, offering a novel approach to combating malignancy. However, the side effect profile associated with this class of agents is distinct from traditional oncology treatments. IrAEs present a unique challenge as they arise directly from the manipulation and stimulation of the immune system. Consequently, managing these toxicities differs significantly from handling side effects of chemotherapy and small-molecule inhibitors.

Unlike toxicities of other oncologic agents, irAEs do not typically resolve with simple withdrawal or dose adjustments. Instead, they demand targeted intervention to modulate the immune response. Administration of steroids and other immunosuppressive agents becomes essential to stop the hyperactivity of the immune system and mitigate adverse effects.

As ICI therapy rapidly expands its reach in the treatment of both solid tumors and hematologic malignancies, clinicians must remain vigilant to recognize early signs of irAEs. Swift and appropriate management of these complications is paramount to prevent potentially life-threatening consequences and ensure a better quality of life for patients. The ability to strike a delicate balance between harnessing the immune system's power against cancer while mitigating the risks of irAEs will be crucial for the continued success and advancement of immunotherapy in oncology (Tables 14.1 and 14.2).

Table 14.1 Toxicity Summary (NCCN, 2023)

Toxicity	Signs/symptoms	Work-up
Diarrhea/colitis	Increase in stool frequency abdominal pain blood in stool mucous in stool dehydration	Stool sample for GI pathogen panel, fecal calprotectin, CT abdomen/pelvis, and flexible sigmoidoscopy or colonoscopy
Hepatitis	Elevation in AST, ALT, bilirubin, fever, fatigue, and jaundice	Acute hepatitis profile, HSV, EBV, CMV, and liver ultrasound with doppler to evaluate for metastases and clot review medications Consider liver biopsy
Dermatitis	Rash and/or itching	Full skin exam biopsy Consider clinical photographs
Hyperthyroidism	Weight loss increased appetite irritability, anxiety, diaphoresis, palpitations, tachycardia, and tremor	TSH and free T4 thyroid antibody testing
Hypothyroidism	Fatigue, cold sensitivity, constipation, and weight gain	TSH and free T4 thyroid antibody testing
Hypophysitis	Headache, nausea/vomiting, and fatigue, often profound: "run over by a truck"	MRI brain with pituitary views a.m. cortisol, ACTH, TSH, T4, LH in males, and FSH and estrogen in premenopausal females
Adrenal insufficiency	Volume depletion, electrolyte derangements, fatigue, nausea, generalized weakness, arthralgias, and myalgias	a.m. cortisol, ACTH, basic metabolic panel, renin, and aldosterone Consider CT to evaluate for metastasis and hemorrhage
Diabetes mellitus	Polyuria, polydipsia, polyphagia, and unintentional weight loss fatigue	Fasting glucose, serum electrolytes and anion gap, hemoglobin A1c, C-peptide, and diabetes auto-antibody profile (anti-GAD and anti-islet cell)
Pneumonitis	Cough and shortness of breath	CT chest, pulse oximetry at rest and with ambulation, PFTs, and bronchoscopy with bronchoalveolar lavage
Nephritis	Commonly asymptomatic azotemia, acid-base imbalance, electrolyte abnormalities, and decreased urine output	Creatinine with eGFR and CRP Random urinalysis for the following: Microscopy Protein/creatinine ratio Retinol binding protein Bilateral kidney ultrasound evaluating for obstruction and clot review medications Consider kidney biopsy
GBS	Progressive ascending muscle weakness, extremity tingling, and decreased deep tendon reflexes pain	Spine MRI, EMG, LP, GBS variants, and PFTs

(continued)

Table 14.1 (continued)

Toxicity	Signs/symptoms	Work-up
MG	Muscle weakness, fatigue, ptosis, diplopia, and dysphagia	Neurologic physical exam, PFTs, EMG, MRI brain, ESR, CRP, CK, aldolase, and MG antibody panel *Rule out myocarditis and myositis
Ocular	Blurred vision/vision changes, diplopia, dry eyes, and conjunctivitis	Refer to ophthalmology for slit lamp evaluation
Arthritis	Joint pain, joint swelling, and joint erythema	Physical examination, with count of involved joints, assessing for tenderness, swelling, and range of motion, ESR, CRP, RF, ANA, anti-CCP, and x-rays of affected joints Consider joint aspiration for analysis of synovial fluid
Myositis	Muscle weakness	Physical exam, including muscle strength, swallowing and respiratory assessment, CMP, CK, aldolase, EMG, ALT, AST, ESR, and CRP Consider that muscle biopsy may be indicated in severe cases *Rule out MG and myocarditis
Myocarditis	Fatigue, muscle weakness, arrhythmia, increased troponin, chest pain, and shortness of breath	Standard cardiac work-up for ischemia troponin, CK, BNP, ESR, and CRP ECG may show ST-T wave abnormalities and new arrhythmias (heart block or ectopy) Echocardiogram may show diffuse LV systolic dysfunction, RWMA, increased wall thickness, pericardial effusion, and strain abnormalities If echocardiogram inconclusive, consider cardiac MRI and cardiac biopsy *Rule out MG and myositis

Table 14.2 Glossary

ACTH	Adrenocorticotropic hormone. Hormones made by the pituitary gland instruct adrenal glands to secrete cortisol
Acute hepatitis panel	Battery of blood tests drawn to detect acute liver infection with hepatitis virus(es)
ADL	Activities of daily living
Adrenal insufficiency, primary	Occurs when adrenal glands are injured and do not make enough hormone (cortisol and aldosterone)
Adrenal insufficiency, secondary	Occurs when the pituitary gland is injured and does not make enough ACTH. Subsequently, adrenal glands do not make enough cortisol.
AI	Adrenal insufficiency

(continued)

Table 14.2 (continued)

AIN	Acute interstitial nephritis. A kidney lesion that generally causes decrease in kidney function. AIN may be caused by drugs or autoimmune diseases, among other causes.
AKI	Acute kidney injury
Aldolase	A blood test that can indicate muscle damage
ALT	Alanine transaminase also known as alanine aminotransferase. An enzyme found in the liver and other organs that can be measured with a blood test. Elevation of ALT may suggest injury to the liver.
ANA	Antinuclear antibodies
Anemia	Lower than normal red blood cells or hemoglobin to carry oxygen to body tissues and organs. Anemia is assessed with a blood test.
Anti-CCP	Anti-cyclic citrullinated peptide. A blood test that can be useful in diagnosis of inflammatory arthritis
Arthralgia	Joint pain
Arthritis	Joint swelling and stiffness. Arthritis may affect a single joint, few joints, or multiple joints.
AST	Aspartate transferase also called aspartate aminotransferase. An enzyme found in the liver and other organs that can be measured with a blood test. Elevation of AST may suggest injury to the liver.
Azotemia	Condition in which there is too much nitrogen, creatinine, and other waste products in the blood caused by injury or disease in the kidney(s).
BSA	Body surface area. Used to determine grade of dermatologic toxicity
CBC	Complete blood count. Blood test that measures red blood cells and characteristics of red blood cells, white blood cells and white blood cell subtypes, and platelets
CK	Creatine kinase. A blood test that provides information about muscle inflammation
Chemotherapy	Cancer treatment using medicines to stop growth of cancer cells. Chemotherapy either kills cancer cells or stops cancer cells from dividing.
C-peptide	Measured in the blood or urine, this test can help to distinguish between type I and type II diabetes mellitus.
CMV	Cytomegalovirus
CNS	Central nervous system. This includes the brain and spinal cord.
Colitis	Inflammation and swelling of the colon lining
Conjunctivitis	Inflammation of the conjunctiva of the eye (transparent membrane that lines the eyelid and eyeball)
CRP	C-reactive protein. A marker of inflammation measured in blood
CT	Computed tomography
CTCAE	Common Terminology Criteria for Adverse Events published by National Cancer Institute. A system for grading severity of side effects of cancer therapy
CTLA-4	Cytotoxic T lymphocyte-associated protein 4. Anti-CTLA4 drugs include ipilimumab and tremelimumab.
Diaphoresis	Excessive sweating

(continued)

Table 14.2 (continued)

Diarrhea	Passage of loose or watery stools, typically occurring more frequently than an individual's usual bowel habit
Diplopia	Double vision
DRESS	Drug reaction with eosinophilia and systemic symptoms. A severe drug reaction with symptoms including extensive skin rash, organ involvement, enlarged lymph nodes, and elevated eosinophils and lymphocytes in the blood
Dual ICI therapy	Treatment with both an anti-CTLA-4 agent and PD-1 or PD-L1 inhibitor
Dysphagia	Difficulty swallowing
EBV	Epstein-Barr virus
ECG	Electrocardiogram. Also called EKG
echocardiogram	Test that uses sound waves to create pictures of the heart and shows blood flow through the heart and heart valves. Also called echo
eGFR	Estimated glomerular filtration rate
EMG	Electromyography. A test that evaluates health and function of muscles and the nerve cells controlling them
Encephalitis	Inflammation of the brain
Episcleritis	Inflammation of the episclera (thin layer of tissue between the conjunctiva and sclera)
FDA	Food and Drug Administration
Flexible sigmoidoscopy	A test in which a scope is inserted into the lower colon (called sigmoid colon) and is used to evaluate the rectum and sigmoid colon
GBS	Guillain-Barré syndrome. A neurological disorder in which the body's immune system attacks the peripheral nervous system, the part of the nervous system outside the brain and spinal cord. Also called acute inflammatory-demyelinating polyradiculoneuropathy (AIDP)
GI	Gastrointestinal. The gastrointestinal tract runs from the mouth to anus.
Hematochezia	Blood in the stool. Blood appears fresh, bright red.
Hematuria	Blood in the urine
Hepatitis	Inflammation of the liver
HSV	Herpes simplex virus
Hyperthyroidism	Overproduction of hormones by the thyroid gland. Symptoms of weight loss, increased appetite, irritability, anxiety, diaphoresis, palpitations, and tachycardia
Hypoxemia	Oxygen level in the blood lower than normal
Hypokalemia	Low potassium in the blood
Hyponatremia	Low sodium in the blood
Hypophysitis	Inflammation of the pituitary gland
Hypothyroidism	Underproduction of hormones by the thyroid gland. Symptoms may include fatigue, cold sensitivity, constipation, and weight gain.
IBD	Inflammatory bowel disease
ICI	Immune checkpoint inhibitor
irAE	Immune-related adverse effects. Side effects of immunotherapy

(continued)

Table 14.2 (continued)

Iritis	Inflammation or swelling of the iris of the eye (the colored ring around the pupil)
IVIG	Intravenous immunoglobulin
LAG-3	Lymphocyte activation gene 3. Relatlimab is a LAG-3 inhibitor.
LFT	Liver function tests. Blood tests
LP	Lumbar puncture
MG	Myasthenia gravis. An autoimmune neuromuscular disorder characterized by muscle weakness and fatigue. Symptoms can manifest as ptosis, diplopia, dysphagia, and weakness in limb muscles.
mg/kg	Milligram of medication per kilogram of patient's body weight. This is the measurement most often used to dose corticosteroids for the treatment of immunotherapy side effects.
MRI	Magnetic resonance imaging
Myalgia	Muscle pain
Myositis	Inflammation of muscles
Nephritis	Inflammation of the kidney(s)
Neuritis	Inflammation of peripheral nerve(s)
Neutropenia	Lower than normal neutrophils
NSAID	Nonsteroidal anti-inflammatory drug
Pallor	Unusual or excessive paleness. Often refers to the skin, mucous membranes, and conjunctiva
Paraneoplastic	Signs and symptoms caused by cancer indirectly by substances produced by cancer or as part of the body's immune response to cancer
Peripheral neuropathy	Damage to nerves outside of the brain and spinal cord. Peripheral neuropathy may cause pain, numbness/tingling, and weakness.
PD-1	Programmed death receptor 1. PD-1 inhibitors include cemiplimab, pembrolizumab, and nivolumab.
PD-L1	Programmed death ligand 1. PD-L1 inhibitors include atezolizumab, avelumab, and durvalumab.
PFT	Pulmonary function tests
Plasmapheresis	Process by which plasma (the liquid part of the blood) is separated from blood cells. Plasmapheresis can be used to treat a variety of autoimmune disorders and may be used to treat neurologic irAEs. Also called plasma exchange or PLEX
PGA axis	Pituitary-gonad-adrenal axis
PJP	Pneumocystis Jirovecii pneumonia. An opportunistic infection, patients with decreased immune systems (such as those with HIV or those taking corticosteroids or other immunomodulating medications) are at risk for developing this rare fungal pneumonia.
PMR	Polymyalgia rheumatica. Classically, bilateral joint pain, weakness, and morning stiffness involving hips and shoulders
PN	Peripheral neuropathy
Polydipsia	Excessive thirst
Polyuria	Excessive urination

(continued)

Table 14.2 (continued)

Pneumonitis	Inflammation of the lung(s)
Proteinuria	Protein in the urine
Pruritus	Itching
Ptosis	Drooping eyelid(s)
RF	Rheumatoid factor. A blood test that may be helpful in diagnosis of inflammatory arthritis
SJS	Stevens-Johnson syndrome. A severe skin reaction that can cause rashes that blister and peel
Small-molecule therapy	Cancer therapy developed to target a specific alteration in a cancer cell. Commonly administered as pills or capsules. Also called targeted therapy
Steroid-dependent toxicity	An initial remission followed by two or more relapses during the steroid diminution period or within 15 days after tapering of prednisone
Steroid refractory	Immune-related adverse events that do not respond to steroids and require additional immunosuppression
Sweet syndrome	Skin condition characterized by abrupt onset of fever and painful skin lesions. Also called acute febrile neutrophilic dermatosis
TEN	Toxic epidermal necrolysis. A severe form of Stevens-Johnson syndrome (SJS). It is a rare, and potentially life-threatening, skin reaction, usually caused by a medication.
Thrombocytopenia	Lower than normal platelets
Thyroiditis	Inflammation of the thyroid
Triple "M" syndrome	Concurrent myocarditis, myositis, and myasthenia gravis as side effects of immunotherapy. This is a rare and often fatal syndrome.
Troponin	Protein found in the heart muscle. This can be measured in the blood. Increased level of troponin in blood may indicate injury or inflammation of the heart muscle.
TSH	Thyroid-stimulating hormone
ULN	Upper limit normal
Uveitis	Inflammation of the uvea, part of the eye (middle layer of tissue in the eye wall). Symptoms can include eye redness, eye pain, and blurred vision or vision change.

Adapted from mayoclinic.org

References

Abdel-Rahman, O., et al. (2017). Immune-related ocular toxicities in solid tumor patients treated with immune checkpoint inhibitors: A systematic review. *Expert Review of Anticancer Therapy, 17*, 387–394.

Azer, S. A., & Sun, Y. (2023). Colitis. In *StatPearls*.

Beck, K. E., et al. (2006). Enterocolitis in patients with cancer after antibody blockade of cytotoxic T-lymphocyte-associated antigen 4. *Journal of Clinical Oncology, 24*, 2283–2289.

Bertrand, A., Kostine, M., Barnetche, T., Truchetet, M. E., & Schaeverbeke, T. (2015). Immune related adverse events associated with anti-CTLA-4 antibodies: Systematic review and meta-analysis. *BMC Medicine, 13*, 211.

Bompaire, F., et al. (2012). Severe meningo-radiculo-neuritis associated with ipilimumab. *Investigational New Drugs, 30*, 2407–2410.

Bot, I., Blank, C. U., Boogerd, W., & Brandsma, D. (2013). Neurological immune-related adverse events of ipilimumab. *Practical Neurology, 13*, 278–280.

Brahmer, J. R., et al. (2012). Safety and activity of anti-PD-L1 antibody in patients with advanced cancer. *The New England Journal of Medicine, 366*, 2455–2465.

Brahmer, J. R., et al. (2021). Society for Immunotherapy of Cancer (SITC) clinical practice guideline on immune checkpoint inhibitor-related adverse events. *Journal for Immunotherapy of Cancer, 9*(6), e002435.

Corsello, S. M., et al. (2013). Endocrine side effects induced by immune checkpoint inhibitors. *The Journal of Clinical Endocrinology and Metabolism, 98*, 1361–1375.

Eggermont, A. M., et al. (2015). Adjuvant ipilimumab versus placebo after complete resection of high-risk stage III melanoma (EORTC 18071): A randomised, double-blind, phase 3 trial. *The Lancet Oncology, 16*, 522–530.

Eigentler, T. K., et al. (2016). Diagnosis, monitoring and management of immune-related adverse drug reactions of anti-PD-1 antibody therapy. *Cancer Treatment Reviews, 45*, 7–18.

Elia, G., et al. (2020). New insight in endocrine-related adverse events associated to immune checkpoint blockade. *Best Practice & Research. Clinical Endocrinology & Metabolism, 34*, 101370.

Fadel, F., El Karoui, K., & Knebelmann, B. (2009). Anti-CTLA4 antibody-induced lupus nephritis. *The New England Journal of Medicine, 361*, 211–212.

Gonzalez-Rodriguez, E., Rodriguez-Abreu, D., & Spanish Group for Cancer Immuno-Biotherapy (GETICA). (2016). Immune checkpoint inhibitors: Review and management of endocrine adverse events. *The Oncologist, 21*, 804–816.

Grover, S., Rahma, O. E., Hashemi, N., & Lim, R. M. (2018). Gastrointestinal and hepatic toxicities of checkpoint inhibitors: Algorithms for management. *American Society of Clinical Oncology Educational Book, 38*, 13–19.

Haanen, J., et al. (2022). Management of toxicities from immunotherapy: ESMO clinical practice guideline for diagnosis, treatment and follow-up. *Annals of Oncology, 33*, 1217–1238.

Hamid, O., et al. (2013). Safety and tumor responses with lambrolizumab (anti-PD-1) in melanoma. *The New England Journal of Medicine, 369*, 134–144.

Hodi, F. S., et al. (2003). Biologic activity of cytotoxic T lymphocyte-associated antigen 4 antibody blockade in previously vaccinated metastatic melanoma and ovarian carcinoma patients. *Proceedings of the National Academy of Sciences of the United States of America, 100*, 4712–4717.

Hodi, F. S., et al. (2010). Improved survival with ipilimumab in patients with metastatic melanoma. *The New England Journal of Medicine, 363*, 711–723.

Hodi, F. S., et al. (2014). Ipilimumab plus sargramostim vs ipilimumab alone for treatment of metastatic melanoma: A randomized clinical trial. *JAMA, 312*, 1744–1753.

Huffman, B. M., Kottschade, L. A., Kamath, P. S., & Markovic, S. N. (2018). Hepatotoxicity after immune checkpoint inhibitor therapy in melanoma: Natural progression and management. *American Journal of Clinical Oncology, 41*, 760–765.

Hunter, G., Voll, C., & Robinson, C. A. (2009). Autoimmune inflammatory myopathy after treatment with ipilimumab. *The Canadian Journal of Neurological Sciences, 36*, 518–520.

Johnson, D. B., et al. (2013). Severe cutaneous and neurologic toxicity in melanoma patients during vemurafenib administration following anti-PD-1 therapy. *Cancer Immunology Research, 1*, 373–377.

Johnson, D. B., et al. (2019). Neurologic toxicity associated with immune checkpoint inhibitors: A pharmacovigilance study. *Journal for Immunotherapy of Cancer, 7*, 134.

Kim, K. W., et al. (2013). Ipilimumab associated hepatitis: Imaging and clinicopathologic findings. *Investigational New Drugs, 31*, 1071–1077.

Kottschade, L., et al. (2016). A multidisciplinary approach to toxicity management of modern immune checkpoint inhibitors in cancer therapy. *Melanoma Research, 26*, 469–480.

Larkin, J., et al. (2015). Combined nivolumab and ipilimumab or monotherapy in untreated melanoma. *The New England Journal of Medicine, 373*, 23–34.

Li, H., Fu, Z. Y., Arslan, M. E., Cho, D., & Lee, H. (2021). Differential diagnosis and management of immune checkpoint inhibitor-induced colitis: A comprehensive review. *World Journal of Experimental Medicine, 11*, 79–92.

Luo, J., et al. (2021). Beyond steroids: Immunosuppressants in steroid-refractory or resistant immune-related adverse events. *Journal of Thoracic Oncology, 16*, 1759–1764.

Mahmood, S. S., et al. (2018). Myocarditis in patients treated with immune checkpoint inhibitors. *Journal of the American College of Cardiology, 71*, 1755–1764.

Martins, F., et al. (2019). Adverse effects of immune-checkpoint inhibitors: Epidemiology, management and surveillance. *Nature Reviews. Clinical Oncology, 16*, 563–580.

National Comprehensive Cancer Network. Management of immmunotherapy-related toxicities (Version 2.2023). https://www.nccn.org/professionals/physician_gls/pdf/immunotherapy.pdf. Accessed June 6, 2024.

Nemeth, V., & Pfleghaar, N. (2023). Diarrhea. In *StatPearls*.

Postow, M. A., et al. (2015). Nivolumab and ipilimumab versus ipilimumab in untreated melanoma. *The New England Journal of Medicine, 372*, 2006–2017.

Ramos-Casals, M., et al. (2020). Immune-related adverse events of checkpoint inhibitors. *Nature Reviews. Disease Primers, 6*, 38.

Remash, D., et al. (2021). Immune checkpoint inhibitor-related hepatotoxicity: A review. *World Journal of Gastroenterology, 27*, 5376–5391.

Robinson, M. R., et al. (2004). Cytotoxic T lymphocyte-associated antigen 4 blockade in patients with metastatic melanoma: A new cause of uveitis. *Journal of Immunotherapy, 27*, 478–479.

Ross, D. S. (2023). Treatment of primary hypothyroidism in adults. Douglass S. Ross

Ryder, M., Callahan, M., Postow, M. A., Wolchok, J., & Fagin, J. A. (2014). Endocrine-related adverse events following ipilimumab in patients with advanced melanoma: A comprehensive retrospective review from a single institution. *Endocrine-Related Cancer, 21*, 371–381.

Schneider, B. J., et al. (2021). Management of Immune-Related Adverse Events in patients treated with immune checkpoint inhibitor therapy: ASCO guideline update. *Journal of Clinical Oncology, 39*, 4073–4126.

Seethapathy, H., Herrmann, S. M., & Sise, M. E. (2021). Immune checkpoint inhibitors and kidney toxicity: Advances in diagnosis and management. *Kidney Medicine, 3*, 1074–1081.

Sznol, M., et al. (2017). Pooled analysis safety profile of nivolumab and ipilimumab combination therapy in patients with advanced melanoma. *Journal of Clinical Oncology, 35*, 3815–3822.

Wang, D. Y., Ye, F., Zhao, S., & Johnson, D. B. (2017). Incidence of immune checkpoint inhibitor-related colitis in solid tumor patients: A systematic review and meta-analysis. *Oncoimmunology, 6*, e1344805.

Wang, Y., et al. (2019). Treatment-related adverse events of PD-1 and PD-L1 inhibitors in clinical trials: A systematic review and meta-analysis. *JAMA Oncology, 5*, 1008–1019.

Weber, J. S., et al. (2013). Patterns of onset and resolution of immune-related adverse events of special interest with ipilimumab: Detailed safety analysis from a phase 3 trial in patients with advanced melanoma. *Cancer, 119*, 1675–1682.

Wilgenhof, S., & Neyns, B. (2011). Anti-CTLA-4 antibody-induced Guillain-Barre syndrome in a melanoma patient. *Annals of Oncology, 22*, 991–993.

Wolchok, J. D., et al. (2010). Ipilimumab monotherapy in patients with pretreated advanced melanoma: A randomised, double-blind, multicentre, phase 2, dose-ranging study. *The Lancet Oncology, 11*, 155–164.

Wolchok, J. D., et al. (2013). Nivolumab plus ipilimumab in advanced melanoma. *The New England Journal of Medicine, 369*, 122–133.

Chapter 15
Immunotherapy for Head and Neck Cancer

Patrick McGarrah, Harry Fuentes Bayne, Casey Fazer-Posorske, and Katharine Price

Abstract Head and neck cancer refers to malignancies originating mainly from the mucosal surfaces of the nose, mouth, and throat. Squamous cell carcinoma is by far the most common type of head and neck cancer, and immunotherapy is a core component of treatment for advanced and metastatic disease. Large clinical trials have demonstrated that the checkpoint inhibitors pembrolizumab and nivolumab extend the survival of patients compared to traditional chemotherapy regimens. Immunotherapy seems to work best in head and neck cancers where the tumor and immune cells express the PD-L1 protein. There have been significant efforts exploring how to use immunotherapy for early-stage and curable head and neck cancers. Thus far, large trials have not shown a benefit to adding immunotherapy in this setting. Future efforts investigating immunotherapy for head and neck cancers are using cancer vaccines, engineered viruses, and therapies targeting the human papilloma virus (HPV)—a virus known to cause many cases of head and neck cancer.

Keywords Head and neck cancer · Head and neck squamous cell carcinoma · Oropharynx cancer · Larynx cancer · Oral cavity cancer · Human papilloma virus · HPV · Mouth cancer · Throat cancer · Pembrolizumab · Nivolumab · Checkpoint inhibitors · PD-L1

Introduction

Head and neck cancer typically refers to malignancies that originate outside of the skull from epithelial surfaces of the oral cavity, sinonasal cavity, pharynx, larynx, and salivary glands. The seventh most common cancer worldwide, there are 660,000 new cases of head and neck cancer each year and 325,000 deaths (Gormley et al., 2022). The great majority (~90%) of these are head and neck squamous cell

P. McGarrah (✉) · H. Fuentes Bayne · C. Fazer-Posorske · K. Price
Division of Medical Oncology, Mayo Clinic, Rochester, MN, USA
e-mail: mcgarrah.patrick@mayo.edu

205

carcinoma (HNSCC) (Pai & Westra, 2009). The incidence of head and neck cancer is increasing, with an expected global annual rate increase of 30% by 2030 compared to 2020. In Western countries, oropharyngeal cancer driven by human papilloma virus (HPV) infection comprises most new cases. HPV-driven HNSCC is also increasing in other parts of the world, but additional risk factors such as betel nut chewing in Southeast Asian populations drive non-virally mediated HNSCC. Tobacco and alcohol, especially in combination, are universal risk factors for head and neck cancer. Each of the causative agents of HNSCC (HPV, smoking, betel, etc.) differentially influences the tumor microenvironment and systemic immune response. This has important ramifications for how to employ immunotherapy as a therapeutic intervention.

Nonsquamous neoplasms (e.g., adenocarcinoma, adenoid cystic carcinoma), especially from salivary glands, the sinonasal cavity, and the thyroid, are also frequently classified as head and neck cancer. Because most head and neck cancer morbidity and mortality worldwide is attributable to HNSCC, the bulk of the research and clinical experience with immunotherapy in head and neck cancer has been with HNSCC. The literature describing immunotherapy in nonsquamous head and neck malignancies is comparatively limited. Therefore, this chapter will focus exclusively on immunotherapy for HNSCC.

The Tumor Microenvironment, Tumor Antigens, and Therapeutic Targets for Immunotherapy in HNSCC

As in other malignancies, the immune system responds to the presence of HNSCC with local infiltration by the innate and adaptive systems. The degree of infiltration in terms of sheer number of immune cells as well as the cell types is highly dependent on whether the tumor is driven by HPV infection (Ruffin et al., 2023). HPV-positive tumors tend to have a greater total number of infiltrating immune cells present in the tumor microenvironment. This increase is seen for a broad range of immune cell types including cytotoxic CD8+ T cells, CD4+ T helper cells, NK cells, B cells, and plasma cells (Mito et al., 2021). Not only are HPV-positive tumors more immune infiltrated, but the immune cells are also more "activated" as evidenced by expression of higher levels of effector proteins such as granzymes and perforin (Mandal et al., 2016). HPV-positive HNSCC carries a more favorable prognosis than HPV-negative disease (Chaturvedi et al., 2011), and increased and more activated immune infiltration accounts for some but not all of this difference. HNSCC patients with high levels of CD8+ T cell infiltration, total T cell infiltration, and overall high immune cell infiltration have all independently correlated with improved survival irrespective of HPV status (Mandal et al., 2016).

As HPV status is not wholly determinative of the immunologic response to HNSCC, behavioral factors such as smoking have been shown to impact the tumor microenvironment. Smoking causes characteristic gene mutations in a variety of cancers (Alexandrov et al., 2013), and models exist to assess whether a patient's tumor harbors a molecular "smoking signature." HNSCC tumors with this gene signature have decreased total infiltrating immune cells, T cells, and interferon-gamma signaling. This remains true in both HPV-positive and HPV-negative tumors (Mandal et al., 2016). The smoking signature is also associated with a high number of total tumor mutations. This finding might be expected to result in a higher number of presented tumor antigens that can be recognized by the immune system. However, not all mutations will result in a successfully presented antigen that in turn leads immune cell infiltration (Zou et al., 2021). This may partially explain how it is possible for tumors with a smoking signature to have decreased immune infiltration. Smoking itself can have local immunosuppressive effects (Stämpfli & Anderson, 2009). Taking this into account, it follows that patients with HNSCC with *high* T cell infiltration but also *low* markers of molecular smoking signature have the best survival, independent of HPV status. This tumor microenvironment promotes the highest level of intrinsic, treatment-naïve anticancer immunity and enables more effective therapeutic intervention with immunotherapy.

Immunotherapy targets described and utilized in other cancers are also present in HNSCC. The immune checkpoint axis PD-1/PD-L1 is expressed by HNSCC tumor cells and by infiltrating immune cells. The majority of patients have some detectable level of PD-L1 expression (Kim et al., 2015). In a patient cohort treated prior to the availability of FDA-approved PD-(L)-1 inhibitors, PD-L1 expression was not significantly associated with patient outcome (Kim et al., 2015). As will be discussed, PD-(L)-1 inhibitors were found in large clinical trials to improve survival in HNSCC. Both HPV-positive and HPV-negative HNSCC tumors express PD-L1, though there is conflicting data regarding whether HPV-positive tumors express PD-L1 more frequently and on a higher percentage of total tumor and infiltrating immune cells (Mandal et al., 2016; Kim et al., 2015; Veigas et al., 2021; Tosi et al., 2022). Another well-described target, the CTLA-4 immune checkpoint surface molecule is expressed in HNSCC. Interestingly, a study of 86 patient samples found that the absolute amount of CTLA-4 expression does not correlate with survival, but the ratio of CD8+ T cells to CTLA-4 expression was positively correlated with a better prognosis (Yu et al., 2016). This suggests that a decreased immunosuppressive effect of CTLA-4 accompanied by sufficient amount of cytotoxic T cell infiltration is important for effective immune response against HNSCC. In this cohort of patients, there was not a statistically significant difference in the CD8+/CTLA-4 ratio between HPV-positive and HPV-negative tumors.

Immunotherapy for Relapsed or Metastatic Disease

Patients initially diagnosed with HNSCC confined to the primary site or with metastasis limited to cervical lymph nodes are considered to have curable disease. These patients can be treated with various combinations of surgery, radiation, and chemotherapy (Pfister & Sharon, n.d.). The precise treatment selected depends on the size

of the primary tumor, the extent of involvement of regional lymph nodes, the anticipated morbidity of treatment, and patient comorbidities. Based on data from 2013
to 2019, 87% of patients with localized-only and 69% of those with regional lymph
node spread of oral cavity and pharynx cancer were alive 5 years after diagnosis
(SEER*Explorer, 2023). For HPV-positive oropharynx cancers, a large dataset
where most patients (~90%) had locally advanced disease still showed that many
patients are cured with a 5-year survival rate of 81% (Mehanna et al., 2023). For
those patients who either have distant metastasis at the time of diagnosis, or those
who have recurrence after initial aggressive treatment, the disease is typically considered incurable. In this setting, the treatment goals are palliative and focus on
controlling cancer growth and maximizing quality and quantity of life.

The cornerstone of treatment for relapsed or metastatic HNSCC that is no longer
considered curable is systemic therapy. Prior to 2008, this had traditionally been
composed of either single-agent or combination cytotoxic chemotherapy regimens.
After 2008, the standard first-line therapy for recurrent or metastatic HNSCC was
platinum-based chemotherapy with the epidermal growth factor receptor monoclonal antibody cetuximab (EXTREME regimen) (Vermorken et al., 2008). The first
licensed immunotherapy drug in HNSCC was the PD-1 inhibitor pembrolizumab,
approved on a conditional basis by the FDA in 2016 (Pembrolizumab (KEYTRUDA),
2023). Nivolumab, another PD-1 inhibitor, was approved just 3 months later
(Nivolumab for SCCHN, 2023). These two agents have become part of the standard
of care for managing relapsed or metastatic HNSCC.

Second-Line Immunotherapy in HNSCC

Pembrolizumab was granted accelerated FDA approval in 2016 based on the results
of the KEYNOTE-012 trial. This nonrandomized study evaluated 174 patients with
recurrent or metastatic HNSCC who had progressed on platinum chemotherapy.
The response rate of 16.1% was superior to historical alternatives, but most impres-
sively, many patients that responded had long-term responses exceeding 12 months.
These promising results prompted early FDA approval contingent on confirmation
of an overall survival benefit in the randomized phase 3 KEYNOTE-040 trial
(Larkins et al., 2017). This trial randomized 495 patients to pembrolizumab versus
standard of care choice of methotrexate, docetaxel, or cetuximab. Despite initially
not reaching the prespecified threshold for statistical significance and delaying full
FDA approval, in the final analysis, the median overall survival improvement was
confirmed at 8.4 months for the pembrolizumab group versus 6.0 months in the
control arm (Cohen et al., 2019; Gyawali et al., 2019).

Nivolumab was studied in the phase 3 CheckMate141 clinical trial which served
as the basis for its FDA approval (Ferris et al., 2016). The trial randomized 361
patients who had recurrent or metastatic HNSCC who had disease progression after
platinum chemotherapy, to either nivolumab or a standard of care choice of cetuximab, methotrexate, or docetaxel. The primary outcome was overall survival, and

nivolumab showed a statistically significant improvement—7.5 months versus 5.1 months. In a subsequent long-term analysis of the trial, the survival benefit was even more substantial—7.7 versus 3.3 months (Gillison et al., 2022). Quality of life was also significantly improved in the nivolumab cohort, with patient level of functioning and symptoms stabilizing with immunotherapy but declining in the chemotherapy-cetuximab group (Harrington et al., 2017). Importantly, there was a small but distinct population of patients who received a sustained benefit from nivolumab. At the 2-year mark, 14.8% of nivolumab patients were still alive without any progression of disease, compared to zero patients in the standard of care group. This highlights an important theme in cancer immunotherapy—some patients will mobilize a sustained immune response to their malignancy after checkpoint inhibitor treatment. The duration of response is often much greater than that seen with conventional cytotoxic chemotherapy.

First-Line Immunotherapy in HNSCC

The first FDA approvals for nivolumab and pembrolizumab in HNSCC were for patients who had progressive disease after receiving platinum chemotherapy. Subsequently, pembrolizumab was tested in the first-line setting for patients previously untreated in the recurrent or metastatic setting. The phase 3 KEYNOTE-048 trial randomized 882 patients with relapsed or metastatic HNSCC to either pembrolizumab alone, pembrolizumab plus 5-fluorouracil (5-FU) and platinum, or the standard of care cetuximab plus 5-FU and platinum (Burtness et al., 2019). In a long-term follow-up analysis, pembrolizumab plus chemotherapy resulted in a median survival of 13.0 months compared to 10.7 months for cetuximab plus chemotherapy (Harrington et al., 2023). Pembrolizumab monotherapy also resulted in a numerically larger median survival of 11.5 months versus 10.7 months for cetuximab plus chemotherapy, but this did not reach the prespecified statistical cutoff for superiority. When groups were stratified according to PD-L1 expression, patients whose tumors and immune infiltrates expressed PD-L1 had better survival with both pembrolizumab alone and pembrolizumab plus chemotherapy compared to cetuximab plus chemotherapy. Based on the results of KEYNOTE-048, the FDA approved pembrolizumab as a first-line treatment for recurrent or metastatic HNSCC in 2019. The approval endorsed pembrolizumab plus chemotherapy for all patients and pembrolizumab alone for patients whose tumors express PD-L1 (FDA, 2023).

Dual Immunotherapy in HNSCC

As the PD-1 inhibitors nivolumab and pembrolizumab became standard treatment options in recurrent or metastatic HNSCC, clinical trials sought to test the benefit of adding CTLA-4 inhibitors to PD-1 inhibition. This was a rational question based on the demonstrated added efficacy of dual checkpoint inhibition in several other solid tumors including non-small cell lung cancer (Brahmer et al., 2023), renal cell carcinoma (Grimm et al., 2021), and melanoma (Wolchok et al., 2022). Furthermore, because response rates for single agent PD-1 inhibitors were in the range of 15–20%, there was a need to expand the proportion of patients that could benefit from immunotherapy. Unfortunately, at present, clinical trials combining PD-1 inhibition with CTLA-4 inhibition in HNSCC have not yielded a positive trial. The CheckMate 651 phase 3 trial randomized 947 patients to the dual immunotherapy nivolumab plus ipilimumab (CTLA-4 inhibitor) versus cetuximab plus chemotherapy (Haddad et al., 2023). There was no difference in overall survival between the groups, though the median duration of response was 32.6 months for dual immunotherapy compared to 7.0 months for cetuximab plus chemotherapy. Two other phase 3 trials, KESTREL and EAGLE, evaluated the combination of the PD-1 inhibitor durvalumab with the CTLA-4 inhibitor tremelimumab compared to chemotherapy and cetuximab combinations in the first and second lines, respectively (Psyrri et al., 2023; Ferris et al., 2020). Both of these trials also failed to meet specified endpoints for survival benefit of the dual immunotherapy regimen. With three negative phase 3 trials, the available data indicates that dual checkpoint inhibition in HNSCC does not have a significant benefit over PD-1 inhibition alone. While some of the analysis suggests that the response rate is augmented, this is not sufficient to meet the high standard needed for regulatory approval.

Immunotherapy in the Curative Intent Setting

With the established clinical benefit and improved survival from immunotherapy in recurrent or metastatic HNSCC, a logical next step is to explore checkpoint inhibitors for locally advanced tumors where the goal of therapy is cure. As locally advanced HNSCC is treated with a combination of surgery, radiation, and chemotherapy, there are multiple options for incorporating immunotherapy into the multimodal treatment approach. Clinical trials have explored adding checkpoint inhibitors prior to surgical resection, after resection, as well as before, during, and after chemoradiation. Multiple phase 1 and phase 2 trials have shown clinical activity in terms of radiographic and pathologic tumor response, as well as safety, when adding checkpoint inhibitors to multimodal, curative intent HNSCC (Ferris et al., 2021; Juloori et al., 2023; Schoenfeld et al., 2020; Zuur et al., 2020). A systematic review of 10 early phase trials including 344 total patients came to a similar conclusion regarding antitumor activity and safety (Masarwy et al., 2021). Two trials using dual immunotherapy prior to surgical resection reported major pathologic response rates of approximately 20% and 30% (Schoenfeld et al., 2020; Zuur et al., 2020). However, two phase 3 trials that were designed to test the more clinically meaningful endpoints such as progression-free survival and overall survival failed to confirm benefit (Lee et al., 2021; Machiels et al., 2022). These two negative trials tested the addition of PD-(L)-1 inhibition during and after chemoradiation. The first, JAVELIN

Head and Neck 100, tested the addition of the PD-L1 inhibitor avelumab versus placebo during chemoradiation, followed by maintenance avelumab/placebo. The primary objective of improving progression-free survival was not met. The second, KEYNOTE-412, was similarly designed, adding pembrolizumab or placebo to chemoradiation, but also fell short of its goal of prolonging time until recurrence or progression. The IMSTAR-HN trial is a phase 3 study exploring the addition of single and dual immunotherapy to both pre- and postsurgical resection of HNSCC (Zech et al., 2020). The results of this trial are eagerly awaited, but at present, there is not yet a consensus standard of care role for immunotherapy in curable HNSCC. It has been postulated that some of the trials failed to show benefit due to the immunosuppressive effects of chemoradiation given simultaneously with immunotherapy. That is, the antitumor T cell response was diminished by chemotherapy-induced bone marrow suppression as well as radiation to involved lymph nodes. Based on this hypothesis, prioritizing adding single-agent immunotherapy either *before* or *after* (but not during) chemoradiation is a rational design for future clinical trials using immunotherapy in curative-intent HNSCC.

Markers to Predict Benefit from Immunotherapy

Modern cancer immunotherapy trials typically include extensive tissue testing of tumor samples to evaluate characteristics that are predictive of either response or resistance to immunotherapy. The most studied marker is protein expression of PD-L1 on the surface of tumor cells and infiltrating immune cells. This has yielded useful selection criteria for immunotherapy candidates, particularly in lung, upper gastrointestinal, breast, cervical, and head and neck cancers. For the phase 3 trials that led to FDA approval of PD-1 inhibitors in HNSCC, expression of PD-L1 on at least 1% of tumor or infiltrating immune cells was highly correlated with increased survival compared to the control arms not using checkpoint inhibitors (Cohen et al., 2019; Ferris et al., 2016; Burtness et al., 2019). While PD-L1 expression is only required for official FDA labeling indications when using pembrolizumab *monotherapy* in the *first-line* setting, expert guidelines emphasize that PD-L1 expression is associated with better outcomes when giving immunotherapy as a single agent in any line of treatment (Pfister & Sharon, n.d.). Hence, single-agent immunotherapy is generally not appropriate for PD-L1-negative tumors, although response can still be seen in PD-L1-negative tumors. It should be noted that in these trials, more than 50% of specimens had PD-L1 expression on the tumor cells and more than 75% had expression on either immune or tumor cells. Despite the correlation of PD-L1 with response and survival, the need for a more precise and accurate biomarker of response to immunotherapy remains.

Tumor mutational burden (TMB) and high microsatellite instability (MSI) from DNA mismatch repair deficiency are two additional markers for immunotherapy benefit. These were evaluated in the nonrandomized phase 2 KEYNOTE-158 trial that enrolled patients with multiple primary tumor types. Approximately, one-third of patients in the trial showed objective response in both the TMB-high and MSI-high cohorts. This led to accelerated FDA approval in 2020 that is subject to future confirmatory analysis of additional patients. The trial, however, only included one patient with HNSCC and that patient was in the MSI-H cohort. There is additional evidence, though, supporting TMB as a predictive marker for response to pembrolizumab. In an exploratory analysis of 257 patients treated in early phase trials with pembrolizumab, TMB, PD-L1, and a T cell-inflamed gene expression profile (Tcell$_{inf}$GEP) were each independent predictors of response (Pfister et al., 2023). This is of particular importance for patients without PD-L1 expression, as TMB (which is commonly obtained on tumor genetic panels) can be used to support pembrolizumab monotherapy where it would otherwise not be recommended. Less commonly available markers, such as Tcell$_{inf}$GEP, require further validation and then broader incorporation into standard tumor testing panels before they can be applied to standard clinical practice. Additional data from large, randomized trials on biomarkers to better predict immunotherapy response are expected, but at present, the most validated tools in HNSCC aid PD-L1, with TMB and MSI being validated biomarkers of immunotherapy response across multiple solid tumor types.

Future Directions

While immunotherapy already has an established role in the treatment of HNSCC, there is a great need to increase the proportion of patients who benefit. Currently, the only setting with proven benefit is in those with advanced disease that is recurrent or metastatic. While those with localized disease often can be cured with standard non-immunotherapeutic approaches, there is strong early-stage data to justify pursuing immunotherapy, in specifically checkpoint inhibitors, to improve cure rates. Additional efforts are underway to improve responses to PD-1 inhibition, with encouraging results particularly from novel HPV-based vaccines and T cell stimulators to augment the antitumor immune response in HPV-positive HNSCC (Price et al., 2023; Chung et al., 2023). Some early phase trials have also reported the feasibility of engineering T cells to target HPV-positive HNSCC, but large randomized trials using cell therapy have not yet begun (Wang et al., 2023). While much of the research and success has been heavily focused on cytotoxic T cells as therapeutic targets, a broader investigation of the tumor microenvironment will facilitate the development of new therapies directed at natural killer cells, B cells, regulatory T cells, and lymph node architectures. Furthermore, personalized evaluation of individual patient tumors and immune signatures will become more feasible as technologies such as single cell RNA sequencing and immune gene expression profiles become more readily available. This will allow for optimized patient selection, an increased proportion of patients who are candidates for immunotherapy, and improved outcomes.

References

Alexandrov, L. B., Nik-Zainal, S., Wedge, D. C., et al. (2013). Signatures of mutational processes in human cancer. *Nature, 500*(7463), 415–421. https://doi.org/10.1038/nature12477

Brahmer, J. R., Lee, J. S., Ciuleanu, T. E., et al. (2023). Five-year survival outcomes with nivolumab plus ipilimumab versus chemotherapy as first-line treatment for metastatic non-small-cell lung cancer in CheckMate 227. *Journal of Clinical Oncology, 41*(6), 1200–1212. https://doi.org/10.1200/jco.22.01503

Burtness, B., Harrington, K. J., Greil, R., et al. (2019). Pembrolizumab alone or with chemotherapy versus cetuximab with chemotherapy for recurrent or metastatic squamous cell carcinoma of the head and neck (KEYNOTE-048): A randomised, open-label, phase 3 study. *Lancet, 394*(10212), 1915–1928. https://doi.org/10.1016/s0140-6736(19)32591-7

Chaturvedi, A. K., Engels, E. A., Pfeiffer, R. M., et al. (2011). Human papillomavirus and rising oropharyngeal cancer incidence in the United States. *Journal of Clinical Oncology, 29*(32), 4294–4301. https://doi.org/10.1200/jco.2011.36.4596

Chung, C. H., Colevas, A. D. D., Adkins, D., et al. (2023). A phase 1 dose-escalation and expansion study of CUE-101, a novel HPV16 E7-pHLA-IL2-Fc fusion protein, given as monotherapy and in combination with pembrolizumab in patients with recurrent/metastatic HPV16+ head and neck cancer. *Journal of Clinical Oncology, 41*(16_suppl), 6013. https://doi.org/10.1200/JCO.2023.41.16_suppl.6013

Cohen, E. E. W., Soulières, D., Le Tourneau, C., et al. (2019). Pembrolizumab versus methotrexate, docetaxel, or cetuximab for recurrent or metastatic head-and-neck squamous cell carcinoma (KEYNOTE-040): A randomised, open-label, phase 3 study. *Lancet, 393*(10167), 156–167. https://doi.org/10.1016/s0140-6736(18)31999-8

FDA approves pembrolizumab for first-line treatment of head and neck squamous cell carcinoma. Accessed 8/18/2023. https://www.fda.gov/drugs/resources-information-approved-drugs/fda-approves-pembrolizumab-first-line-treatment-head-and-neck-squamous-cell-carcinoma

Ferris, R. L., Blumenschein, G., Fayette, J., et al. (2016). Nivolumab for recurrent squamous-cell carcinoma of the head and neck. *New England Journal of Medicine, 375*(19), 1856–1867. https://doi.org/10.1056/nejmoa1602252

Ferris, R. L., Haddad, R., Even, C., et al. (2020). Durvalumab with or without tremelimumab in patients with recurrent or metastatic head and neck squamous cell carcinoma: EAGLE, a randomized, open-label phase III study. *Annals of Oncology, 31*(7), 942–950. https://doi.org/10.1016/j.annonc.2020.04.001

Ferris, R. L., Spanos, W. C., Leidner, R., et al. (2021). Neoadjuvant nivolumab for patients with resectable HPV-positive and HPV-negative squamous cell carcinomas of the head and neck in the CheckMate 358 trial. *Journal for ImmunoTherapy of Cancer, 9*(6). https://doi.org/10.1136/jitc-2021-002568

Gillison, M. L., Blumenschein, G., Fayette, J., et al. (2022). Long-term outcomes with nivolumab as first-line treatment in recurrent or metastatic head and neck cancer: Subgroup analysis of CheckMate 141. *Oncologist, 27*(2), e194–e198. https://doi.org/10.1093/oncolo/oyab036

Gormley, M., Creaney, G., Schache, A., Ingarfield, K., & Conway, D. I. (2022). Reviewing the epidemiology of head and neck cancer: Definitions, trends and risk factors. *British Dental Journal, 233*(9), 780–786. https://doi.org/10.1038/s41415-022-5166-x

Grimm, M.-O., Esteban, E., Barthélémy, P., et al. (2021). Efficacy of nivolumab/ipilimumab in patients with initial or late progression with nivolumab: Updated analysis of a tailored approach in advanced renal cell carcinoma (TITAN-RCC). *Journal of Clinical Oncology, 39*(15_suppl), 4576. https://doi.org/10.1200/JCO.2021.39.15_suppl.4576

Gyawali, B., Hey, S. P., & Kesselheim, A. S. (2019). Assessment of the clinical benefit of cancer drugs receiving accelerated approval. *JAMA Internal Medicine, 179*(7), 906–913. https://doi.org/10.1001/jamainternmed.2019.0462

Haddad, R. I., Harrington, K., Tahara, M., et al. (2023). Nivolumab plus ipilimumab versus EXTREME regimen as first-line treatment for recurrent/metastatic squamous cell carcinoma of the head and neck: The final results of CheckMate 651. *Journal of Clinical Oncology, 41*(12), 2166–2180. https://doi.org/10.1200/jco.22.00332

Harrington, K. J., Ferris, R. L., Blumenschein, G., Jr., et al. (2017). Nivolumab versus standard, single-agent therapy of investigator's choice in recurrent or metastatic squamous cell carcinoma of the head and neck (CheckMate 141): Health-related quality-of-life results from a randomised, phase 3 trial. *The Lancet Oncology, 18*(8), 1104–1115. https://doi.org/10.1016/s1470-2045(17)30421-7

Harrington, K. J., Burtness, B., Greil, R., et al. (2023). Pembrolizumab With or Without Chemotherapy in Recurrent or Metastatic Head and Neck Squamous Cell Carcinoma: Updated Results of the Phase III KEYNOTE-048 Study. *Journal of Clinical Oncology, 41*(4), 790–802. https://doi.org/10.1200/jco.21.02508

Juloori, A., Agrawal, N., Cursio, J., et al. (2023). Neoadjuvant nivolumab, paclitaxel, and carboplatin followed by response-stratified chemoradiation in locoregionally advanced HPV negative head and neck squamous cell carcinoma (HNSCC): The DEPEND trial. *Journal of Clinical Oncology, 41*(16_suppl), 6007. https://doi.org/10.1200/JCO.2023.41.16_suppl.6007

Kim, H. S., Ham, J., Byeon, S., et al. (2015). The prevalence and prognostic relevance of PD-L1 expression in patients with HPV-negative and HPV-positive oropharyngeal cancer. *Journal of Clinical Oncology, 33*(15_suppl), e14003. https://doi.org/10.1200/jco.2015.33.15_suppl.e14003

Larkins, E., Blumenthal, G. M., Yuan, W., et al. (2017). FDA approval summary: Pembrolizumab for the treatment of recurrent or metastatic head and neck squamous cell carcinoma with disease progression on or after platinum-containing chemotherapy. *The Oncologist, 22*(7), 873–878. https://doi.org/10.1634/theoncologist.2016-0496

Lee, N. Y., Ferris, R. L., Psyrri, A., et al. (2021). Avelumab plus standard-of-care chemoradiotherapy versus chemoradiotherapy alone in patients with locally advanced squamous cell carcinoma of the head and neck: A randomised, double-blind, placebo-controlled, multicentre, phase 3 trial. *The Lancet Oncology, 22*(4), 450–462. https://doi.org/10.1016/s1470-2045(20)30737-3

Machiels, J. P., Tao, Y., Burtness, B., et al. (2022). Primary results of the phase III KEYNOTE-412 study: Pembrolizumab (pembro) with chemoradiation therapy (CRT) vs placebo plus CRT for locally advanced (LA) head and neck squamous cell carcinoma (HNSCC). Meeting abstract. *Annals of Oncology, 33*(7), S1399–S1399. https://doi.org/10.1016/j.annonc.2022.08.029

Mandal, R., Şenbabaoğlu, Y., Desrichard, A., et al. (2016). The head and neck cancer immune landscape and its immunotherapeutic implications. *JCI Insight, 1*(17). https://doi.org/10.1172/jci.insight.89829

Masarwy, R., Kampel, L., Horowitz, G., Gutfeld, O., & Muhanna, N. (2021). Neoadjuvant PD-1/PD-L1 inhibitors for Resectable head and neck cancer: A systematic review and meta-analysis. *JAMA Otolaryngology and Head and Neck Surgery, 147*(10), 871–878. https://doi.org/10.1001/jamaoto.2021.2191

Mehanna, H., Taberna, M., Von Buchwald, C., et al. (2023). Prognostic implications of p16 and HPV discordance in oropharyngeal cancer (HNCIG-EPIC-OPC): A multicentre, multinational, individual patient data analysis. *The Lancet Oncology, 24*(3), 239–251. https://doi.org/10.1016/s1470-2045(23)00013-x

Mito, I., Takahashi, H., Kawabata-Iwakawa, R., Ida, S., Tada, H., & Chikamatsu, K. (2021). Comprehensive analysis of immune cell enrichment in the tumor microenvironment of head and neck squamous cell carcinoma. *Scientific Reports, 11*(1). https://doi.org/10.1038/s41598-021-95718-9

Nivolumab for SCCHN. Accessed 8/18/2023. https://www.fda.gov/drugs/resources-information-approved-drugs/nivolumab-scchn

Pai, S. I., & Westra, W. H. (2009). Molecular pathology of head and neck cancer: Implications for diagnosis, prognosis, and treatment. *Annual Review of Pathology: Mechanisms of Disease, 4*(1), 49–70. https://doi.org/10.1146/annurev.pathol.4.110807.092158

Pembrolizumab (KEYTRUDA). Accessed 8/18/2023. https://www.fda.gov/drugs/resources-information-approved-drugs/pembrolizumab-keytruda

Pfister DG, & Sharon S. (n.d.). *NCCN clinical practice guidelines in oncology – Head and neck cancers version 2.2023.* https://www.nccn.org/professionals/physician_gls/pdf/head-and-neck.pdf

Pfister, D. G., Haddad, R. I., Worden, F. P., et al. (2023). Biomarkers predictive of response to pembrolizumab in head and neck cancer. *Cancer Medicine, 12*(6), 6603–6614. https://doi.org/10.1002/cam4.5434

Price, K. A., Kaczmar, J. M., Worden, F. P., et al. (2023). Safety and efficacy of immune checkpoint inhibitor (ICI) Naïve cohort from study of PDS0101 and pembrolizumab in HPV16-positive head and neck squamous cell carcinoma (HNSCC). *American Society of Clinical Oncology.*

Psyrri, A., Fayette, J., Harrington, K., et al. (2023). Durvalumab with or without tremelimumab versus the EXTREME regimen as first-line treatment for recurrent or metastatic squamous cell carcinoma of the head and neck: KESTREL, a randomized, open-label, phase III study. *Annals of Oncology, 34*(3), 262–274. https://doi.org/10.1016/j.annonc.2022.12.008

Ruffin, A. T., Li, H., Vujanovic, L., Zandberg, D. P., Ferris, R. L., & Bruno, T. C. (2023). Improving head and neck cancer therapies by immunomodulation of the tumour microenvironment. *Nature Reviews. Cancer, 23*(3), 173–188. https://doi.org/10.1038/s41568-022-00531-9

Schoenfeld, J. D., Hanna, G. J., Jo, V. Y., et al. (2020). Neoadjuvant nivolumab or nivolumab plus ipilimumab in untreated Oral cavity squamous cell carcinoma: A phase 2 open-label randomized clinical trial. *JAMA Oncologia, 6*(10), 1563–1570. https://doi.org/10.1001/jamaoncol.2020.2955

SEER*Explorer. Accessed 8/17/2023. https://seer.cancer.gov/statistics-network/explorer/application.html

Stämpfli, M. R., & Anderson, G. P. (2009). How cigarette smoke skews immune responses to promote infection, lung disease and cancer. *Nature Reviews Immunology, 9*(5), 377–384. https://doi.org/10.1038/nri2530

Tosi, A., Parisatto, B., Menegaldo, A., et al. (2022). The immune microenvironment of HPV-positive and HPV-negative oropharyngeal squamous cell carcinoma: A multiparametric quantitative and spatial analysis unveils a rationale to target treatment-naïve tumors with immune checkpoint inhibitors. *Journal of Experimental & Clinical Cancer Research, 41*(1). https://doi.org/10.1186/s13046-022-02481-4

Veigas, F., Mahmoud, Y. D., Merlo, J., Rinflerch, A., Rabinovich, G. A., & Girotti, M. R. (2021). Immune checkpoints pathways in head and neck squamous cell carcinoma. *Cancers, 13*(5), 1018. https://doi.org/10.3390/cancers13051018

Vermorken, J. B., Mesia, R., Rivera, F., et al. (2008). Platinum-based chemotherapy plus cetuximab in head and neck cancer. *The New England Journal of Medicine, 359*(11), 1116–1127. https://doi.org/10.1056/NEJMoa0802656

Wang, H. Q., Fu, R., Man, Q. W., Yang, G., Liu, B., & Bu, L. L. (2023). Advances in CAR-T cell therapy in head and neck squamous cell carcinoma. *Journal of Clinical Oncology, 12*(6). https://doi.org/10.3390/jcm12062173

Wolchok, J. D., Chiarion-Sileni, V., Gonzalez, R., et al. (2022). Long-term outcomes with nivolumab plus ipilimumab or nivolumab alone versus ipilimumab in patients with advanced melanoma. *Journal of Clinical Oncology, 40*(2), 127–137. https://doi.org/10.1200/jco.21.02229

Yu, G.-T., Bu, L.-L., Zhao, Y.-Y., et al. (2016). CTLA4 blockade reduces immature myeloid cells in head and neck squamous cell carcinoma. *OncoImmunology, 5*(6), e1151594. https://doi.org/10.1080/2162402x.2016.1151594

Zech, H. B., Moeckelmann, N., Boettcher, A., et al. (2020). Phase III study of nivolumab alone or combined with ipilimumab as immunotherapy versus standard of care in resectable head and neck squamous cell carcinoma. *Future Oncology, 16*(36), 3035–3043. https://doi.org/10.2217/fon-2020-0595

Zou, X. L., Li, X. B., Ke, H., et al. (2021). Prognostic value of neoantigen load in immune checkpoint inhibitor therapy for cancer. *Frontiers in Immunology, 12*, 689076. https://doi.org/10.3389/fimmu.2021.689076

Zuur, L., Vos, J. L., Elbers, J. B., et al. (2020). LBA40 neoadjuvant nivolumab and nivolumab plus ipilimumab induce (near-) complete responses in patients with head and neck squamous cell carcinoma: The IMCISION trial. *Annals of Oncology, 31*, S1169. https://doi.org/10.1016/j.annonc.2020.08.2270

Chapter 16
Resources for Patients

Yiyi Yan and Jessica Lee

Abstract The medical treatment landscape is continually changing. New medications and novel treatment modalities are emerging, thanks to ongoing research endeavors. Notably, immunotherapy has been a recent groundbreaking approach to treating cancer. Over the last few years, immunotherapy has been proven to alter the course of cancer care. It is quickly changing the ways we treat cancer and is bringing hope and optimism to cancer patients. Given the rapid advances in this field, we strongly encourage our patients to engage in conversations about treatment options with their healthcare team to formulate an individualized treatment plan, including potential participation in ongoing clinical trials.

Keywords Resources · Immunotherapy · Education

The medical treatment landscape is continually changing. New medications and novel treatment modalities are emerging, thanks to ongoing research endeavors. Notably, immunotherapy has been a recent groundbreaking approach to treating cancer. Over the last few years, immunotherapy has been proven to alter the course of cancer care. It is quickly changing the ways we treat cancer and is bringing hope and optimism to cancer patients. Given the rapid advances in this field, we strongly encourage our patients to engage in conversations about treatment options with their healthcare team to formulate an individualized treatment plan, including potential participation in ongoing clinical trials.

Immunotherapies to treat cancer have a unique side effect profile compared to other conventional cancer therapies, such as chemotherapy. It is important to have thorough patient education prior to the initiation of treatment. Equally vital is communicating with the healthcare team to inform the providers about the onset of side

Y. Yan
Division of Medical Oncology, Mayo Clinic, Rochester, MN, USA

J. Lee (✉)
Department of Medical Oncology, Mayo Clinic, Rochester, MN, USA
e-mail: lee.jessica@mayo.edu

effects or any new symptoms. Early recognition and prompt treatment of immunotherapy-related side effects are critical to ensure the best possible outcomes for patients. It is imperative not to self-medicate for common symptoms, such as diarrhea, as this may inadvertently exacerbate potential complications. The health-care team will help you navigate the complexities of immunotherapy side effects.

Recognizing the limitations of this book in covering all aspects of cancer immu-notherapy, we have compiled a list of additional resources for those seeking further information. Additionally, you can visit the website specific to your immunotherapy for more information. While the Internet can provide a lot of great resources and knowledge, we again encourage continuing conversations with your healthcare pro-vider to address any specific questions related to your treatment.

We hope that these resources will assist you in gaining insights into cancer immunotherapy and its potential benefits.

List of Resources
- American Cancer Society: www.cancer.org
American Society of Clinical Oncology: www.cancer.net
American Society of Hematology: www.hematology.org
Cancer Research Institute: www.cancerresearch.org
Chemocare: www.chemocare.com
Clinical Trial Information: www.clinicaltrials.gov
Intravenous Cancer Treatment Education: www.ivcanceredsheets.com
Leukemia and Lymphoma Society: www.lls.org
National Cancer Institute: www.cancer.gov
National Comprehensive Cancer Network: www.nccn.org

Index